I0034398

Scientific Researches in Health Sciences II

Fatma Eti Aslan
Gökay Kurtulan
Hayat Yalın
(Editors)

Scientific Researches in

Health Sciences II

PETER LANG

**Bibliographic Information published by the
Deutsche Nationalbibliothek**

The Deutsche Nationalbibliothek lists this publication in the Deutsche Nationalbibliografie; detailed bibliographic data is available online at http://dnb.d-nb.de.

Library of Congress Cataloging-in-Publication Data

A CIP catalog record for this book has been applied for at the Library of Congress.

The chapters in this book are first reviewed by the independent reviewers and then proof-read and edited by the editors. The opinions and views expressed in the articles are not necessarily those of the editors. All the views expressed in the book are purely that of the authors themselves and may not in any circumstances be regarded as stating an official position of Bahçeşehir University nor that of the editors of the book.

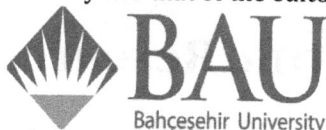

Bahçeşehir University

ISBN 978-3-631-84377-2 (Print)
E-ISBN 978-3-631-84835-7 (E-PDF)
E-ISBN 978-3-631-84836-4 (EPUB)
E-ISBN 978-3-631-84837-1 (MOBI)
DOI 10.3726/b18089
© Peter Lang GmbH
Internationaler Verlag der Wissenschaften
Berlin 2021
All rights reserved.

Peter Lang – Berlin · Bern · Bruxelles · New York · Oxford · Warszawa · Wien

All parts of this publication are protected by copyright. Any utilisation outside the strict limits of the copyright law, without the permission of the publisher, is forbidden and liable to prosecution. This applies in particular to reproductions, translations, microfilming, and storage and processing in electronic retrieval systems.

This publication has been peer reviewed.

www.peterlang.com

Foreword

We are very happy and proud to publish our second book "Scientific Researches in Health Sciences II" in a very short time after our first book "Scientific Researches in Health Sciences" published in 2019.

After the COVID pandemic in 2020, the importance of health services was once again understood by the whole world. Scientific research in the field of health services contributes greatly to the development of health services. In this book, there are a total of 26 chapters in 4 different scientific fields: 6 in nutrition and dietetics, 11 in nursing, 6 in physiotherapy and rehabilitation and 3 in health management. We hope our book will contribute to the development of health sciences around the world and the quality of healthcare services.

Fifty-one researchers/authors, who have chapters in this book, prepared their chapters with a great effort and meticulousness and contributed to the preparation of the book for publication. We thank our peer team (Hayat Yalın, Hasan Kerem Alptekin, Can Ergün and Mustafa Çiçek) for their tremendous contribution to the book.

Editors
Prof. Dr. Fatma Eti Aslan
Assist. Prof. Dr. Gökay Kurtulan
Assist. Prof. Dr. Hayat Yalın

Contents

8   Contents

Contents 9

List of Contributors

Ahu Kürklü
Bahçeşehir University, Faculty of
Health Sciences, Department of
Nursing, İstanbul, Turkey

Beyza İnce
Bahçeşehir University, Faculty of
Health Sciences, Department of
Physiotherapy and Rehabilitation,
İstanbul, Turkey

Burcu Ceylan
Necmettin Erbakan University,
Faculty of Nursing, Department
of Mental Health and Psychiatric
Nursing, Konya, Turkey

Can Ergün
Bahçeşehir University, Faculty
of Health Sciences, Department
of Nutrition and Dietetics,
İstanbul, Turkey

Çiğdem Çelebi
Bahçeşehir University, Faculty
of Architecture and Design,
Department of Architecture,
İstanbul, Turkey

Dilara Güler
Bahçeşehir University, Graduate
Education Institute, Chiropractic
Master of Science Program,
İstanbul, Turkey

Dilay Hacıdursunoğlu Erbaş
Sancaktepe Şehit Prof.Dr. İlhan
Varank Training and Research
Hospital, İstanbul, Turkey

Dilber Karagözoğlu Coşkunsu
Bahçeşehir University, Faculty of
Health Sciences, Department of
Physiotherapy and Rehabilitation,
İstanbul, Turkey

Dilek Arduzlar Kağan
Bahçeşehir University, Faculty
of Health Sciences, Department
of Nutrition and Dietetics,
İstanbul, Turkey

Ecenur Özkul
Bahçeşehir University, Faculty
of Health Sciences, Department
of Nutrition and Dietetics,
İstanbul, Turkey

Emine Özdemir Aslan
Bahçeşehir University, Faculty of
Health Sciences, Department of
Nursing, İstanbul, Turkey

Emre Batuhan Kenger
Bahçeşehir University, Faculty
of Health Sciences, Department
of Nutrition and Dietetics,
İstanbul, Turkey

Esin Koç
Gazi University, Neonatal Science
Branch, Ankara, Turkey

Esra Atılgan
İstanbul Medipol University, Faculty
of Health Sciences, Department of
Physiotherapy and Rehabilitation,
İstanbul, Turkey

Evrim Karadağ Saygı
Ministry of Health, İstanbul
Provincial Health Directorate,
Marmara University İstanbul Pendik
Education and Research Hospital,
İstanbul, Turkey

Fadime Çınar
İstanbul Sebahattin Zaim University,
Faculty of Health Sciences,
İstanbul, Turkey

Fatma Eti Aslan
Bahçeşehir University, Faculty of
Health Sciences, Department of
Nursing, İstanbul, Turkey

Gamze Zengin
İstanbul Bakırköy Dr. Sadi Konuk
Training and Research Hospital,
İstanbul, Turkey

Gökay Kurtulan
Bahçeşehir University, Faculty
of Health Sciences, Department
of Health Management,
İstanbul, Turkey

Gökçen Garipoğlu
Bahçeşehir University, Faculty
of Health Sciences, Department
of Nutrition and Dietetics,
İstanbul, Turkey

Gülderen Yentür
Gazi University, Faculty of
Pharmacy, Department of
Food Analysis and Nutrition,
Ankara, Turkey

Hakan Güveli
Bahçeşehir University, Faculty
of Health Sciences, Department
of Nutrition and Dietetics,
İstanbul, Turkey

Hasan Kerem Alptekin
Bahçeşehir University, Faculty of
Health Sciences, Department of
Physiotherapy and Rehabilitation,
İstanbul, Turkey

Hayat Yalın
Bahçeşehir University, Faculty of
Health Sciences, Department of
Nursing, İstanbul, Turkey

Hazal Genç
Bahçeşehir University, Faculty of
Health Sciences, Department of
Physiotherapy and Rehabilitation,
İstanbul, Turkey

İbrahim Elmas
Ministry of Health, Ankara, Turkey

İlayda Öztürk
Bahçeşehir University, Faculty
of Health Sciences, Department
of Nutrition and Dietetics,
İstanbul, Turkey

İlkay Öztürk
Bahçeşehir University, Vocational
School of Health Services,
İstanbul, Turkey

İrem Sarıhan
Bahçeşehir University, Faculty
of Health Sciences, Department
of Health Management,
İstanbul, Turkey

Kardelen Besen
Bahçeşehir University, Faculty of
Health Sciences, Department of
Physiotherapy and Rehabilitation,
İstanbul, Turkey

Leyla Ataş Balcı
Bahçeşehir University, Faculty of
Health Sciences, Department of
Physiotherapy and Rehabilitation,
İstanbul, Turkey

Merve İlker
Bahçeşehir University, Graduate
Education Institute, Nutrition and
Dietetics Master of Science Program,
İstanbul, Turkey

Merve Tarhan
İstanbul Medipol University, Faculty
of Health Sciences, Department of
Nursing, İstanbul, Turkey

Mirsad Alkan
Bahçeşehir University, Vocational
School of Health Services,
İstanbul, Turkey

Murat Dündar
Bahçeşehir University, Faculty
of Architecture and Design,
Department of Architecture,
İstanbul, Turkey

Muzaffer Saraç
İstanbul Metropolitan Municipality,
İstanbul, Turkey

Neriman Özge Çalışkan
Bahçeşehir University, Graduate
Education Institute, Nursing
Doctor of Philosophy Program,
İstanbul, Turkey

Neslihan Bektaş
Bahçeşehir University, Vocational
School of Health Services, İstanbul,
Turkey

Nilgün Altunbaş
Bahçeşehir University, Graduate
Education Institute, Nursing Master
of Science Program, İstanbul, Turkey

Nurşah Büyükçamsarı Şanlıer
Acıbadem Maslak Hospital,
İstanbul, Turkey

Pelin Pişirici
Bahçeşehir University, Faculty of
Health Sciences, Department of
Physiotherapy and Rehabilitation,
İstanbul, Turkey

Pelin Velioğlu
Bahçeşehir University, Graduate
Education Institute, Nutrition and
Dietetics Master of Science Program,
İstanbul, Turkey

Pınar Doğan
İstanbul Medipol University, Faculty
of Health Sciences, Department of
Nursing, İstanbul, Turkey

Şebnem Çalkavur
Dr. Behçet Uz Children Hospital,
Neonatology Department,
İzmir, Turkey

Seda Akkoyun
Bahçeşehir University, Faculty of
Health Sciences, Department of
Physiotherapy and Rehabilitation,
İstanbul, Turkey

Selda Polat
Bahçeşehir University, Faculty of
Health Sciences, Department of
Nursing, İstanbul, Turkey

Semih Özdemir
Bahçeşehir University, Graduate
Education Institute, Osteopathy
Manual Therapy Master of Science
Program, İstanbul, Turkey

Semra Bülbüloğlu
Gaziosmanpaşa University,
Erbaa Faculty of Health Sciences,
Department of Surgical Nursing,
Tokat, Turkey

Taner Özgürtaş
Health Science University,
Medical Biochemistry Branch,
İstanbul, Turkey

Tuğçe Özlü
Bahçeşehir University, Faculty
of Health Sciences, Department
of Nutrition and Dietetics,
İstanbul, Turkey

Yonca Sevim
Bahçeşehir University, Faculty
of Health Sciences, Department
of Nutrition and Dietetics,
İstanbul, Turkey

Dilek Arduzlar Kağan, Ecenur Özkul, and Pelin Velioğlu

Assessment of Consumption Frequency of Cereal Products by Adults and Some Factors Affecting Consumption

Abstract

Objective: The majority of daily energy requirements are provided by cereals. With different recipes and uses, cereal products have an important place in daily diet due to being generally cheap, easy to obtain, their nutrient content and neutral flavor. Apart from these characteristics, the fiber content is an important quality criterion for cereal products. As the product diversity increases, cereal products which can be evaluated as functional foods increase.

Materials and Methods: The aim of the study is to investigate the frequency and diversity of cereal products consumed by adult individuals and effective factors. From March to April 2018, İstanbul province was accepted as population, with the sample comprising 299 women and 151 men, for a total of 450 individuals, aged from 18 to 65 years living in İstanbul. Survey questioned demographic features, health knowledge, habits and participant's consumption frequency and choices in relation to cereal products.

Results: The 450 adults participating in this study consumed white bread (45.5 %) and wholewheat bread at least once per day (38 %), while most did not consume bran bread (52 %), rye bread (56 %) and multigrain bread (53 %). It was identified that most ate phyllo pastry at least once per month, white rice 1-2 times per week and did not consume brown rice (81 %). They ate bulgur at least once every 15 days (26.8 %), ate pasta 1-2 times per week (36.5 %), and mostly did not consume brown pasta (79 %), muesli (72.5 %), breakfast cereals (59.7 %), wholegrain biscuits (49.5 %) and cereal bars (65 %).

Conclusion: It was observed that differences in sex and educational level change choice of food and knowledge level about nutrition. Generally, when cereal product consumption and factors affecting choices of participants are assessed, high rates of individuals chose white bread which can be assessed as being a traditional flavor and did not appear to choose foods like brown rice and rye with higher dietary fiber but more foreign flavor. It was concluded that women and individuals with higher educational level had higher healthy product choices.

Keywords: Dietary Fiber, Fiber Sources, Wholegrain, Edible Cereal

Introduction

Currently linked to the increase in knowledge levels among consumers, interest in healthy eating has increased (1). Related to this, consumer's expectations from food are not just that it will be tasty, but that it will also be safe and have nutritional features. For balanced and sufficient nutrition of the growing population, the quality characteristics of cereals and cereal products with an important place in daily diet, as in our country, are important (2). The amount of energy provided, dietary fiber they contain, protein, vitamin and mineral amounts are important quality criteria for cereal products.

Considering these features, interest was observed to increase especially related to dietary fiber within the last quarter century (3). Studies performed with this interest have developed the hypothesis that there is a correlation between fiber consumption in developed countries with frequently encountered diseases (4). Research has shown that dietary fiber operates with different mechanisms in the body. The basic mechanisms may be assessed as increased volume in feces and formation of short-chain fat acids with colon fermentation (5). Short-chain fat acids are important energy sources for mucosa. A high fiber and low-fat diet provided by cereals assists in protecting the body against chronic diseases like heart disease, stroke, and some cancers (6).

The strengthening relationship between eating habits and health has encouraged research into functional food (7). Adding the bioactive food component with proven effects of dietary fiber to foods may make the foods more functional. Dried bread products using resistant starch may be shown as an example of this research (8). For assessment of dietary fiber consumption and functional foods, along with portion size and consumption frequency, the first group that comes to mind is cereals (9). Cereals are a good source of fiber, while they are widely used in traditional eating styles due to being cheap, easy to obtain, their nutrient content and neutral flavor (10).

The aim of this study is to assess the frequency and diversity of consumption of cereal products by adult individuals from 18 to 65 years living in İstanbul province and investigate factors affecting choices.

Materials and Methods

From March to April 2018, İstanbul province was accepted as population, with the sample comprising 299 women and 151 men, for a total of 450 individuals, aged from 18 to 65 years living in İstanbul. The study was performed with the aim of researching knowledge levels about dietary fiber and consumption frequency of cereal products. For the research, permission was obtained from Bahçeşehir University Scientific Research and Publication Ethics Committee at a meeting on 19 February 2020. The researchers prepared a survey with 3 sections based on the literature and similar studies. The survey form was completed by participants using the face-to-face technique. The first section of the survey questioned demographic features, health knowledge and habits with 19 questions. The second section included 17 questions aiming to identify knowledge levels about dietary fiber. The third section questioned participant's consumption frequency and choices in relation to cereal products. The study used the statistical program SPSS (Statistical Package for Social Sciences) v22.0 program. Analysis of data benefitted from descriptive statistics like frequency, percentage (%), arithmetic mean, standard deviation (+SD), minimum and maximum. Analysis of data used parametric tests. Comparison of means in 2 independent groups used the independent samples t test, while comparison of more than 2 independent groups used the one-way ANOVA test and correlation of 2 categoric variables used the chi-square correlation test. Correlation analysis for measures used the Pearson correlation coefficient. Tests were assessed at 0.05 significance level.

Results

As shown in Table 1, 76.5 % of participants in the study were 18-54 years of age, 66 % were women and 34 % were men. Among these people, 83 % lived in households of 3 or more people, 30 % earned from 2,000 to 4,000 TL, and 64 % had family income above 4,000 TL. When educational level is assessed, the majority of people (69 %) had received education at university level. Among participants, 15 % were office workers, 10 % were self-employed, 9 % were retired and 35 % were students, while 7 % of people were not employed. When body mass index is assessed, 5 % were underweight, 54 % had normal weight, 29 % were overweight and 11.5 % were obese.

Table 2 investigates the cereal product consumption of participants. The most frequent consumption level was 2-3 times per day for white bread identified at high rates of 25.9 %. After white bread came whole-wheat bread at 23.7 %, bran bread at 6.3 % and rye and multigrain breads at 6.2 %. When the consumption once per day is investigated, 19.6 % consumed white bread followed by whole-wheat bread at 14.3 %. When cereal consumption apart from bread, like rice and bulgur, are considered, 41.8 % ate bulgur 2-3 times per week, followed by pasta (36.5 %), white rice (33.4 %) and phyllo (14.4 %). The highest rate of consumption of other cereal products that can be considered in the breakfast and snack class was wholegrain biscuits (14.1 %), followed by breakfast cereals (12.7 %), cereal bars (8.4 %) and muesli (7.8 %). When general consumption of products is investigated, participants consumed white bread (45.5 %) and whole-wheat bread (38 %) at least once per day, while most did not consume bran bread (52 %), rye bread (56 %) and multigrain bread (53 %). They ate phyllo pastry at least once per month, white rice at least 1-2 times per week and did not consume brown rice (81 %). They ate bulgur at least once every 15 days (26.8 %), white pasta (36.5 %) at least 1-2 times per week and did not consume brown pasta (79 %), muesli (72.5 %), breakfast cereals (59.7 %), wholegrain biscuits (49.5 %) and cereal bars (65 %).

As shown in Table 3, men participating in the study had significantly higher mean consumption of white bread, phyllo pastry, and white rice compared to consumption by women (p<0.05). Women had higher mean consumption of rye bread, muesli and cereal bars compared to consumption by men (p<0.05).

Correlation analysis between participants' consumption of cereal and bread group foods with educational level is assessed in Table 4. There was a negative linear correlation between white bread, phyllo pastry and white rice consumption with educational level and a positive linear and significant correlation between whole-wheat, brown pasta, muesli, breakfast cereal, wholegrain biscuits and cereal bar consumption with educational level (p<0.05). In other words, as educational level increased, consumption of white bread, phyllo pastry and rice reduced, while consumption of whole-wheat, brown rice, muesli, breakfast cereal, wholegrain biscuits and cereal bars increased. There was a positive linear correlation between points for dietary fiber knowledge levels of people with whole-wheat bread, rye bread, multigrain bread and muesli consumption and a negative linear and significant correlation with white bread, phyllo pastry, white rice and pasta consumption (p<.01).

Participants with health problems and underweight according to BMI consumed white bread 1-2 times per week, white rice, and pasta 3-4 times per week and phyllo pastry once every 15 days. People with normal weight consumed white bread 1-2 times per week, white rice, and pasta 3-4 times per week, and phyllo pastry once every 15 days. Individuals in the overweight group ate white pasta 3-4 times per week, and white rice and white pasta once every 15 days. In the obese class, people with 1st degree obesity ate white bread, white rice, and white pasta once every 15 days and phyllo pastry once every month, while those with 2nd degree obesity ate white bread 1-2 times per week, white rice, phyllo pastry and white pasta 3-4 times per week. People with health problems and in the underweight group according to BMI classification ate bran and rye bread and brown pasta once per month. People in the normal weight class

Tab. 1: Sociodemographic and BMI Information for Participants

Sociodemographic and BMI Information		n	%
	18-25 years	178	39.6
	26-35 years	97	21.6
Age	36-45 years	69	15.3
	46-55 years	61	13.6
	56-65 years	45	10.0
Sex	Female	299	66.0
	Male	151	34.0
	1 person	14	3.0
	2 people	63	14.0
Number of people in household	3 people	111	25.0
	4 people	181	40.0
	5 or more	80	18.0
	Less than 2,000 TL	27	6.0
Family income	2,000-4,000 TL	130	30.0
	4,000 TL and above	280	64.0
	Illiterate	3	1.0
	Primary school graduate	19	4.0
Education Level	Middle school graduate	18	4.0
	High school graduate	99	22.0
	University	309	69.0
	Unemployed	30	7.0
	Student	155	35.0
	Retired	41	9.0
Occupation	Office worker	67	15.0
	Self-employed	46	10.0
	Other	106	24.0
	Low (<18.50)	23	5.1
	Normal (18.50 - 24.99)	243	54
BMI	Overweight (25.00 - 29.99)	131	29.1
	Obese I (30.00 - 34.99)	42	9.3
	Obese II (35 or more)	11	2.4

ate bran bread once every 15 days, rye bread once per month and additionally did not consume brown pasta. People with 1st degree obesity ate whole-wheat bread 2-3 times per day, bran, and rye bread once every 15 days and brown pasta once per month. People with 2nd degree obesity ate whole-wheat bread

Tab. 2: Consumption Frequency of Cereal Product Foods

	Never		Once per month		Once every 15 days		3-4 times per week		1-2 times per week		2-3 times per day		Once per day	
	n	%	n	%	n	%	n	%	n	%	n	%	n	%
White bread	111	25.9	26	6.1	24	5.6	20	4.7	52	12.1	111	25.9	84	19.6
Whole-wheat bread	113	26.5	23	5.4	23	5.4	21	4.9	85	19.9	101	23.7	61	14.3
Bran bread	214	52.1	35	8.5	32	7.8	20	4.9	55	13.4	26	6.3	29	7.1
Rye bread	225	56	36	9	38	9.5	12	3	50	12.4	25	6.2	16	4
Multigrain bread	213	53	45	11.2	28	7	16	4	53	13.2	25	6.2	22	5.5
Phyllo	111	27	122	29.7	100	24.3	7	1.7	59	14.4	3	0.7	9	2.2
White rice	74	17.1	66	15.2	77	17.7	35	8.1	145	33.4	16	3.7	21	4.8
Brown rice	323	81.6	24	6.1	22	5.6	5	1.3	18	4.5	2	0.5	2	0.5
Bulgur	32	7.3	49	11.1	118	26.8	37	8.4	182	41.4	8	1.8	14	3.2
White pasta	63	14.5	57	13.2	104	24	31	7.2	158	36.5	7	1.6	13	3
Wholegrain pasta	321	79.1	27	6.7	32	7.9	1	0.2	20	4.9	3	0.7	2	0.5
Muesli	298	72.5	31	7.5	22	5.4	12	2.9	32	7.8	4	1	12	2.9
Breakfast cereal	253	59.7	30	7.1	45	10.6	5	1.2	54	12.7	9	2.1	28	6.6
Wholegrain biscuits	211	49.5	69	16.2	63	14.8	11	2.6	60	14.1	4	0.9	8	1.9
Cereal bars	270	64.9	48	11.5	47	11.3	8	1.9	35	8.4	1	0.2	7	1.7

Tab. 3: Comparison of Cereal Product Food Consumption According to Sex

	Sex				T	p
	Female		Male			
	Mean	S.D.	Mean	S.D.		
White bread	4.09	2.40	4.63	2.20	-2.236	0.026*
Wholewheat bread	4.47	2.16	3.50	2.31	4.262	0.000*
Bran bread	2.68	2.07	2.62	2.12	0.284	0.776
Rye bread	2.59	1.95	2.06	1.83	2.597	0.010*
Multigrain bread	2.66	2.02	2.28	1.95	1.803	0.072
Phyllo	2.47	1.42	2.79	1.60	-2.068	0.039*
White rice	3.29	1.65	4.09	1.81	-4.578	0.000*
Brown rice	1.41	1.02	1.52	1.28	-0.863	0.389
Bulgur	3.85	1.37	3.81	1.62	0.238	0.812
White pasta	3.44	1.57	3.76	1.66	-1.950	0.052
Wholegrain pasta	1.55	1.12	1.39	1.18	1.360	0.175
Muesli	1.98	1.67	1.45	1.25	3.269	0.001*
Breakfast cereal	2.39	1.90	2.21	2.04	0.930	0.353
Wholegrain biscuits	2.34	1.61	2.09	1.58	1.519	0.130
Cereal bars	1.96	1.48	1.62	1.29	2.280	0.023*

*Independent samples t test, *p<0.05*

once every 15 days, bran, and rye bread once per month and additionally did not consume brown pasta.

Discussion

Currently the rates of some disorders like cardiovascular diseases, digestive system diseases, obesity, diabetes, and intestinal diseases are increasing. However, common disorders were reduced with dietary fiber consumption in western countries and dietary fiber consumption was observed to protect against metabolic disorders. As a result, studies have focused on the metabolic importance of dietary fiber and benefit in terms of health (11,12). High intake of dietary fiber is known to have inverse correlation with cardiovascular disease (CVD) and myocardial infarcts (MI) risk. Additionally, prospective data generally recommended that the primary protective precaution against CVD is increased consumption of wholegrains, fruit, and vegetables rich in fiber (13). One of the disorders considered to be associated with dietary fiber is diabetes. High rates of dietary fiber consumption are known to benefit diabetic

Tab. 4: Correlation of Cereal Product Food Consumption with Educational Level and Dietary Fiber Knowledge Level

	Education Level		Dietary Fiber Knowledge Level	
	R	p	R	p
White bread	-.132**	0.006	-0.253	0.00
Whole-wheat bread	.126**	0.009	0.373**	0.00
Bran bread	0.041	0.413	0.086	0.081
Rye bread	0.027	0.591	.173**	0.00
Multigrain bread	0.071	0.155	.212**	0.00
Phyllo	-.132**	0.008	-0.154	0.002
White rice	-.116*	0.016	-.220**	0.00
Brown rice	0.078	0.121	-0.007	0.892
Bulgur	-0.016	0.732	0.024	0.623
White pasta	-0.025	0.611	-.192**	0.00
Wholegrain pasta	.183**	0.00	.099*	0.046
Muesli	.205**	0.00	.161**	0.001
Breakfast cereal	.174**	0.00	0.088	0.071
Wholegrain biscuits	.174**	0.00	0.039	0.425
Cereal bars	.152**	0.002	0.023	0.648

*Pearson correlation, *p<0.05, **p<.01*

individuals by lowering serum glucose levels and insulin requirements (14). A broad-scale study of 65,173 women aged from 40 to 65 years investigated the correlation between type 2 diabetes risk and diet. They found a positive correlation between diabetes and glycemic load and an inverse correlation between diabetes risk and cereal fiber intake. The combination of high cereal consumption and low glycemic load was shown to further reduce diabetes risk. Globally, nearly 2 million people are affected by inflammatory bowel diseases (IBD) including Crohn disease (CD) and ulcerative colitis (UC) (15). A study by Pituch identified long-term dietary fiber consumption was associated with a 40 % reduction in Crohn disease (CD) risk; however, there was no correlation with ulcerative colitis (UC). A study of children with inflammatory bowel disease observed that total dietary fiber consumption was largely effective on ameliorating the disease (16). There is strong epidemiological evidence that dietary fiber is protective against being overweight and obesity. Thompson et al. assessed results related to weight management, body weight, body fat percentage and waist circumference with randomized controlled studies with isolatable soluble fiber supplements in overweight and obese adults. This study observed findings for 2-17 weeks. The results of the study observed that soluble fiber supplementation caused a reduction in BMI, body weight, body fat, fasting glucose and insulin values of 0.84, 2.52 kg, 0.41 %, 0.17 mmol/L and 15.88 pmol/L, respectively (17). Our study was identified to support studies in the literature. As the BMI of individuals increases, it was observed they oriented toward foods with lower dietary fiber rates. Brown pasta may be assessed as functional; however, they were identified not to choose foods which did not appeal to the traditional palate.

Among cereals, which are the main consumption source of dietary fiber, the product consumed most frequently and in largest amounts was bread. In Turkey, the daily consumption per person was determined to be 333 g (18). Globally, the annual bread consumption per person was identified as 180 kg in Egypt, 150 kg in Iran, 73 kg in Italy, 44 kg in Australia, 98 kg in Kuwait, 130 kg in Syria and 34 kg in USA (19). According to study results by Dölekoğlu et al., though the diversity of bread products is increasing, white bread consumption preserves its importance and has high consumption. According to the study results, consumption of bran bread in Antalya province was identified to be 2 times the rate in other provinces (20). Considering eating habits, availability and taste factors in the assessment results, foods like white bread, pasta and rice containing lower fiber appear to be consumed more compared to other cereal products. In our study, results were obtained which support the literature. According to BMI assessment, people with normal weight consumed whole-wheat bread 3-4 times per week, bran bread once every 15 days, and rye bread and brown pasta once per month. People who were overweight consumed whole-wheat bread 1-2 times per week, bran bread once every 15 days and rye bread once per month, while they did not consume brown pasta at all. Obese people ate whole-wheat bread once every 15 days, bran, and rye bread once per month and additionally did not eat brown pasta. According to these results, as the degree of obesity increased, the consumption of cereal products containing dietary fiber was observed to reduce. Participants consumed high rates of white bread once per day, while they were identified to choose whole-wheat bread in second place. When basic cereals apart from bread are investigated, it was found they consumed phyllo pastry once per month, white rice, and white pasta 1-2 times per week. Bulgur, a rich source in terms of dietary fiber, was consumed at least once every 15 days. Muesli, breakfast cereals, wholegrain biscuits and cereal bars are foods which were not consumed by the majority. According to the results, individuals' choice of cereal products is thought to be generally shaped by palate as a result of traditional eating habits.

Sex is known to be an important factor among factors affecting healthy food choices. Monneuse et al. identified that women were aware individuals in research assessing adult eating behavior and attitudes, beliefs and knowledge related to food. Women are reported to have healthier habits compared to men in relation to topics like avoiding excess sugar consumption, not consuming animal fat and eating more dietary fiber (21). Research investigating differences in eating behavior according to sex determined women abided by healthy food and eating behavior more than men. The results of the research observed that women were more willing to change eating habits compared to men (22). In Turkey, Ergün performed research with the aim of identifying the healthy eating concept and consumer perceptions of 494 adults aged 25 years and older. They identified that women (63.2 %) attached more importance to healthy eating compared to men (46.3 %) (23). When the sex factor is investigated in our study, studies in the literature were supported. Men participating in the study had significantly high mean consumption of white bread, rye bread, phyllo pastry and white rice compared to mean consumption by women, while women had higher mean consumption of muesli and cereal bars compared to consumption by men. Similarly, when points for knowledge about dietary fiber are examined, women were identified to have higher mean points compared to men.

The increase in educational level, ease of access to information, widespread use of communication tools, change in women's social position, and increased awareness of healthy eating have led to differences in cereal product consumption by consumers (24). Currently, eating problems were revealed to be closely associated with lack of education and lack of knowledge in a variety of research. In order to protect health and ensure enough and balanced eating, individuals and society must be informed about eating (25). Currently, cereal products are no longer single-type foods like bread and rice but meet variable consumer choices with differentiated products. This differentiation is thought to be a factor making it more difficult to choose correct/healthy food products. One of the important factors in order to make correct choice of education is notable. As the educational level of individuals increase, they orient toward more correct choices and acquire the habit of reading labels (26). When the study is investigated in line with this, there were negative linear correlations between white bread, phyllo pastry and white rice consumption with educational level. As educational level increased, consumption of white bread, phyllo pastry and rice reduced; while consumption of whole wheat, brown pasta, muesli, breakfast cereal, wholegrain biscuits and cereal bars increased.

Currently, a variety of research has revealed a close correlation between eating problems with lack of education and information. The increase in nutritional information level is accepted as directly proportional to preserving health and ensuring sufficient and balanced nutrition (27). A study was performed with 148 chefs with the aim of determining the nutritional (nutrient) knowledge levels of chefs working in kitchens in holiday villages in holiday resorts, starred hotels, and public organizations. With ages from 18 to 55 years, participants were asked which food contained highest dietary fiber. While only 25 % of participants gave the correct answer, 48.6 % stated they did not know the answer to the question. The results of the research revealed that 64.9 % of chefs had insufficient nutritional (nutrient) knowledge levels (25). Deniz and Alsaffar included 360 people in a study with the aim of investigating the validity and reliability of a dietary fiber information survey among university students and identifying the knowledge levels of the sample group. They divided participants into two groups as those receiving nutrition lessons and those who did not. The basis of the study was to answer the question: "is the knowledge level about dietary fiber higher among those attending nutrition lessons than for those not attending nutrition lessons?" The results of the study found the score for the group attending nutrition lessons was higher than the other group and the difference between the two groups was significant (27). When the knowledge level about dietary fiber is assessed among participants in this study, high rates stated that fiber-rich food contained beneficial elements, were effective in treating diseases and protecting against diseases, that consumption of fruit and vegetables with skin was rich in terms of dietary fiber, while less than 50 % stated they were undecided about whether dietary fiber reduced vitamin and mineral requirements. The results of the study show the need for more comprehensive information studies related to dietary fiber and cereal consumption.

Conclusion

When cereal product consumption and factors affecting choices by participants are assessed, men were observed to choose higher rates of products with low dietary fiber content obtained from white flour compared to women. More than 50 % of participants did not consume bran, rye and multigrain breads and the majority stated they ate white bread at least once per day. As a result of this, the bread consumed was identified to be insufficient in terms of dietary fiber. Meeting the majority of daily energy requirements from foods rich in complex carbohydrates (breakfast cereal products, bran, oat breads, bulgur, starch-rich foods like brown pasta, brown rice, etc.) will increase dietary fiber consumption. The study observed that individuals will orient toward healthier food choices with nutritional education. In line with this, in the name of increasing nutritional knowledge levels, health policies should be created to increase the knowledge levels and consumption of dietary fiber by individuals. For example, public notices about dietary fiber can be created explaining the positive effects of dietary fiber to society. Providing information about foods containing dietary fiber to individuals will increase dietary fiber consumption levels of individuals and ensure more inclusion of cereal products in nutritional programs and new recipes suitable for traditional diet flavors should be developed to encourage consumption of foods with high fiber content but low consumption.

References

1. Sonnenberg, L., Gelsomin, E., Levy, D. E., Riis, J., Barraclough, S., & Thorndike, A. N. (2013). A traffic light food labeling intervention increases consumer awareness of health and healthy choices at the point-of-purchase. *Preventive Medicine, 57*(4), 253–257. doi:10.1016/j.ypmed.2013.07.001

2. Demirbas, N., & Atis, E. (2005). Examining the food security problem of Turkish agriculture at the wheat case. *Ziraat Fakültesi Dergisi, 42*(1), 179-190.

3. Morley, B., Scully, M., Martin, J., Niven, P., Dixon, H., & Wakefield, M. (2013). What types of nutrition menu labelling lead consumers to select less energy-dense fast food? An experimental study. *Appetite, 67*, 8-15. doi:10.1016/j.appet.2013.03.003

4. Causey, J. L., Feirtag, J. M., Gallaher, D. D., Tungland, B. C., & Slavin, J. L. (2000). Effects of dietary inulin on serum lipids, blood glucose and the gastrointestinal environment in hypercholesterolemic men. *Nutrition Research, 20*(2), 191-201. doi:10.1016/S0271-5317(99)00152-9

5. Post, R. E., Mainous III, A. G., Diaz, V. A., Matheson, E. M., & Everett, C. J. (2010). Use of the nutrition facts label in chronic disease management: Results from the national health and nutrition examination survey. *Journal of the American Dietetic Association, 110*(4), 628-632. doi:10.1016/j.jada.2009.12.015

6. Janssen, I., Katzmarzyk, P. T., Boyce, W. F., Vereecken, C., Mulvihill, C., Roberts, C., ... Health Behavior in School-Aged Children Obesity Working Group. (2005). Comparison of overweight and obesity prevalence in school-aged youth from 34 countries and their relationships

with physical activity and dietary patterns. *Obesity Reviews*, 6(2), 123-132. doi:10.1111/j.1467-789X.2005.00176.x

7. Dayısoylu, K. S., Gezginç, Y., & Cingöz, A. (2014). Fonksiyonel gıda mı, fonksiyonel bileşen mi? Gıdalarda fonksiyonellik. *Gıda*, 39(1), 57-62. doi:10.5505/gida.03511

8. Garipoğlu, G. (2019). Enzime dirençli nişasta kullanarak fonksiyonel galeta geliştirilmesi. *Avrupa Bilim ve Teknoloji Dergisi*, 15, 375-380. doi:10.31590/ejosat.514165

9. Gray, J., Armstrong, G., & Farley, H. (2003). Opportunities and constraints in the functional food market. *Nutrition & Food Science*, 33(5), 213-218. doi:10.1108/00346650310499730

10. Bilgiçli, N., Elgün, A., & Türker, S. (2006). Effects of various phytase sources on phytic acid content, mineral extractability and protein digestibility of tarhana. *Food Chemistry*, 98(2), 329-337. doi:10.1016/j.foodchem.2005.05.078

11. Merriam, P. A., Persuitte, G., Olendzki, B. C., Schneider, K., Pagoto, S. L., Palken, J. L., ... Ma, Y. (2012). Dietary intervention targeting increased fiber consumption for metabolic syndrome. *Journal of the Academy of Nutrition and Dietetics*, 112(5), 621-623. doi:10.1016/j.jand.2012.01.024

12. Harris, P. J., & Smith, B. G. (2006). Plant cell walls and cell-wall polysaccharides: Structures, properties and uses in food products. *International Journal of Food Science & Technology*, 41, 129-143. doi:10.1111/j.1365-2621.2006.01470.x

13. Liu, S., Buring, J. E., Sesso, H. D., Rimm, E. B., Willett, W. C., & Manson, J. E. (2002). A prospective study of dietary fiber intake and risk of cardiovascular disease among women. *Journal of the American College of Cardiology*, 39(1), 49-56. doi:10.1016/S0735-1097(01)01695-3

14. Köksel, H., & Özboy, Ö. (1993). Besinsel liflerin insan sağlığındaki rolü. *Gıda*, 18(5), 309-314.

15. Elam, M. B., Ginsberg, H. N., Lovato, L. C., Corson, M., Largay, J., Leiter, L. A., ... Friedewald, W. T. (2017). Association of fenofibrate therapy with long-term cardiovascular risk in statin-treated patients with type 2 diabetes. *JAMA Cardiology*, 2(4), 370-380. doi:10.1001/jamacardio.2016.4828

16. Pituch-Zdanowska, A., Albrecht, P., Banasiuk, M., & Banaszkiewicz, A. (2018). Dietary fiber intake in children with inflammatory bowel disease. *Journal of Pediatric Gastroenterology and Nutrition*, 66(4), 624-629. doi:10.1097/MPG.0000000000001736

17. Thompson, S. V., Hannon, B. A., An, R., & Holscher, H. D. (2017). Effects of isolated soluble fiber supplementation on body weight, glycemia, and insulinemia in adults with overweight and obesity: A systematic review and meta-analysis of randomized controlled trials. *The American Journal of Clinical Nutrition, 106*(6), 1514-1528. doi:10.3945/ajcn.117.163246

18. Toprak Mahsulleri Ofisi. (2018). *Ekmek israfı ve tüketici alışkanlıkları raporu.*

19. Koç, B. (2011). *Ekmek tüketiminde tüketici tercihleri: Van ili örneği.* Ankara: Tepge Yayın, Tarımsal Ekonomi ve Politika Geliştirme Enstitüsü Yayını.

20. Dölekoğlu, C. Ö., Giray, F. H., & Şahin, A. (2014). Mutfaktan çöpe ekmek: tüketim ve değerlendirme. *Akademik Bakış Uluslararası Hakemli Sosyal Bilimler Dergisi, 44,* 4-15.

21. Monneuse, M. O., Bellisle, F., & Koppert, G. (1997). Eating habits, food and health related attitudes and beliefs reported by French students. *European Journal of Clinical Nutrition, 51*(1), 46-53.

22. Missagia, S. V., Oliveira, S. R., & Rezende, D. C. (2013). Beauty and the beast: Gender differences in food-related behavior. *Revista Brasileira de Marketing, 12*(1), 149-165. doi:10.5585/remark.v12i1.2441

23. Ergün, C. (2003). *Sağlıklı beslenme kavramı ve tüketici algısı üzerine bir araştırma.* (Unpublished master's thesis). Hacettepe University, Ankara, Turkey.

24. Hasselbalch, A. L. (2010). Genetics of dietary habits and obesity. *Danish Medical Bulletin, 57,* 1-18.

25. Besler, H. T., Buyuktuncer, Z., & Uyar, M. F. (2012). Consumer understanding and use of food and nutrition labeling in Turkey. *Journal of Nutrition Education and Behavior, 44*(6), 584-591. doi:10.1016/j.jneb.2012.01.005

26. Güler, B., & Özçelik, A. Ö. (2002). Çalışan ve çalışmayan kadınların yiyecek satın alma hazırlama davranışları üzerinde bir araştırma. *Ankara Üniversitesi Ev Ekonomisi Mezunları Derneği Yayınları Bilim Serisi, 3,* 1-13.

27. Deniz, M. Ş., & Alsaffar, A. A. (2014). Diyet lifi bilgisi anketinin Türk öğrenci popülasyonunda geçerlilik ve güvenilirliğinin değerlendirilmesi. *9. Uluslararası Beslenme ve Diyetetik Kongresi Yayınları.* 319-320.

Ecenur Özkul and Can Ergün

An Evaluation of Nutritional Supplement Habits of Mothers and Eating Habits of Children Aged 0-6 Years

Abstract

Objective: The breastfeeding and nutritional supplement habits adopted by mothers after childbirth are significant factors in securing the healthy growth and development of infants. Starting from the postpartum sixth month, additional foods that have the required nutrients should be introduced to the nutrition plan of the infant to ensure a healthy transition to an adult diet.

Materials and Methods: This study examines the breastfeeding period of mothers, the postpartum month supplementary feeding was started, the eating behavior of the children, and the changes in the eating behaviors of the children according to the person in charge of feeding them. The study was conducted between the dates of March 2019 and May 2019 with 401 mothers of children who were in the age range of 0-6 years old.

Results: Among the participants who started complementary feeding before postpartum six months, the average breastfeeding time was found to be 13.45±1.13 months, while among those who started complementary feeding at the postpartum sixth month, the average breastfeeding time was found to be 16.33±0.54 months. The vast majority of the participants (99 %) stated that they continued to breastfeed after the infant was six months of age. In terms of the complementary foods the mothers used, 49.6 % of the mothers started complementary feeding with yoghurt, 34.7 % with pureed vegetables, and 31.7 % with ready-to-feed formula. In examining the eating habits of the participants' children in terms of the person in charge of feeding them, when it was the mothers who were in charge, 64.3 % of the children ate their meals at the dinner table without any distractions, while 35.7 % ate their meals in company with a tv/tablet or mobile phone. When it was immediate family or relatives in charge of feeding the children, it was found that 65.9 % ate their meals at the table without any distractions, and that 37.4 % ate their meals with a tv/tablet or mobile phone.

Conclusion: It was observed that the participants generally had high levels of awareness about the benefits of breastfeeding, but that their complementary feeding and meal habits varied according to different factors affecting their behaviors.

Keywords: Mother's Milk, Nutrition Behavior, Complementary Nutrition, Additional Nutrition Habits

Introduction

Nutrition is one of the most important factors affecting the growth and development of children. Particularly from the birth of the child up to 24 months of age, the breastfeeding and complementary breastfeeding habits of mothers are key factors affecting the babies' health status. Proper breastfeeding duration and complementary nutrition habits promote the healthy physiological and psychosocial development of infants (1). If infants continue to regularly gain weight in their first six months, then breastfeeding should be maintained. The World Health Organization (2) and the United Nations Children's Fund (3) suggest that infants should be given nutritious complementary foods and should continue breastfeeding up to the age of two years. The complementary foods given to the infant starting at six months of age should be maintained to support breastfeeding (4). To ensure a healthy transition to an adult diet program, complementary foods should be added at the proper time to the infants' diet to fulfill their necessary nutrient requirements (2). Starting complementary feeding at the proper time and with suitable foods facilitates the development of chewing and biting skills in the infant and serves to familiarize them with different types of food that have different textures and tastes. Nutrition has an important role in the development of all components of metabolism, including the central nervous system, the endocrine system, and the immune system (5).

The way mothers feed their babies is just as important as the foods they feed their babies. Various factors, such as the attitudes and behaviors exhibited by the caretakers of the children and regular meal hours, are not only socially important but also nutritionally important for a child's development (6). The eating culture of Turkey places high value on children eating together with family, especially the elders of the family, at the dinner table. However, with the growing popularity of technological tools, like tablets and mobile phones, the eating behaviors of children and the perspectives of parents on this subject have been changing (7).

This study examined the breastfeeding period of mothers, the postpartum month supplementary feeding was started, the eating behavior of the children, and the changes in the eating behaviors of the children according to the person in charge of them.

Materials and Methods

This study was conducted from March 2019 to May 2019 with mothers living in İstanbul who had children between the ages of 0-6 years old to evaluate the breastfeeding and complementary nutrition habits of mothers and the eating habits of the children aged 0-6 years old. Based on the objectives of the study, the convenience sampling method was applied to determine the study sample. With convenience sampling, participants are selected from a population easily accessible (8). Accordingly, the sample size was calculated as 384 (margin of error: 5 %; level of confidence: 95 %). A total of 401 mothers were included in the study group to compensate for possible participant withdrawals from the study. Mothers who did not have any children between the ages of 0-6 years old, did not voluntarily agree to participate in the research, or had communication and/or mental problems were excluded from the study. Prior to starting the application, ethical approval to perform the study was granted by the Ethics Committee of Bahçeşehir University Faculty of Medicine (approval number 2018-17/08, dated December 19, 2018), and all the mothers who agreed to participate signed a "Volunteer Consent Form" after being informed about the study. Data were then collected via two formats, face-to-face at a private kindergarten, from which permission was obtained to conduct the study, and from an internet-based survey.

The questionnaire form used as the data collection tool was prepared by the researchers of this study. The form included a total of 20 questions, five of which addressed the socio-demographic characteristics of the participants, and 15 of which addressed the children's weight and height, their eating habits, the duration of breastfeeding, the month supplementary feeding started, type of supplementary feeding, and meal habits, and the primary caretaker of the children during mealtimes since their birth.

The evaluation of the children's body weights was performed by calculating the z-score, which is the most commonly used parameter to evaluate children using the body mass index values specified by the World Health Organization. According to these specifications, a BMI z-score value that is between +1 and +2 standard deviations (+1SD - +2SD) is considered overweight, +2 or more standard deviations (+2SD) is considered obese, between +1 and -2 standard deviations (+1SD - -2SD) is considered normal, between -3 and -2 standard deviations (-3SD - -2SD) is considered thin, and -3 standard deviations and below (-3SD) is considered very thin. The SPSS 21.00 program was used for statistical analyses. After applying the normality test, the differences between the mothers in terms of the study variables were tested. Percentile evaluations of the multiple-choice questions were conducted using the Chi-square test.

Results

It was observed that 66.1 % of the participating mothers were younger than 35 years old, and that 33.9 % were older than 35 years old. Examining their education status, it was found that 10.2 % of the mothers were primary school graduates, 7.5 % were secondary school graduates, 18 % were high school graduates, 49.4 % were university graduates, and 15 % had master's or PhD degrees. While 97.3 % of the mothers were married to the fathers of their children, 2.7 % were divorced from their husbands, and 51.6 % of the mothers were housewives, 47.6 % were employed, and 1 % were retired. Regarding the income status of the mothers, it was seen that 1 % had no income, 5 % had income less than or equal to 1,600 TL, 15.7 % had an income of between 1,601 TL and 3,000 TL, 27.2 % had an income of between 3,001 TL and 5,000 TL, 21.7 % had an income of between 5,001 TL and 7,000 TL, and 29.4 % had an income higher than or equal to 7,001 TL. Finally, 56.1 % of the mothers had male children, while 43.9 % had female children (Table 1).

For the participants who started complementary feeding before six months, the average breastfeeding time was found to be 13.45±1.13 months, while for

Tab. 1: General Information of the Participants

General Information		n	%
Mothers' Ages	Young mothers<35 years	265	66.1
	Mature mothers≥35 years	136	33.9
Education Status	Primary school	41	10.1
	Secondary school	30	7.5
	High school	72	18.0
	University	198	49.4
	Master's degree-PhD	60	15.0
Marital Status	I live with my child's father	390	97.3
	My child's father and I are divorced	11	2.7
Employment Status	Housewife	207	51.6
	Employed	190	47.4
	Retired	4	1.0
Income Status	No income	4	1.0
	Less than or equal to 1,600 TL	20	5.0
	1,601-3,000 TL	63	15.7
	3,001-5,000 TL	109	27.2
	5,001-7,000 TL	87	21.7
	More than or equal to 7,001 TL	118	29.4
Gender of the Child	Male	225	56.1
	Female	176	43.9

Tab. 2: The Breastfeeding Period According to the Start Month of Complementary Feeding

The Start Time of Complementary Feeding	n	The Average Breastfeeding Time	Standard Deviation	Inter-Group Significance
The participants who started complementary feeding before the age of six months	65	13.45	1.13	
The participants who started complementary feeding by the age of six months	327	16.33	0.54	0.026
Total	392			

the participants who started complementary feeding by the sixth month, the average breastfeeding time was found to be 16.33±0.54 months. The significance level between groups was found 0.026 ($p < 0.05$) (Table 2). Sixty-three of the participating mothers stated that they continued to breastfeed their children. Of the participants who had stopped breastfeeding, 24.9 % stated that they breastfed between 0 and 6 months, while 75.1 % stated that they breastfed for at least 7 months. In regard to the time of starting complementary feeding, 12 participants reported that they had not yet started any complementary feeding, and 16.6 % of the 327 who had started complementary feeding stated that they had started before six months. It was determined that 83.4 % of the participants started complementary feeding by the sixth month (These data are not presented in a table.).

Nearly all the participants (99 %) stated that they continued to breastfeed after six months of age. In terms of the complementary foods used, it was found that 49.6 % of the mothers started complementary feeding with yoghurt, 34.7 % with pureed vegetables, 31.7 % with ready-to-feed formula, 26.4 % with water, and 7.2 % with fruit juices (Table 3).

In examining the eating habits of the children of the participants according to the person who cares for their children, it was found that when it was the mothers who were caring for their children, 64.3 % of the children ate their meals at the table without any distractions or movement, 35.7 % ate while watching a tv/tablet or mobile phone, 17.5 % ate while playing games, and 19.9 % were always moving about when they ate. When the children were cared for by immediate family or relatives, it was determined that 65.9 % of the children ate their meals at the table without any distractions or movement, 37.4 % ate while watching a tv/tablet or mobile phone, 26.8 % ate while playing games, and 22.8 % were always moving

Tab. 3: Complementary Food Given to the Infants from the Sixth Month of Age

Complementary Foods	n	%	Total %
Mother's milk	397	39.8	99.0
Formula	127	12.7	31.7
Water	106	10.6	26.4
Yoghurt	199	20.0	49.6
Pureed vegetables	139	13.9	34.7
Fruit juices	29	2.9	7.2
Total	997	100.0	248.6

Tab. 4: The Evaluation of Eating Habits According to the Person Who Cares for the Child

The Person Who Cares for the Child		At Dinner Table	With TV/ Tablet/ Mobile Phone	Plays	Always Moves	Total
Mother	n	220	122	60	68	342
	%	64.3	35.7	17.5	19.9	
	Total %	55.1	30.6	15.0	17.0	85.7
Immediate Family & Relatives	n	81	46	33	28	123
	%	65.9	37.4	26.8	22.8	
	Total %	20.3	11.5	8.3	7.0	30.8
Paid Babysitter	n	27	17	8	4	43
	%	62.8	39.5	18.6	9.3	
	Total %	6.8	4.3	2.0	1.0	10.8
Kindergarten	n	70	44	12	27	111
	%	63.1	39.6	10.8	24.3	
	Total %	17.5	11.0	3.0	6.8	27.8

about when eating. When the children were cared for by a paid babysitter, 62.8 % ate their meals at the table without any distractions or movement, 39.5 % ate while watching a tv/tablet or mobile phone, 18.6 % ate while playing games, and 9.3 % were always moving about when eating. Finally, when the children were under the care of a kindergarten, 63.1 % ate their meals at the table without any distractions or movement, 39.6 % ate while watching a tv/tablet or mobile phone, 10.8 % ate while playing games, and 24.3 % were always moving about while eating (Table 4).

In comparing the determination of the mealtimes of the children of the participants according to their weight level, it was found that, of the mothers of obese children, 19.7 % regulated the mealtimes of their children, 13.8 % fed

Tab. 5: How Mealtimes of the Children Are Determined and Its Relationship to Their Weight Levels

Weight Evaluation of Children		I regulate mealtimes	I feed my child when he/she is hungry	I do not have a regular feeding routine	Other	Total
Obese	n	24	12	5	4	45
	%	19.7	13.8	15.2	30.8	17.6
	Total %	9.4	4.7	2.0	1.6	17.6
Overweight	n	21	18	6	3	48
	%	17.2	20.7	18.2	23.1	18.8
	Total %	8.2	7.1	2.4	1.2	18.8
Normal	n	72	43	20	4	139
	%	59.0	49.4	60.6	30.8	54.5
	Total %	28.2	16.9	7.8	1.6	54.5
Thin	n	5	13	2	2	22
	%	4.1	14.9	6.1	15.4	8.6
	Total %	2.0	5.1	0.8	0.8	8.6
Very Thin	n	0	1	0	0	1
	%	0.0	1.1	0.0	0.0	0.4
	Total %	0.0	0.4	0.0	0.0	0.4
Total	n	122	87	33	13	255
	%	100.0	100.0	100.0	100.0	100.0
	Total %	47.8	34.1	12.9	5.1	100.0

their children when their children were hungry, 15.2 % did not follow a specific routine, and 30.8 % regulated the feeding of their children in a variety of ways. Among the mothers of overweight children, 17.2 % regulated the mealtimes of their children, 20.7 % fed their children when their children were hungry, 18.2 % did not follow a specific routine, and 23.1 % regulated the feeding of their children in a variety of ways. Among the mothers of normal weight children, 59 % regulated the mealtimes of their children, 49.4 % fed their children when their children were hungry, 60.6 % did not follow a specific routine, and 30.8 % regulated the feeding of their children in a variety of ways. Among the mothers of thin children, 4.1 % regulated the mealtimes of their children, 14.9 % fed their children when their children were hungry, 6.1 % did not follow a specific routine, and 15.4 % regulated the feeding of their children in a variety of ways. Finally, among the mothers of very thin children, 1.1 % fed their children when their children were hungry and 0.4 % regulated the feeding of their children in a variety of ways (Table 5).

Discussion

Introducing complementary foods is an important step for ensuring the physical and mental development of babies and their formation of proper nutritional habits. The types of complementary food selected by mothers during this period are important as well. The first foods given to infants in the complementary feeding period can vary due to a number of reasons. In a review of the studies conducted in Turkey on this subject, it was observed that Yücecan et al. reported that the foods preferred by mothers to introduce complementary feeding were fruit juice, formula, cow's milk, and pudding, in respective order of most to least preferred (9); Gürakan et al. indicated that the foods preferred by mothers when starting nutritional supplements were formula, pudding (rice flour and milk), yoghurt, and cow's milk, in respective order of most to least preferred (10); Öztürk and Öktem, in their study, reported that the first complementary foods given to infants were formula, pudding, fruit juice, and yoghurt, in respective order of most to least preferred (11); and finally Kaya et al. stated that the first complementary foods preferred by mothers were home-made soups (28.4 %), ready-to-feed yoghurt (24 %), home-made yoghurt (12.4 %), fruit (10 %), ready-to-feed formula (8.8 %), breakfast-type foods (crumbs and cheese with tea, biscuit with tea or cow's milk, etc.) (7.6 %), pudding (6.8 %), and ready-to-feed soup (2 %) (12). In the present study, 39.8 % of the mothers were still breastfeeding their infants, and as complementary feeding, they preferred yoghurt (20 %), pureed vegetables (13.9 %), ready-to-feed formula (12.7 %), water (10.6 %), and fruit juices (2.9 %).

In this study, it was observed that all the mothers breastfed their infants. Similarly, Şahin and Özyurt reported in their study that 96.4 % of the mothers breastfed their children (13), Yetim et al. indicated this rate to be 99.5 % in their study (14), Yıldız et al. reported a 100 % rate in their study (15), and according to the 2013 Turkey Demographic and Health Survey, 96.09 % of mothers breastfed their children (13). Evaluating the mothers in terms of the continuity of breastfeeding, this study found the average breastfeeding period to be 15.85±2.2 months. Şahin and Özyurt indicated that the average breastfeeding period was 8.5±6.2 months in their study(13), Gün et al., 11.0±4.4 months, in their study (16), Kutlu et al., 10.6±5.7 months in their study (17), Ünsal et al., 8.5±5.9 months in their study (18), and Açık et al., 10.4±6.4 months in their study (19). These differences could be attributed to the different locations from which the samples were drawn, the homogeneity of the participant population, or education level.

Complementary feeding has major impacts on both the physiological and the psychological development of babies. It is important to note here that the early or late introduction of complementary foods may cause harm to babies. In this study, it was found that the mothers who started complementary feeding before six months breastfed their babies for a significantly shorter amount of time. Yılmazbaş et al. reported that the reasons the mothers gave for starting complementary feeding before six months was that they believed breastfeeding alone was not enough to meet the hunger and nutritional needs of their babies, and that they wanted their babies to acquire new tastes (20). In a review of the worldwide research on this subject, it was seen that there are very high rates of mothers who are prompted to start complementary foods under the belief that the breast milk is no longer sufficient (21-25). This belief, however, is not driven by apparent insufficient weight gain of the infant, but rather, by the subjective feelings of the mothers.

To learn new tastes was stated to be another reason the mothers introduced complementary feeding before six months. Yet, given that the baby is introduced to different tastes by virtue of the mother's diet, it is unnecessary for mothers to begin complementary feeding during the breastfeeding period. In fact, evidence has shown that continuing to breastfeed babies during the complementary feeding period reduces the possibility of babies having adverse reactions to new foods (26).

How children eat is equally as important as what children eat. According to the findings reported by Dereli, 57.3 % of children eat in front of the TV, and 31.3 % eat while wandering about (7). Oğuz and Derin found that 34.7 % of children eat in front of the TV, 3.6 % eat while playing, and 7.2 % eat while being chased around (27). Kobak and Pek compared children who applied to the Mother and Child Health Center and preschool children who attend a nursery school in terms of who were the primary caretakers of the children and reported that 30 % of the latter were cared for by their mothers, and 70 % by paid babysitters, whereas 100 % of the children who applied to the Mother and Child Health Center were cared for by their mothers primarily. It was further found that 42.3 % of these children ate at the dinner table, 20.0 % ate in front of the TV, 8.5 % ate while listening to a story, 13.8 % ate while playing, and 15.4 % ate while being chased around (6). In a study by Terzi, it was reported that 24 % of children ate at the dinner table and/or in front of the TV, 17.3 % ate only at the dinner table, 12.5 % ate in front of the TV, and 5.8 % ate while being chased around (28). The present study evaluated the eating habits of children according to the person who cared with them and found that regardless of who this person was, most of the children ate at the dinner table, while the second most prominent eating habit of the children was to eat while watching a tv/tablet/telephone. In the food culture of Turkey, eating meals is an important activity that functions to bring families together. Considering the high value placed on this function, it would be expected that families teach their children to acquire these cultural habits. However, as a result of the growing popularity of technological devices and the appeal they have for children, families need to have a better awareness of their impact on the eating habits of children in order to reduce the rates of feeding children in company with these devices. It has been shown that acclimatizing children in early ages to eating at the dinner table without any technological devices to distract them is beneficial, insofar as it allows families to better monitor what and how much the children eat, both of which are important factors that affect long-term nutritional habits (29).

Regulating the mealtimes of children is also considered to be a significant factor in terms of establishing healthy nutritional habits in children. In a study by Güneyli, it was found that 31.9 % of children were fed at times determined by their mothers, whereas 16.9 % were fed when they felt hungry (30). Dereli stated in her study, that of the participating mothers, 72.4 % fed their children at regular intervals, 18.9 % fed their children when their children were hungry, and 8.7 % fed their children without following any fixed schedule (7). The present study compared the data on the children in terms of the Z-score and the children's mealtimes. No significant relationship was found between mealtime regulation and the children's weight levels. There is no study found in the literature comparing the obesity evaluation and mealtime routines of children. Further studies, therefore, are required on this subject.

Conclusion

Nutrition is a process that starts in the mother's womb. The food consumption habits adopted by mothers in the maternal period are determinant factors for their babies' health status during and after delivery. In addition, the nutrition process, which starts with breastfeeding after delivery, has various physiological and psychological effects on both the child and the mother. This study examined the feeding habits of mothers with children between the ages of 0-6 years old, starting from delivery and the eating behaviors of children according to the person primarily responsible for caring for them. Results from the study showed that the mothers were strongly aware of the value of breastfeeding. However, their reasons for starting complementary feeding and the foods they chose to start with suggest that more studies are needed on this subject to raise awareness on this issue. The mothers cited different reasons for starting early complementary feeding and for the amount of complementary feeding they preferred. In examining the eating style habits of the children, the influence of technology on these habits needs to be taken into account. Although parents use technological devices as an alternative, easy method to facilitate the feeding of their children, the potential negative impact this can have on their future eating habits, including risks like obesity, needs to be taken seriously, especially considering that the healthy dining habits acquired at younger ages can help to mitigate eating behavior conducive to obesity.

References

1. Gür, E. (2006). Tamamlayıcı beslenme. *Türk Pediatri Arşivi, 41*, 181-8.
2. World Health Organization. (n.d.). Breastfeeding. Retrieved from https://www.who.int/topics/breastfeeding/en/
3. UNICEF Publications. (2018). Breastfeeding: A mother's gift, for every child. Retrieved from https://data.unicef.org/resources/breastfeeding-a-mothers-gift-for-every-child/
4. Bhandari, N., Kabir, A. K., & Salam, M. A. (2008). Main streaming nutrition in to maternal and child health programmes: Scaling up of exclusive breastfeeding. *Maternal & Child Nutrition, 4*(s1), 5-23. doi:10.1111/j.1740-8709.2007.00126.x
5. Victora, C. G., Bahl, R., Barros, A. J., França, G. V., Horton, S., & Krasevec, J. (2016). Breastfeeding in the 21st century: Epidemiology, mechanisms, and lifelong effect. *The Lancet, 387*(10017), 475-490. doi:10.1016/S0140-6736(15)01024-7
6. Kobak, C., & Pek, H. (2015). Okul öncesi dönemde (3-6 yaş) ana çocuk sağlığı ve anaokulundaki çocukların beslenme özelliklerinin karşılaştırılması. *Hacettepe Üniversitesi Eğitim Fakültesi Dergisi, 30*(2), 42-55.
7. Dereli, F. (2006). *2-5 yaş arası sağlıklı çocukların beslenme özellikleri ve aile etkileşimi.* (Unpublished master's thesis). Marmara University, İstanbul, Turkey.
8. Chin, M. K., & Siew, N. M. (2015). The development and validation of a figural scientific creativity test for preschool pupils. *Creative Education, 6*(12), 1391-1402. doi:10.4236/ce.2015.612139
9. Yücecan, S., Pekcan, G., & Akal, E. (1993). Ankara, İstanbul, Muğla, Yozgat, Sivas ve Tokat illerinde 0-2 yaş grubu çocuk sahibi annelerin beslenme bilgi düzeyi ve uygulamalarının saptanmasına yönelik bir araştırma. *Beslenme ve Diyet Dergisi, 22*(1), 27-42.
10. Gürakan, B., Özcebe, H., & Bertan, M., (1993). Multipar annelerin anne sütü ile ilgili deneyimleri. *Çocuk Sağlığı ve Hastalıkları Dergisi, 36*, 1-10.

11. Öztürk, M., & Öktem, F. (2000). Isparta Yedişehitler sağlık ocağı bölgesi'ndeki 4-24 aylık çocuklarda ek besinlere geçiş döneminin incelenmesi. *Süleyman Demirel Üniversitesi Tıp Fakültesi Dergisi*, 7(1), 53-58.

12. Kaya, Z., Yiğit, Ö., Erol, M., & Bostan Gayret, Ö. (2016). Altı-yirmi dört ay arası yaş grubunda beslenmeyle ilgili anne ve babaların bilgi ve deneyimlerinin değerlendirilmesi. *Med Bull Haseki*, 54, 70-75. doi:10.4274/haseki.2756

13. Bilgin Şahin, B., & Cengiz Özyurt, B. (2017). Manisa'da yarı-kentsel bir bölgede 0-24 ay çocuklarda anne sütü alma durumu ve beslenme alışkanlıkları. *Turkish Journal of Public Health*, 3(15), 164-176. doi:10.20518/tjph.375324

14. Yetim, A., Yetim, Ç., & Devecioğlu, E. (2015). Igdır'da annelerin süt çocugu beslenmesi konusundaki bilgi ve davranışları. *The Journal of Current Pediatrics*, 13(1), 7-12. doi:10.4274/jcp.32032

15. Yıldız, A., Baran, E., Akdur, R., Ocaktan, E., & Kanyılmaz, O. (2008). Bir sağlık ocağı bölgesinde 0-11 aylık bebekleri olan annelerin emzirme durumları ve etkileyen faktörler. *Ankara Üniversitesi Tıp Fakültesi Mecmuası*, 61(2), 9-15.

16. Gün, İ., Yılmaz, M., & Şahin, H. (2009). Kayseri Melikgazi eğitim ve araştırma bölgesi'nde 0-36 aylık çocuklarda anne sütü alma durumu. *Çocuk Sağlığı ve Hastalıkları Dergisi*, 52, 176-182.

17. Kutlu, R., & Marakoğlu, K. (2006). Evaluation of initiating, continuing, and weaning time of breastfeeding. *Marmara Medical Journal*, 19, 121-126.

18. Unsal, H., Atlıhan, F., Ozkan, H., Targan, Ş., & Hassoy, H. (2005). Toplumda anne sütü verme eğilimi ve buna etki eden faktörler. *Çocuk Sağlığı ve Hastalıkları Dergisi*, 48(3), 226-233.

19. Açık, Y., Dinç, E., Benli, S., & Tokdemir, M. (1999). Elazığ İlinde yaşayan 0-2 yaş grubu çocuğu olan kadınların bebek beslenmesi ve anne sütü konusundaki bilgi, tutum ve uygulamaları. *Türkiye Klinikleri Pediatri Dergisi*, 8(2), 53-62.

20. Bilgin, B., & Cengiz, B. (2017). Manisa'da yarı-kentsel bir bölgede 0-24 ay çocuklarda anne sütü alma durumu ve beslenme alışkanlıkları. *Turkish Journal of Public Health*, 3(15), 164-176. doi:10.20518/tjph.375324

21. Thurman, S. E., & Allen, P. J. (2008). Integrating lactation consultants into primary health care services: Are lactation consultants affecting breastfeeding success? *Pediatric Nursing*, 34(5), 419-425.

22. Inoue, M., & Binns, C. W. (2012). Infant feeding practices and breastfeeding duration in japan: A review. *International Breastfeeding Journal*, 7(1), 25-15. doi:10.1186/1746-4358-7-15

23. Bai, D. L., Fong, D. Y., & Tarrant, M. (2015). Factors associated with breastfeeding duration and exclusivity in mothers returning to paid employment postpartum. *Maternal and Child Health Journal, 19*(5), 990-999. doi:10.1007/10995-014-1596-7

24. Newby, R. M., & Davies, P. S. (2015). A prospective study of the introduction of complementary foods in contemporary Australian infants: What, when and why?. *Journal of Paediatrics and Child, 51*(2), 186-191. doi:10.1111/jpc.12699

25. Bagul, A. S., & Supare, M. S. (2012). The infant feeding practices in an urban slum of Nagpur, India. *Journal of Clinical and Diagnostic Research, 6*(9), 1525-1527. doi:10.7860/JCDR/2012/4622.2549

26. Gökçay, G., Kural, B., & Devecioğlu, E. (2014). Anne beslenme özelliklerinin anne sütüne etkisi. *Türkiye Klinikleri Pediatrik Bilimler-Özel Konular, 10*(3), 57-62.

27. Oğuz, Ş., & Derin, D. (2013). An investigation of some nutrition habits of 60-72 month-old children. *Elementary Education Online, 12*(2), 498-511.

28. Terzi, A. Ö. (2005). *Bir-üç yaş grubu sağlıklı çocuklarda beslenme alışkanlıkları ve günlük posa alım düzeyleri.* (Unpublished master's thesis). Hacettepe University, Ankara, Turkey.

29. Watt, R. G., Dykes, J., & Sheiham, A. (2001). Socio-economic determinants of selected dietary indicators in British preschool children. *Public Health Nutrition, 4*(2), 1229-1233. doi:10.1079/PHN2001202

30. Güneyli, U. (1988). 4-6 yaş grubu çocuklarında beslenme alışkanlıkları ve bunu etkileyen etmenler konusunda bir araştırma. *Beslenme ve Diyet Dergisi, 17*(1), 37-45.

Gökçen Garipoğlu, Gülderen Yentür, Esin Koç, and Taner
Özgürtaş

Research into Effect of Nutritional Status in Pregnancy on Breast Milk Lipid Content and Fatty Acid Composition

Abstract

Objective: This study researched the effects of women's eating habits on breast milk fatty acid content.

Materials and Methods: Thirty mothers (15 term, 15 preterm) randomly chosen from Gazi University Faculty of Medicine Neonatal Unit participated in this study. The food consumption choices and eating habits of mothers during pregnancy were identified with a survey method. The obtained data were compared with lipid (cholesterol, triglyceride, EPA, DHA, oleic and arachidonic acid) values in milk samples taken on the 3rd, 7th and 28th days (90 samples). Additionally, the correlation between pregnancy duration (term/preterm) with breast milk lipid content was investigated. Data were analyzed in the SPSS 15.0 statistics program; significance was accepted as $p<0.05$.

Results: While the total fat content of colostrum was higher than mature milk, it was observed to reduce as the duration of lactation continued ($p<0.05$). While milk did not show differences in DHA and oleic acid content in term and preterm milk, preterm milk had lower EPA and arachidonic acid content ($p<0.05$). The n-6/n-3 ratio varied with the lactation duration and was higher in preterm milks ($p<0.05$). According to mothers' food consumption choices, there was no significant correlation between frequency of red meat and cereal consumption with breast milk lipid content ($p>0.05$). Mothers with more frequent fish consumption had higher cholesterol level in breast milk ($p<0.05$). Mothers with higher olive oil and margarine consumption during pregnancy had higher triglyceride level in breast milk, while those consuming oily nuts had higher cholesterol level ($p<0.05$).

Conclusion: The lipid content of breast milk is affected by the mother's food choices during pregnancy. This study will guide future studies investigating infant development and eating habits during the lactation period.

Keywords: Pregnancy, Nutrition, Breast Milk, Lipid, Fatty Acids

Introduction

Pregnancy and lactation are natural physiological events for women. During pregnancy, the fetus grows as a result of nutrients from the mother being transported via the placenta (1). The most natural and most ideal product for neonatal feeding of breast milk is a physiological product responding to the baby's needs. Breast milk meets all the nutrient requirements for normal development of every newborn born at term and with sufficient fetal stores from the mother and is the most basic food sufficient alone for the first 6 months (2).

There are some factors affecting health of mother and infant in the pregnancy and lactation period. These may be listed as the mother giving birth at early or late age, number of pregnancies, duration between the last two pregnancies, infections during pregnancy, medications used, chronic diseases of the mother, smoking, alcohol and drug used, radiation exposure, intake of mold, fungus and pesticide residue in foods and most importantly, adequate and balanced diet (3).

Nutrient requirements in pregnancy are linked to many factors like age, physical activity level, and weight before pregnancy. Additionally, pregnancy increases the basal metabolic rate (BMR). Meeting the nutrients required by this increase is mandatory for the mother's own health, just as it is important for normal development of the fetus (4).

For children to be born healthy, mothers need to have sufficient and balanced diet during pregnancy for fetal development and milk production. Women with inadequate diet are known to have higher numbers of infants born preterm compared to women with normal diet. Linked to this, the incidence of congenital disorders and mental development retardation increases (1,5).

A variety of studies have shown that significant amounts of omega-3 acid, one of the sufficient and balanced nutrients in diet, consumed by pregnant cases increases pregnancy quality and supports fetal brain development. During pregnancy, beneficial effects of intake of docosahexaenoic acid (DHA) and eicosapentaenoic acid (EPA) may be listed as lengthened mean duration of pregnancy and reduced preterm births, increased birth weight and head circumference, increased visual acuity within the first year after birth, accelerated cognitive development and reduced diseases related to the allergic and immune system (autoimmune) (6,7).

The energy and nutrients in breast milk are provided by what the mother eats and her own body stores. Energy provided by diet is accepted to transform to milk energy at rates of 81 %. As the unsaturated fatty acid proportion in a woman's diet increases, the unsaturated fatty acid proportion in milk increases. Increased consumption of seafood products rich in omega-3 fatty acids, especially, increases the content of this fatty acid in breast milk. Again, a diet rich in water-soluble vitamins increases the vitamin value in milk by an amount. Inadequate and unbalanced diet in the mother lowers milk yield (1,8).

Nearly half of the energy provided by breast milk comes from fats. Triglycerides comprise 98 % of fats in breast milk. Breast milk, and colostrum even more so, is rich in polyunsaturated fatty acids (PUFA) ensuring normal brain development, myelinization, retinal functions and cell proliferation (renewed proliferation). The PUFA amount in breast milk is closely related to the mother's diet (9).

In this study, the aim was to research the food consumption habits of mothers due to the effect of food consumed by pregnant women during pregnancy on breast milk fatty acid content. With this aim, the demographic features and eating habits of 30 randomly chosen mothers in Gazi University Hospital Neonatal Unit were investigated.

Materials and Methods

The research was performed from April-December 2008 in Gazi University Faculty of Medicine Hospital Neonatal Unit. Thirty mothers aged from 21 to 43 years were chosen at random (15 term, 15 preterm) and a survey about frequency of food consumption during pregnancy was applied with the face-to-face interview technique. Mothers provided voluntary consent. On the 3rd, 7th and 28th days of lactation, from 8 to 11 in the morning before breast-feeding, milk samples were taken from a single breast with the aid of a vacuum breast pump (Medela Lactina® Select). The samples were placed in plastic tubes and centrifuged for 15 minutes at 2000 g. The supernatant was obtained by passing the thin layer on the surface with the aid of a needle. The samples were stored at -80 °C until analysis. Within the scope of the "determination and comparison of breast milk content of premature and term neonates" project (Project no: 109S006), the collected samples had total protein, albumin, triglycerides, total cholesterol, fatty acids, iron, iron-binding capacity, magnesium and phosphorus levels measured with the enzymatic colorimetric method on an Olympus AU 2700 (Olympus, Mishima, JAPAN) autoanalyzer with kits in Gülhane Military Medical Academy (GATA) Department of Medical Biochemistry. Among the measured parameters, lipid content was compared with the frequency of food consumption during pregnancy by the mother.

Statistical analysis of data used the SPSS 15.0 statistical program for Windows. Data determined with measurements obtained from participants are given as mean, lower, upper, and standard deviation values along with number and percentage distribution. For identification of differences between groups, the chi-square (x^2) test was used, while comparisons for groups of data with normal distribution used the t test, Fisher Exact chi-square test. Normal distribution was checked with the Kolmogorov-Smirnov test. Comparisons of data without normal distribution used the Mann Whitney U test. Statistical significance was accepted as p<0.05.

Results

The frequency of food consumption during pregnancy by the mothers and the lipid content in breast milk on the 3rd, 7th and 28th days were compared and the effect of eating during pregnancy on breast milk lipid profile was researched.

When the mothers' age interval is investigated, 6.6 % of mothers with pre-term births and 20.0 % of mothers with term births were identified to be in the age interval for risky pregnancy. When assessed in terms of body mass index, 20.0 % of mothers with preterm birth and 16.6 % of mothers with term birth were identified to be overweight. There were no significant correlations between maternal age, height, weight, and BMI values with premature or term birth (p>0.05) (Table 1).

Mothers participating in the study were determined to gain from 4 to 28 kg during pregnancy. The weight gained by both groups was similar (p>0.05). The mean birth weight of preterm neonates was 2.5 kg, while term neonates had mean weight of 3.5 kg. Preterm birth was determined as at least 32 weeks.

Among mothers, 90.0 % used some food supplements during pregnancy. Twenty-six individuals used iron supplements, while 2 individuals used fish

Tab. 1: Distribution According to General Characteristics of Individuals

	Preterm Birth (n:15)		Term Birth (n:15)		Total (n: 30)	
	n	%	n	%	n	%
Age Interval						
21-25 years	3	20.0	2	13.3	5	16.6
26-30 years	6	40.0	5	33.3	10	33.3
31-35 years	5	33.3	5	33.3	10	33.3
36-40 years	-	-	3	20.0	3	10.0
41-45 years	1	6.6	-	-	1	3.3
BMI (kg/m²)						
18.5-24.9	10	66.6	11	73.3	21	70.0
25.0-29.9	2	13.3	2	13.3	4	13.3
30.0-35.9	3	20.0	2	13.3	5	16.6

Tab. 2: Variables Related to Pregnancy Status of Mothers

	Preterm (n=15)	Term (n=15)	P
Weight at end of pregnancy (kg)	79.7±11.5	78.6±7.4	0.752
Weight gained during pregnancy (kg)	16.6±6.9	15.7±5.9	0.686
Pregnancy duration (weeks)	35.8±1.7	39.13±1.06	0.690

oil supplements. There was no difference between the two groups in terms of nutritional supplements used (p>0.05). Only 2 mothers were observed to use fish oil supplements during pregnancy. One of these individuals had preterm birth and the neonate weighed 2.1 kg. The other individual gave birth at term and the neonate weighted 3.3 kg. The effect of fish oil use was not found to be significant, but no statistical data can be given due to the very low number of individuals using this supplement.

When activity levels are assessed, 53.0 % of individuals did not change their daily activities, while 36.0 % reduced activity. Among the 18 individuals with weight gain above 15 kg during pregnancy, 8 stated they reduced activity.

It appeared that 56.0 % of mothers changed their eating habits during pregnancy, and stated they especially increased fruit and milk consumption. In both groups, eating habits were similar (p>0.05) (Table 2).

When the most frequently consumed foods are investigated in the mothers' food consumption, 53.3 % of mothers with preterm birth and 33.3 % of mothers with term birth consumed milk/yogurt 2-3 times per day. Cheese was consumed once per day by 86.7 % of preterm mothers and 73.3 % of term mothers. Mothers generally were seen to consume meat like red meat, chicken, and fish 1-2 times per week. In the preterm group 53.3 % of mothers consumed egg once per day, while in the term group this rate was 26.7 %. Consumption of meat products like salami and sausages was very low. The most frequent consumption in the term group was 1-2 times per week for 53.3 %. Dried pulses and cereals were consumed at most 1-2 times per week while bread consumption was 2-3 times per day. Vegetable consumption frequency was once per day at most for 33.3 % in the preterm group and 40.0 % in the term group. Olive oil consumption was 2-3 times per day for 33.3 % of the preterm group and 60.0 % of the term group, while margarine and butter consumption had low rates of once per day (Table 3).

Breast milk samples taken on the 3rd, 7th and 28th days after birth and analyzed in terms of total lipid content and fatty acids were shown to have

Tab. 3: Food Consumption Frequency of Mothers with Preterm and Term Birth

Foods	1 time per day				2-3 times per day				1-2 times per week				3-4 times per week			
	n		%		n		%		n		%		n		%	
	P	T	P	T	P	T	P	T	P	T	P	T	P	T	P	T
Milk/yogurt	4	10	26.7	66.7	8	5	53.3	33.3	2	-	13.3	-	1	-	6.7	-
Cheese	13	11	86.7	73.3	1	4	6.7	26.7	-	-	-	-	1	-	6.7	-
Red meat	2	3	13.3	20.0	-	-	-	-	8	7	53.3	46.7	3	3	20.0	20.0
White meat (turkey, chicken)	1	-	6.7	-	-	-	-	-	11	11	73.3	73.3	2	1	13.3	6.7
Fish	-	-	-	-	-	-	-	-	8	12	53.3	80.0	-	-	-	-
Eggs	8	4	53.3	26.7	-	1	-	6.7	3	5	20.0	33.3	4	5	26.7	33.3
Meat products (salami, sausage etc.)	1	-	6.7	-	-	-	-	-	1	8	6.7	53.3	-	1	-	6.7
Oily nuts (walnut, hazelnut etc.)	5	4	33.3	26.7	1	-	6.7	-	-	-	-	-	-	-	-	-
Dried pulses	-	-	-	-	-	-	-	-	11	13	73.3	86.7	-	3	-	20.0
Vegetables	5	6	33.3	40.0	-	7	-	46.7	3	-	20.0	-	2	-	13.3	-
Fruits	2	5	13.3	33.3	13	10	86.7	66.7	-	-	-	-	7	2	46.7	13.3
Bread	5	3	33.3	20.0	9	11	60.0	73.3	-	-	-	-	-	-	-	-
Rice, pasta, bulgur	2	1	13.3	6.7	-	1	-	6.7	9	10	60.0	66.7	1	1	6.7	6.7
Olive oil	4	3	26.7	20.0	5	9	33.3	60	1	1	6.7	6.7	3	3	20.0	20.0
Margarine	3	2	20.0	13.3	-	-	-	-	3	-	20.0	-	1	-	6.7	-
Butter	4	5	26.7	33.3	-	-	-	-	1	5	6.7	33.3	1	1	6.7	6.7

P=Preterm, T=Term

Tab. 4: Assessment of Biochemical Analysis of Breast Milk According to Group

Biochemical findings	Preterm (n:15) Mean±SD	Term (n:15) Mean±SD	t	p
Triglycerides (mg/dL)				
3rd day	315.6±180.2	337.4±138.1	0.371	0.714
7th day	375.1±246.6	282.2±129.2	-1.292	0.207
28th day	194.8±92.2	164.6±61.8	-1.053	0.301
Total Cholesterol (mg/dL)				
3rd day	10.9±7.5	10.2±5.0	-0.285	0.778
7th day	9.0±84	6.2±3.1	-1.200	0.240
28th day	1.8±1.7	1.5±1.3	-0.580	0.567
EPA (mg/dL)				
3rd day	4.1±5.1	3.7±2.3	-0.242	0.811
7th day	5.6±4.6	5.6±2.6	0.022	0.983
28th day	4.3±2.8	8.9±6.9	2.376	0.025
DHA (mg/dL)				
3rd day	44.2±38.5	57.3±34.9	0.976	0.337
7th day	48.2±36.4	54.8±34.6	0.510	0.614
28th day	46.3±34.0	46.3±34.8	0.003	0.997
Oleic Acid (mg/dL)				
3rd day	678.8±437.1	880.9±263.2	1.533	0.136
7th day	717.8±352.5	692.6±258.1	-0.224	0825
28th day	758.5±235.1	854.5±251.6	1.080	0.289
Arachidonic Acid (mg/dL)				
3rd day	68.8±54.2	76.0±29.1	0.452	0.655
7th day	121.9±176.3	80.9±35.3	-0.883	0.385
28th day	97.2±45.1	70.2±19.3	-2.130	0.042

reducing cholesterol and triglyceride levels which were similar in both groups of both preterm and term birth ($p > 0.05$). In terms of DHA and oleic acid levels, the 3 sample times had similar levels with no clear reduction or increase in both groups ($p > 0.05$). The fatty acids of EPA and arachidonic acid had close levels at the 3 sample times. However, milk samples from mothers with preterm birth were observed to contain lower levels of EPA and arachidonic acid on the 3rd day compared to women with term birth and this situation was statistically significant ($p < 0.05$) (Table 4).

When lipid content of breast milk is assessed according to food consumption frequency, while there was no significant correlation between red meat consumption frequency and breast milk lipid content, there was a significant correlation found between frequency of chicken/turkey meat consumption and breast milk arachidonic acid (AA) levels. Milk from mothers who consumed chicken once or more per week were found to have lower AA levels on the 7th day. Mothers who consumed fish once or more per week were found to have higher cholesterol level in milk samples from the 28th day compared to mothers who consumed fish less than once per week. According to the frequency of eating meat products like sausages and salami, milk from mothers consuming these meat products once or more per week had lower cholesterol levels on the 3rd day, and higher EPA levels on the 28th day.

The 3rd day milk samples from mothers who consumed olive oil once or more per week had higher triglyceride levels. Mothers eating oily nuts like walnut and hazelnut once or more per week had higher cholesterol levels in milk samples from the 28th day. Again, mothers who consumed margarine once or more per week had higher triglyceride levels in 28th day samples, while the frequency of butter consumption did not have a significant effect on breast milk lipid content.

Mothers eating dried pulses once a week or more had higher cholesterol levels in breast milk samples from the 28th day, while mothers eating cereal foods like rice and pasta did not have a significant effect on breast milk lipid content (Table 5).

Discussion

In this study planned with the aim of seeing the effect of food consumption frequencies on breast milk lipid content, the lipid content (cholesterol, triglyceride, EPA, DHA, oleic and arachidonic acid) in 90 breast milk samples from 15 preterm and 15 term mothers in Gazi University Neonatal Unit taken on the 3rd, 7th and 28th days of lactation were compared with food consumption during pregnancy.

When the age distribution of individuals is investigated, 10 % were in the 36-40-year group and 3.3 % were in the 40-45-year group, for a total of 13.3 % geriatric pregnancies (36-45 years), while other individuals experienced pregnancy during the normal age interval. When individuals are investigated according to BMI, 70.0 % had normal weight, 13.3 % were overweight and 16.0 % were obese. There was no statistically significant correlation found between BMI with preterm or term birth ($p > 0.05$) (Table 1).

Excess weight at the start of pregnancy may affect the development of some diseases like hypertension and gestational diabetes. Weight gained during

Tab. 5: Effect of Consumption Frequency of Some Foods on Breast Milk Lipid Content

Lipid content	Foods									
	Red Meat	Chicken/Turkey meat	Fish	Meat products (salami, sausage, etc.)	Olive Oil	Oily Nuts	Margarine	Butter	Dried Pulses	Cereals (rice, pasta, etc.)
	p	p	p	p	p	p	p	p	p	p
Triglycerides										
3rd	0.807	0.760	0.708	0.636	0.012*	0.870	0.836	0.302	0.272	0.775
7th	0.647	0.344	0.281	0.098	0.590	0.116	0.407	0.731	0.211	0.454
28th	0.376	0.502	0.523	0.763	0.467	0.888	0.029*	0.413	0.927	0.676
Cholesterol										
3rd	0.142	0.392	0.567	0.036*	0.638	0.481	0.421	0.983	0.783	0.290
7th	0.111	0.902	0.757	0.092	0.410	0.832	0.677	0.829	0.878	0.365
28th	0.377	0.468	0.022*	0.082	0.981	0.027*	0.748	0.306	0.020*	0.856
EPA										
3rd	0.760	0.300	0.058	0.254	0.639	0.079	0.604	0.667	0.669	0.982
7th	0.669	0.077	0.187	0.451	0.223	0.348	0.325	0.683	0.222	0.660
28th	0.152	0.542	0.253	0.004*	0.888	0.511	0.959	0.780	0.179	0.676
DHA										
3rd	0.272	0.583	0.792	0.621	0.574	0.453	0.351	0.237	0.360	0.379
7th	0.360	0.360	0.403	0.220	0.708	0.399	0.254	0.846	0.625	0.660
28th	0.428	0.669	0.333	0.683	0.778	0.101	0.325	0.401	0.807	0.895
Oleic acid										
3rd	0.300	0.088	0.455	0.715	0.511	0.851	0.604	0.747	0.807	0.455
7th	0.393	0.855	0.567	0.846	0.963	0.708	0.300	0.478	0.329	0.758
28th	0.329	0.583	0.159	0.533	0.223	0.708	0.276	0.189	0.464	0.965
Arachidonic acid										
3rd	0.625	0.180	1.000	0.561	0.482	0.925	0.378	0.505	0.714	0.826
7th	0.222	0.010*	0.860	0.055	0.111	0.606	0.678	0.983	0.127	0.291
28th	0.161	0.360	0.202	0.312	0.348	0.189	0.233	0.715	0.113	0.567

*$p<0.05$

pregnancy is very important for the baby's health. Inappropriate weight gain may cause low birth weight or stillbirth (10). Weight at the end of pregnancy showed that the total weight gained during pregnancy was mean 16 kg in both groups. When preterm or term births are compared in terms of weight gain, there was no significant difference found (p>0.05) (Table 2). A study monitored 3511 pregnant cases and showed that low weight gain during pregnancy increased the risk of early birth (11). In our study, weight gain of mothers in both groups was within normal values. There appeared to be no correlation between preterm birth and weight gain.

The amount of fat contained in breast milk varies according to the mother's BMI before pregnancy, weight gained during pregnancy, income level, educational level, and lactation time (12). A breast milk study in Germany found that the cholesterol and triglyceride levels in breast milk increase with advancing lactation time. It is thought that food consumption not just during pregnancy but during the lactation period affects lipid profile (13).

A study in America examined food consumption by pregnant cases and observed the basic fat sources in diet were pastries, snack drinks, fast food, and margarines (14). In our study, consumption of food like margarine and fast food was very limited. A study found that breast milk analysis after birth for pregnant cases with excess carbohydrate consumption had low total cholesterol and higher PUFA. High carbohydrates are considered to increase PUFA biosynthesis (15).

Fish are first place in the list of foods risk in unsaturated fatty acids. When mothers living in regions with high fish consumption and American mothers were compared, mothers living in the region with fish consumption were found to have higher DHA amounts in breast milk (16). DHA supplementation increased the DHA level of breastfeeding women, the DHA level in breast milk, in addition to increasing the infant's lipid DHA level (17). In our study, when fish consumption of individuals is investigated, 53.0 % of mothers with preterm birth ate fish 1-2 times per week, while 20.0 % did not consume it at all. Among mothers with term birth, 80 % were observed to eat fish 1-2 times per week (Table 3).

Biochemical analyses of breast milk found that total cholesterol level and triglyceride content in the preterm group reduced from the 3rd day to the 7th and 28th days (10.9±7.5; 9.0±8.4; 1.8±1.7 mg Kol/dL and 315.6±180.2; 375.1±246.6; 194.8±92.2 mg Trg/dL, respectively). The EPA, DHA and arachidonic acid content increased on the 7th day and reduced again by the 28th day (4.1±5.1; 5.6±4.6; 4.3±2.8 mg EPA/dL, 44.2±38.5; 48.2±36.4; 46.3±34.0 mg DHA/dL and 68.8±54.2; 121.9±176.3; 97.2±45.1 mg Ars/dL, respectively). The oleic acid increased continuously (678.8±437.1; 717.8±352.5; 758.5±235.1 mg Ole/dL) (Table 4). For the term group, the total cholesterol, triglyceride and DHA contents reduced from the 3rd day to the 7th and 28th days (10.2±5.0; 6.2±3.1; 1.5±1.3 mg Kol/dL, 337.4±138.1; 282.2±129.2; 164.6±61.8 mg Trg/dL, and 57.3±34.9; 54.8±34.6; 46.3±34.8 mg DHA/dL, respectively). The EPA content continuously increased (3.7±2.3; 5.6±2.6; 8.9±6.9 mg EPA/dL). The oleic acid content reduced on the 7th day and increased again on the 28th day (880.9±263.2; 692.6±258.1; 854.5±251.6 mg Ole/dL), while the arachidonic acid content increased on the 7th day and reduced on the 28th day (76.0±29.1; 80.9±35.3; 70.2±19.3 mg Ars/dL) (Table 4).

According to data from 55 studies investigating the lipid content of breast milk sampled after 4374 term and 1017 preterm births, linoleic and oleic acid levels did not change during lactation, while the long-chain fatty acid content (arachidonic acid, DHA, etc.) reduced and short-medium chain fatty acid levels increased (18).

When biochemical analyses are compared in the two groups, the EPA level in breast milk from the preterm group on the 28th day was lower compared to the term group, while the arachidonic acid level was identified to be higher in the preterm group and these differences were statistically significant (p≤0.05). In our study, the total fat content in colostrum was higher compared to mature breast milk and was observed to reduce as lactation continued.

A study by Weber et al. (19) showed that total lipids in breast milk reduced during lactation, similar to our study. Similarly, a study of breast milk samples from Spanish women found mature milk had lower triglyceride amounts than colostrum (20). It was concluded that triglyceride and cholesterol contents vary during lactation.

After birth, infants continue to receive unsaturated fatty acids from breast milk and begin to synthesize the acids themselves. However, preterm birth may cause inability to feed with breast milk and these fatty acids may be deficient in premature infants due to insufficient synthesis (21). In our study, comparison of fatty acid content in breast milk found no difference between term and preterm milk in terms of DHA and oleic acid content, while EPA and arachidonic acid levels were different.

A study by Kovacs et al. (22) found that preterm breast milk was high in arachidonic acid in addition to DHA. Different to our study, another study investigating fatty acids found DHA level was high in breast milk from women with preterm births, while similar to our study arachidonic acid levels were higher in preterm milk (23).

Among fatty acids in breast milk, the omega-6 (arachidonic acid) and omega-3 (EPA, DHA) fatty acid ratio is very important. If the n-6 amount is higher inflammation increases, while if the n-3 acid amount is higher anti-inflammatory effect is observed (24). The World Health Organization recommends the n-6/n-3 ratio should be 1 in breast milk (25). Breast milk from mothers eating diets rich in n-6 fatty acids during pregnancy and mothers with inadequate n-3 acid intake has low DHA levels throughout lactation (26). Another study found that pregnant cases consuming excess food containing carbohydrates had high n-6 and low n-3 levels in breast milk (21). In our study, this ratio varied during lactation and was found to be 1.3:1-2.3:1 with breast milk having high n-6. This ratio was higher in the preterm group, especially. It is known that omega-3 fatty acids are stored in the last 3 months of pregnancy (27). This rate is high in our study, which shows inadequate consumption of foods like fish and oily nuts which have high n-3 content (Table 5).

According to food consumption records in our study, the high or low consumption frequencies for red meat, cereals (rich, pasta, etc.) and butter by mothers had no significant effect on breast milk lipids (p≥0.05) (Table 5). Mothers reduced consumption of these foods during pregnancy.

White meat (chicken, turkey), fish, meat products (salami, sausage, etc.), oily nuts, dried pulses, olive oil and margarine consumption frequencies were identified to have significant effect on breast milk lipid content (p≤0.05). In the group with frequent chicken and turkey consumption, arachidonic acid levels were higher on the 7th day, while the group with frequent consumption of meat products like salami and sausage had lower cholesterol and EPA levels on the 3rd day, and the group with frequent fish consumption had higher cholesterol level in breast milk on the 28th day (Table 5). It is known that the fatty acid in meat and meat products is affected by the animal's nutrition. Feeding animals with natural fodder or artificial feed changes the arachidonic acid and omega-3 amounts (28). Similarly, fish from the sea fed with seaweed and algae from deep waters have increased EPA and DHA contents, while farmed fish have much lower levels. Additionally, the form of cooking (frying, etc.) is important, as is the species of fish. For example, sardines have highest PUFA contents, while the fish with highest EPA and DHA content is mackerel (29). A study found that pregnant cases consuming fish had higher DHA amounts in breast milk compared to those who did not consume fish (30).

The group with frequent consumption of oily nuts had higher cholesterol level in milk from the 28th day, while the group with frequent olive oil consumption had higher triglyceride levels in milk from the 3rd day, and the group with frequent margarine consumption had higher triglyceride amounts in milk from the 28th day (Table 5). Margarines are generally made from sunflower oil and corn oil with high n-6 content. As a result, excess margarine consumption affects triglyceride level. A study researching the breast milk profile with food consumption in pregnancy showed that the α-linolenic fatty acid content in breast milk reduced related to margarine consumption (31). Additionally, when fats are heated to high temperatures, the structures degrade and degradation products form. As a result, fats used during cooking are important, just as the cooking method affects the fatty acid content in food.

The group with frequent dried pulse consumption had higher cholesterol level in breast milk from the 28th day (Table 5). It was observed that breast milk from the 28th day was affected by feeding during lactation. Additionally, the form of cooking foods; for example, adding meat or type of oil used during cooking affect these results. Most studies directly comparing foods consumed with breast milk profile focus on fish consumption and DHA level due to effects on brain development and many vital functions in the neonate (30,32,33).

Though significant results were found between breast milk lipid content and foods consumed, breast milk samples taken on 3 different days are affected by the mother's nutrition during lactation. As a result, it is considered more significant to assess according to n-6/n-3 ratio. In order to preserve this ratio, it is recommended to consume at least 300-450 g of fish every week. However, as bottom-feeding fish like haddock and sea bass may contain heavy metals like mercury and cadmium, surface fish like anchovy and mackerel should be chosen (34).

Conclusion

The results of our study found statistically significant effect on breast milk lipid content with food consumption frequency and general nutritional status during pregnancy. The consumption frequency of some foods (red meat, cereals, butter) was identified not to affect the breast milk lipid content (p>0.05).

Due to important known effects, it is recommended to consume mean 650 mg/day unsaturated fatty acids during pregnancy and that at least 300 mg of this be DHA.

References

1. Baysal, A. (2002). *Beslenme*. Ankara: Hatipoğlu Yayınevi.
2. Irmak, N. (2016). Anne sütünün önemi ve ilk 6 ay sadece anne sütü vermeyi etkileyen unsurlar. *The Journal of Turkish Family Physician, 7*(2), 27-31. doi:10.15511/tjtfp.16.02627

3. Balkaya, N. A., Vural, G., & Eroğlu, K. (2014). Gebelikte belirlenen risk faktörlerinin anne ve bebek sağlığı açısından ortaya çıkardığı sorunların incelenmesi. *Düzce Üniversitesi Sağlık Bilimleri Enstitüsü Dergisi*, *1*(1), 6-16.

4. Kominiarek, M. A., & Rajan, P. (2016). Nutrition recommendations in pregnancy and lactation. *The Medical Clinics of North America*, *100*(6), 1199-1215. doi:10.1016/j.mcna.2016.06.004

5. Thiele, K., Diao, L., & Arck, P. C. (2017). Immunometabolism, pregnancy, and nutrition. *Seminars in Immunopathology*, *40*(2), 157-174. doi:10.1007/s00281-017-0660-y

6. Lauritzen, L., Brambilla, P., Mazzocchi, A., Harsløf, L. B., Ciappolino, V., & Agostoni, C. (2016). DHA effects in brain development and function. *Nutrients*, *8*(6). doi:10.3390/nu8010006

7. Nordgren, T. M., Anderson Berry, A., Van Ormer, M., Zoucha, S., Elliott, E., Johnson, R., . . . Hanson, C. (2019). Omega-3 fatty acid supplementation, pro-resolving mediators, and clinical outcomes in maternal-infant pairs. *Nutrients*, *11*(98). doi:10.3390/nu11010098

8. Bravi, F., Wiens, F., Decarli, A., Dal Pont, A., Agostoni, C., & Ferraroni, M. (2016). Impact of maternal nutrition on breast-milk composition: A systematic review. *The American Journal of Clinical Nutrition*, *104*(3), 646-662. doi:10.3945/ajcn.115.120881

9. Andreas, N. J., Kampmann, B., & Mehring Le-Doare, K. (2015). Human breast milk: A review on its composition and bioactivity. *Early Human Development*, *91*(11), 629-35. doi:10.1016/j.earlhumdev.2015.08.013

10. Cheng, Y., Dibley, M. J., Zhang, X., Zeng, L., & Yan, H. (2009). Assessment of dietary intake among pregnant women in a rural area western China. *BMC Public Health*, *9*(1), 222.

11. Al-Saleh, A., & Di Renzo, G. C. (2009). Actions needed to improve maternal health. *International Journal of Gynecology and Obstetrics*, *106*, 115–119.

12. Hahn-Holbrook, J., Fish, A., & Glynn, L. M. (2019). Human milk omega-3 fatty acid composition is associated with infant temperament. *Nutrients*, *11*(2964), 1-12. doi:10.3390/nu11122964

13. Schweigert, F. J., Bathe, K., Chen, F., Büscher, U., & Dudenhausen, J. W. (2014). Effects of the stage of lactation in humans on carotenoid levels in milk, blood plasma and plasma lipoprotein fractions. *European Journal of Nutrition*, *43*(1), 39-44. doi:10.1007/s00394-004-0439-5

14. Innis, S. M., & Elias, S. M. (2003). Intakes of essential n_6 and n_3 polyunsaturated fatty acids among pregnant Canadian women. *The*

American Journal of Clinical Nutrition, 77(2), 473–478. doi:10.1093/ajcn/77.2.473

15. Thiombiano-Coulibaly, N., Rocquelin, G., Eymard-Duvernay, S., Kiffer-Nunes, J., Tapsoba, S., & Traoré, S. A. (2007). Seasonal and environmental effects on breast milk fatty acids in Burkina Faso and the need to improve the omega 3 PUFA content. *Acta Paediatrica, 92*(12). doi:10.1111/j.1651-2227.2003.tb00820.x

16. Denomme, J., Stark, K. D., & Holub, B. J. (2005). Directly quantitated dietary (n-3) fatty acid intakes of pregnant Canadian women are lower than current dietary recommendations. *The Journal of Nutrition, 135*(2), 206–211. doi:10.1093/jn/135.2.206

17. Deng, J., Li, X., Ding, Z., Wu, Y., Chen, X., & Xie, L. (2017). Effect of DHA supplements during pregnancy on the concentration of PUFA in breast milk of Chinese lactating mothers. *Journal of Perinatal Medicine, 45*(4), 437-441. doi:10.1515/jpm-2015-0438

18. Floris, L. M., Stahl, B., Abrahamse-Berkeveld, M., & Teller, I. C. (2019). Human milk fatty acid profile across lactational stages after term and preterm delivery: A pooled data analysis. *Prostaglandins, Leukotrienes and Essential Fatty Acids, 156*, 102023. doi:10.1016/j.plefa.2019.102023

19. Weber, A., Loui, A., Jochum, F., Bührer, C., & Obladen, M. (2001). Brest milk from mothers of very low birth weight infants: Variability in fat and protein content. *Acta Paediatrica, 90*(7), 720-723.

20. Minda, H., Kovacs, A., Funke, S., Szasz, M., Burus, I., Molnar, S., . . . Desci, T. (2004). Changes of fatty acid composition of human milk during the first month of lactation: A day-to-day approach in the first week. *Annals of Nutrition and Metabolism, 48*(3), 202-209. doi:10.1159/000079821

21. Helland, I. B., Saugstad, O. D., Saarem, K., Van Houwelingen, A. C., Nylander, G., & Drevon, C. A. (2006). Supplementation of n-3 fatty acids during pregnancy and lactation reduces maternal plasma lipid levels and provides DHA to the infants. *Journal of Maternal-Fetal and Neonatal Medicine, 19*(7), 397-406. doi:10.1080/14767050600738396

22. Kovacs, A., Funke, S., Marosvölgyi, T., Burus, I., & Desci, T. (2005). Fatty acids in early human milk after preterm and full-term delivery. *Journal of Pediatric Gastroenterology and Nutrition, 41*(4), 454-459. doi:10.1097/01.mpg.0000176181.66390.54

23. Al-Tamer, Y. Y., & Mahmood, A. A. (2006). The influence of Iraqi mothers' socioeconomic status on their milk lipid content. *European Journal of Clinical Nutrition, 60*(12), 1400-1405. doi:10.1038/sj.ejcn.1602470

58   Gökçen Garipoğlu, Gülderen Yentür, Esin Koç, and Taner Özgürtaş

24. Koletzko, B. (2016). Human milk lipids. *Annals of Nutrition & Metabolism, 69*(2), 28-40. doi:10.1159/000452819

25. T.C. Sağlık Bakanlığı. (2002). Toplumun beslenmede bilinçlendirilmesi. Saha personeli için toplum beslenmesi programı eğitim materyali. Ankara.

26. Barrera, C., Valenzuela, R., Chamorro, R., Bascuñán, K., Sandoval, J., Sabag, N., ... Valenzuela, A. (2018). The impact of maternal diet during pregnancy and lactation on the fatty acid composition of erythrocytes and breast milk of Chilean women. *Nutrients, 10*(7). doi:10.3390/nu10070839

27. McCann, J., & Ames, B. N. (2005). Is docosahexaenoic acid, an n-3 long-chain polyunsaturated fatty acid, required for development of normal brain function? An overview of evidence from cognitive and behavioral tests in humans and animals. *The American Journal of Clinical Nutrition, 82*(2), 281-295.

28. Çakmakçı, S., & Tahmas-Kahyaoğlu, D. (2012). Yağ asitlerinin sağlık ve beslenme üzerine etkilerine genel bir bakış. *Akademik Gıda, 10*(1), 103-113.

29. Öksüz, A., Alkan, Ş. B., Taşkın, H., & Ayranc, M. (2018). Yaşam boyu sağlıklı ve dengeli beslenme için balık tüketiminin önemi. *Food and Health, 4*(1), 43-62. doi:10.3153/JFHS18006

30. Wong, V. W., Ng, Y. F., Chan, S. M., Su, Y. X., Kwok, K. W., Chan, H. ... Wong, M. S. (2019). Positive relationship between consumption of specific fish type and n-3 PUFA in milk of Hong Kong lactating mothers. *The British Journal of Nutrition, 121*(12), 1431-1440. doi:10.1017/S0007114519000801

31. Anderson, N. K., Beerman, K. A., McGuire, M. A., Dasgupta, N., Griinari, J. M., Williams, J., & McGuire, M. K. (2005). Dietary fat type influences total milk fat content in lean women. *The Journal of Nutrition, 135*(3), 416-421. doi:10.1093/jn/135.3.416

32. Çelik, F., & Büyüktuncer Demirel, Z. (2012). Omega-3 yağ asitlerinin nörolojik ve görsel gelişim üzerindeki etkileri. *Beslenme ve Diyet Dergisi, 40*(3), 266-272.

33. Carlson, S. E. (2001). Docosahexaenoic acid and arachidonic acid in infant development. *Seminars in Neonatology, 6*(5), 437-449.

34. Can, E., Cömert, S. Uslu, S. Bülbül, A., Bolat, F., & Nuhoğlu, A. (2009). Uzun zincirli çoklu doymamış yağ asitlerinin yenidoğan beslenmesindeki rolü. *Kartal Eğitim ve Araştırma Hastanesi Tıp Dergisi, 20*(2):108-112.

Hakan Güveli, Merve İlker, Emre Batuhan Kenger, and
Tuğçe Özlü

The Importance of Medical Nutrition Treatment and Determinants of Its Effects of in Non-alcoholic Fatty Liver Disease Patients

Abstract

Objective: Non-alcoholic fatty liver disease (NAFLD) is histologically identified as lipid accumulation of more than five percent in liver. NAFLD, which is the most common chronic liver disease in the world, is a clinical and pathological status related to abdominal obesity, insulin resistance, type-2 diabetes, hypertension, dyslipidemia and gut dysbiosis. The purpose of this study is to determine the effects of medical nutrition treatment and education on NAFLD patients' eating habits, anthropometric and biochemical findings.

Materials and Methods: A total of 50 NAFLD-diagnosed participants in this study were separated into two groups of 25 patients randomly. The standardized nutrition treatment protocol accompanied by nutrition education was implemented to the intervention group in twice a month for 3 months.

Results: It was observed a significant difference in anthropometric findings in the intervention group (p<0.05) while no significant differences were found in the control group (p>0.05). The AST and ALT levels showed a significant decrease in the intervention group (p>0.05); however, no significant difference was found in the control group (p<0.05).

Conclusion: It was observed that well-planned nutritional treatment and nutrition education have a crucial contribution to patients' anthropometric measurements and biochemical parameters within the scope of NAFLD treatment.

Keywords: Non-alcoholic Fatty Liver Disease, Nutritional Status, Eating Habits, Medical Nutrition

Introduction

Non-alcoholic fatty liver disease (NAFLD), which is a chronic liver disease involving non-inflammatory steatosis, steatohepatitis, and cirrhosis, occurs in individuals who do not drink alcohol or use it a little (1). Non-alcoholic steatohepatitis (NASH) is known as a clinical status which inflammation and liver fibrosis occur along with NAFLD. Cirrhosis, liver failure and hepatocellular carcinoma (HCC) can be seen if NASH is not been treated in time (2). Changing eating habits and sedentary lifestyle causes an increment in NAFLD and the prevalence in the general population varies by 20-30 % (3). Obesity, type-2 diabetes, dyslipidemia, metabolic syndrome is known as the risk factors that affect the development of NAFLD (4-7). Recently, it has been determined a relationship between gut microbiota and NAFLD that gut-liver axis can play in the pathogenesis and progression of NAFLD (8,9). Although many alternative medications have been assessed; unfortunately, there is no licensed medication use for NAFLD treatment (10). Providing weight loss with adequate nutrition and physical activity, decreasing the liver enzyme and liver-fat amounts, improving insulin sensitivity and reducing the hepatic fibrosis and inflammation levels are accepted the gold standard for the diagnosis and evaluation of NAFLD (11). Uncontrolled weight loss in NAFLD can cause worse prognosis that increases free-fatty acids flowing into the liver (12). Therefore, the medical nutrition treatment, which is accepted as a gold standard, comes into prominence more.

The main aim of this study is to determine the effects of medical nutrition treatment and education on NAFLD patients' eating habits, anthropometric and biochemical findings. In addition, this study purposes to create important awareness of nutritional treatment in NAFLD.

Materials and Methods

Participants and Method

A case-control study was aimed to investigate the importance and effects of medical nutritional treatment and nutrition education in NAFLD patients. The participants in this study were recruited from a private clinic with an institutional permit between January 2018 and September 2018. The sample was selected on the basis of the NAFLD-diagnosed patients by a gastroenterologist. Fifty patients who matched the selection criteria were identified. Criteria for selecting the subjects were as follows: aged between 20 and 75, body mass index (BMI) between 25.0 and 40.0 kg/m². The randomized study was divided into two groups of 25 people as an intervention and a control group. The exclusion criteria for the patients were as follows: alcohol use (women; >20 g/day, men; >30 g/day); pregnancy and lactation; viral hepatitis; autoimmune hepatitis; Wilson disease; constant medication use such as corticosteroids, methotrexate, tamoxifen and oral contraceptive; patients who diagnosed jejunoileal bypass or large and small bowel resection, heart-renal failure and

Tab. 1: The General Implementation Plan of the Study

	Before Treatment	During Treatment	After Treatment (after 12 weeks)
Control Group	Questionnaire Form Anthropometric measurements Biochemical measurements Dietary Record		Anthropometric measurements Biochemical measurements Dietary Record
Intervention Group	Questionnaire Form Anthropometric measurements Biochemical measurements Dietary Record	Nutrition education every 2 weeks for 3 months	Anthropometric measurements Biochemical measurements Dietary Record

other chronic liver diseases. Ethical approval was obtained from Bahçeşehir University Clinical Research Ethics Committee. A face-to-face interview was conducted with voluntary patients and they were informed in detail. The consent form was signed by the patients. Table 1 demonstrates a general plan for the implementation of the research.

Questionnaire

The questionnaire asked participants their demographic traits such as age, gender, employment status, marital status, and educational status by using the face-to-face interview.

A Dietary Record

Three-day after treatment diet records (2 days from weekday and 1 day from the weekend) were obtained from all patients and their nutritional status was observed. Daily energy and nutrient intake analysis were performed using EBISpro for Windows, Stuttgart, Germany; Turkish version (BeBiS 8).

Biochemical Findings

All the biochemical findings were obtained from Melikgazi Hospital Laboratory. Fasting glucose (FG) and insulin levels, alanine aminotransferase (ALT), aspartate aminotransferase (AST), hemoglobin A1c (HbA1C), total cholesterol, low-density lipoprotein (LDL), high-density lipoprotein (HDL) and triglyceride (TG) levels were investigated.

Anthropometric Measurements

Anthropometric measurements such as weight, BMI, waist-hip circumference, were assessed before and after treatment. Body compositions were measured by using a bioelectric impedance tool Tanita MC 780 S. In addition, the waist-hip circumference was girthed by using non-stretch tape measure before and after nutrition therapy.

Standardized Nutrition Treatment Protocol

According to standardized nutrition treatment, the daily energy consists of 55-60 % of carbohydrate, 12-15 % of protein, and 25-30 % of fats. Total fat content is arranged as 7-8 % of saturated fat, 13-15 % of monounsaturated fat and 7-8 % of polyunsaturated fat in the nutrition therapy. The daily energy intake was planned as less than 30 kcal/kg for patients. In the standardized nutrition treatment, the consumption of foods high in simple sugar, saturated fat, cholesterol, and trans-fat was restricted. It was recommended the required amount and frequency of consumption of vegetables and fruits consisting vitamin, mineral, fiber, and antioxidant (13).

Data Assessment

Statistical analysis was performed using SPSS software (version 24) and significance levels were set at the 0.05 level. Normal distribution of data was calculated using the Kolmogorov-Smirnov test. Number, percentage, mean, and standard deviation were used as descriptive data. Comparisons between the two groups were made using t-tests.

Results

In this study, 42 % of patients are women and 40 % of women were the age of 40-49. Thirty-eight percent (38 %) of those were participated had type-2 diabetes, hyperlipidemia, hypertension, and hypothyroidism. Table 2 shows the results of the demographic traits.

The table above illustrates the energy and nutrient intake of patients after treatment (Table 3). It was found that there was a significant difference between the control and intervention group in the energy, protein, fat, carbohydrate, fiber, and cholesterol intake (p<0.05).

Table 4 compares the anthropometric measurements of patients before and after treatment between the control and the intervention group. It was detected that the anthropometric measurements, except the waist/hip ratio, showed no

Tab. 2: Demographic Characteristics

	Number (n)	Percentage (%)
Gender		
Women	21	42.0
Men	29	58.0
Age (year)		
20-29	4	8.0
30-39	11	22.0
40-49	20	40.0
50 +	15	30.0
Employment status		
Employed	35	70.0
Unemployed	15	30.0
Educational status		
Primary education	4	8.0
Secondary education	24	48.0
University	22	44.0
Illness		
Yes	19	38.0
No	31	62.0

Tab. 3: The Energy and Nutrient Intake of Patients After Treatment

Energy and Nutrients	Control Group (n=25)	Intervention Group (n=25)	p
	Mean±Standard Deviation		
Energy	2033.30±198.86	1705.20±140.30	0.000*
Protein	71.30±5.43	57.52±4.70	0.000*
Fat	80.20±18.82	52.11±4.27	0.000*
Polyunsaturated fatty acids	22.26±3.71	5.768±0.354	0.000*
Carbohydrate	239.36±20.36	223.97±18.35	0.007*
Fiber	17.77±1.70	27.76±0.92	0.000*
Cholesterol	341.72±87.13	106.77±2.95	0.000*

t-test was used in independent groups.

Tab. 4: Anthropometric Measurements of Patients Before and After Treatment

Anthropometric Measurements	Control Group (n=25) Mean±Standard Deviation			Intervention Group (n=25) Mean±Standard Deviation		
	Before Treatment	After Treatment	p	Before Treatment	After Treatment	p
Weight (kg)	97.72±12.26	98.16±12.35	0.525	105.34±15.46	91.292±13.225	0.000*
BMI (kg/m²)	33.43±2.58	33.24±2.65	0.553	36.51±6.01	31.864±5.288	0.000*
Waist circumference (cm)	97.95±11.98	98.12±12.26	0.733	110.07±16.91	94.140±13.902	0.000*
Hip circumference (cm)	114.68±9.50	114.48±10.00	0.671	124.08±16.69	109.340±12.761	0.000*
Waist/Hip Ratio (cm)	0.847±0.07	0.862±0.07	0.020*	0.852±0.07	0.824±0.066	0.033*
Body Fat Ratio (%)	33.70±4.53	34.01±4.43	0.164	35.42±7.23	29.900±8.194	0.000*
Body Fat Mass (kg)	32.72±4.53	33.14±4.49	0.327	37.43±9.99	27.464±9.237	0.000*

BMI: Body Mass Index; * t-test was used in paired groups.

significant difference between before and after treatment in the control group patients (p>0.05). However, a significant decrease observed in all anthropometric measurements between before and after treatment in the intervention group (p<0.05).

Table 5 demonstrates the overview of the biochemical parameters of patients before and after treatment. It was found that no significant difference in biochemical parameters, except LDL and TG levels between before and after treatment in the control group (p>0.05). In the intervention group, fasting glucose, insulin, alanine aminotransferase, aspartate aminotransferase, hemoglobin A1c, total cholesterol, low-density lipoprotein, triglyceride showed a significant decrement after treatment (p<0.05).

Discussion

It is assumed that the general prevalence of NAFLD is almost 15 % in Asian countries and around 30 % in western countries. Moreover, the prevalence of the disease is affected by gender, age, and chronic diseases such as obesity and type-2 diabetes (14,15). NAFLD has a crucial place in clinics due to the fact that the disease is really common in most communities. In addition, if NAFLD is not treated, cirrhosis, HCC and liver failure can appear among patients (14).

It has been thought that one of the main reasons behind the rapid increase of NAFLD is type-2 diabetes and obesity (16). Bellentani et al. (2010) identified that NAFLD prevalence increased almost 5 times in obese patients (BMI 30 kg/m² and above) (14). One study demonstrated that 69 % of those who were type-2 diabetes was diagnosed NAFLD by the ultrasonographic method (17). Similar to the literature, in this study, the mean BMI values of the control and the intervention group before treatment were 33.43±2.58 and 36.51±6.02 kg/m², respectively. Moreover, the mean fasting glucose levels of the control and the intervention group before treatment were 102.1±38.1 and 102.0±12.5, respectively.

Lifestyle changes such as adequate and balanced nutrition and regular physical activity are determined as the primary treatment in NAFLD to provide moderate weight loss (3,18). In this study, the anthropometric measurements were compared in both groups before and after treatment. Compared with the control group, the intervention group had a significant difference in all the anthropometric measurements (p<0.05). It was determined that patients who had standardized nutrition treatment, had 13.3 % of average body weight loss. In 2018, the American Association for the Study of Liver Diseases (AASLD) indicated that losing at least 3-5 % of body weight is necessary to improve

Tab. 5: Biochemical Parameters of Patients Before and After Treatment

Biochemical Parameters	Control Group (n=25) Mean±Standard Deviation			Intervention Group (n=25) Mean±Standard Deviation		
	Before Treatment	After Treatment	p	Before Treatment	After Treatment	p
FG (mg/dL)	102.16±28.183	102.04±24.701	0.950	102.04±12.54	94.76±7.37	0.001*
Insulin (µU/mL)	7.580±4.457	7.448±4.231	0.380	8.30±4.83	7.21±3.89	0.002*
HbA1c	5.144±1.274	5.164±1.255	0.625	5.22±1.45	4.68±0.62	0.040*
ALT (U/L)	60.96±11.42	61.24±10.91	0.693	64.36±8.66	47.72±8.98	0.000*
AST (U/L)	30.96±9.04	31.20±8.83	0.533	30.28±8.79	26.56±8.70	0.012*
TC (mg/dL)	195.08±40.85	196.48±41.91	0.803	213.32±51.60	182.84±33.10	0.000*
LDL (mg/dL)	115.18±27.19	120.84±29.38	0.040*	121.16±30.13	103.16±22.57	0.000*
HDL (mg/dL)	40.44±9.14	40.32±9.63	0.917	46.24±7.64	46.92±5.72	0.707
TG (mg/dL)	196.08±68.31	213.08±54.84	0.032*	215.08±49.57	187.84±42.46	0.000*

FG: Fasting glucose, ALT: alanine aminotransferase, AST: aspartate aminotransferase, HbA1C: hemoglobin A1c, TC: total cholesterol, LDL: low-density lipoprotein, HDL: high-density lipoprotein, TG: triglyceride * t-test was used in paired groups.

steatosis (1). In addition, AASLD highlighted that losing at least 10 % of body weight help to improve fibrosis in NAFLD (1).

High levels of serum liver enzymes are associated with the NAFLD risk (19). In the study, there was a comparison between the control and the intervention group regarding the biochemical parameters during before and after treatment. Serum AST and ALT levels showed no significant difference both before and after treatment in the control group (p>0.05). However, the intervention group demonstrated a statistical reduction in serum AST and ALT levels both before and after treatment (p<0.05). Cho et al. (2014) indicated that fatty liver patients who lose weight had a significant reduction in AST and ALT levels compared with patients with weight gain or stable weight (20). It has been assumed that a low level of liver enzymes was related to medical nutritional treatment and nutrition education. Although a high level of liver enzymes is associated with the progression of NAFLD, most of NAFLD diagnosed patients have normal liver enzyme levels; thus, this condition complicates the diagnosis of the disease (21). Determining the effectiveness of nutrition therapy on the disease with biochemical findings was one of the limiting factors in this study.

The nutritional profile in NAFLD consists of the excessive consumption of energy, fat, saturated fat and carbohydrates and the low amount of vitamin, mineral and polyunsaturated fatty acid intakes (22). Eating habits should be taken personally in every patient and nutrition education should be counseled to them (22-24). In both groups, nutritional status was assessed with their dietary records after treatment. Carbohydrate consumption was inadequate and fat intake was high in the control group whereas carbohydrate and fat consumption had normal in the intervention group. Besides, compared with the control group, dietary fiber intake was high, and the cholesterol intake was less in the intervention group.

Conclusion

Nutrition has an important role in the formation and the treatment of NAFLD as with many other diseases. Adequate and balanced nutrition along with regular physical activity has a protective effect against the formation of the disease. In this point, it was observed that well-planned nutrition therapy and regular nutrition education has a positive impact on the biochemical and anthropometric measurements. It is believed that nutrition therapy in NAFLD would contribute to the awareness-raising in the community.

References

1. Chalasini, N., Younossi, Z., Lavine, J. E., Charlton, M., Cusi, K., & Rinella, M. (2018). The diagnosis and management of nonalcoholic fatty liver disease: Practice guidance from the American Association for the Study of Liver Diseases. *Hepatology, 67*(1), 328-357. doi:10.1002/hep.29367

2. Loomba, R., & Sanyal, A. J. (2013). The global NAFLD epidemic. *Nature Reviews Gastroenterology & Hepatology, 10*(11), 686-90. doi:10.1038/nrgastro.2013.171

3. Oliveria, C. P., de Lima Sanches, P., de Abreu-Silva, E. O., & Marcadenti, A. (2016). Nutrition and physical activity in nonalcoholic fatty liver disease. *Journal of Diabetes Research, 2016*, 4597246. doi:10.1155/2016/4597246

4. Williams, C. D., Stengel, J., Asike, M. I., Torres, D. M., Shaw, J., Contreras, M., Landt, C. L., & Harrison, S. A. (2011). Clinical advances in liver, pancreas, and biliary tract. *Gastroenterology, 140*, 124-131.

5. Medina, J., Fernandez-Salazar, L., Garcia-Buey, L., & Moreno-Otero, R. (2004) Approach to the pathogenesis and treatment of nonalcoholic steatohepatitis. *Diabetes Care, 27*(8), 2057-2066. doi:10.2337/diacare.27.8.2057

6. Chatrath, H., Vuppalanchi, R., & Chalasani, N. (2012). Dyslipidemia in patients with nonalcoholic fatty liver disease. *Seminars in Liver Disease, 32*(1), 22-29. doi:10.1055/s-0032-1306423

7. Targher, G., Chonchol, M., & Zoppini, G. (2011). Risk of chronic kidney disease in patients with non-alcoholic fatty liver disease: Is there a link? *Journal of Hepatology, 54*(5), 1020-1029.

8. Rabot, S., Membrez, M., Bruneau, A., Gerard, P., Harach, T., Moser, M., . . . Chou, C. J. (2010). Germ-free C57BL/6J mice are resistant to high-fat-diet-induced insulin resistance and have altered cholesterol metabolism. *FASEB Journal, 24*(12), 4948-4959. doi:10.1096/fj.10-164921

9. Henao-Mejia, J., Elinav, E., Thaiss, C. A., Licona Limon, P., & Flavell, R. A. (2013). Role of the intestinal microbiome in liver disease. *Journal of Autoimmunity, 46*, 66-73. doi:10.1016/j.jaut.2013.07.001

10. Bril, F., Ntim, K., Lomonaco, R., & Cusi, K. (2015). Treatment of NAFLD and NASH. In R. A. DeFronzo, E. Ferrannini, P. Zimmet, & G. Alberti G (Eds.), *International Textbook of Diabetes Mellitus* (p. 292) New Jersey, ABD: John Wiley & Sons.

11. Al-Dayyat, H., Rayyan, Y. M., & Tayyem, R. F. (2018). Non-alcoholic fatty liver disease and associated dietary and lifestyle risk factors. *Diabetes & Metabolic Syndrome, 12*(4), 569-575. doi:10.1016/j.dsx.2018.03.016

12. Güngör, H., & Türker, P. F. (2016). Nonalkolik yağlı karaciğer hastalığı ve tıbbi beslenme. *Güncel Gastroenteroloji, 20*(3), 297-304.

13. Naniwadekar, A. S. (2010). Nutritional recommendations for patients with non-alcoholic fatty liver disease: An evidence based review. *Practical Gastroenterology, 34*(2), 8-16.

14. Bellentani, S., Scaglioni, F., Marino, M., & Bedogni, G. (2010). Epidemiology of non-alcoholic fatty liver disease. *Digestive Diseases, 28*(1), 155-161. doi:10.1159/000282080

15. Radu, C., Grigorescu, M., & Crisan, D. (2008). Prevalence and associated risk factors of nonalcoholic fatty liver disease in hospitalized patients. *Journal of Gastrointestinal and Liver Diseases, 1*(3), 255-260.

16. Finelli, C., & Tarantino, G. (2013). What is the role of adiponectin in obesity related non-alcoholic fatty liver disease? *World Journal of Gastroenterology, 19*(6), 802-812. doi:10.3748/wjg.v19.i6.802

17. Vernon, G., Baranova, A., & Younossi, Z. M. (2011). Systematic review: The epidemiology and natural history of non-alcoholic fatty liver disease and non-alcoholic steatohepatitis in adults. *Alimentary Pharmacology & Therapeutics, 34*(3), 274-285. doi:10.1111/j.1365-2036.2011.04724.x

18. Lonardo, M., Nascimbenib, F., Targherc, G., Bernardid, M., Boninoe, F., & Bugianesif, E. (2017). AISF position paper on nonalcoholic fatty liver disease (NAFLD): Updates and future directions. *Digestive and Liver Disease, 49*(5), 471-483. doi:10.1016/j.dld.2017.01.147

19. Elias, M. C., Parise, E. R., de Carvalho, L., Szejnfeld, D., & Netto, J. P. (2010). Effect of 6-month nutritional intervention on non-alcoholic fatty liver disease. *Nutrition, 26*(11-12), 1094-9. doi:10.1016/j.nut.2009.09.001

20. Cho, J. Y., Chung, T. H., Lim, K. M., Park, H. J., & Jang, J. M. (2014). The impact of weight changes on nonalcoholic Fatty liver disease in adult men with normal weight. *Korean Journal of Family Medicine, 35*(5), 243-250. doi:10.4082/kjfm.2014.35.5.243

21. Rinella, M. E. (2015). Nonalcoholic fatty liver disease: A systematic review. *The Journal of the American Medical Association, 313*(22), 2263-73.

22. Yasutake, K., Kohjima, M., & Kotoh, K. (2014). Dietary habits and behaviors associated with nonalcoholic fatty liver disease. *World Journal of Gastroenterology, 20*(7), 1756-1767. doi:10.3748/wjg.v20.i7.1756

23. Zelber-Sagi, S., Godos, J., & Salomone, F. (2016). Lifestyle changes for the treatment of nonalcoholic fatty liver disease: A review of observational studies and intervention trials. *Therapeutic Advances in Gastroenterology, 9*(3), 392-407. doi:10.1177/1756283X16638830

24. George, A., Bauman, A., Johnston, A., Farrell, G., Chey, T., & George, J. (2009). Independent effects of physical activity in patients with nonalcoholic fatty liver disease. *Hepatology, 50*(1), 68-76. doi:10.1002/hep.22940

İlayda Öztürk

The Relationships Between Sleep Patterns, Eating Habits, and Obesity of University Students

Abstract

Objective: This study was conducted to determine the effects of college students' sleeping and late eating habits on BMI, waist circumference, and fat mass measurements, which are less studied in than other age groups.

Materials and Methods: During the study period, participants' body mass indexes and fat masses were measured with a body composition analyzer (InBody 230) and their waist circumference was measured with a non-flexible meter. A questionnaire was designed and used to question sleeping habits, eating behaviors, and accommodation status and exercise habits of participants.

Results: According to the results obtained, no significant relationship was found between university students in the age range of 18-25, for their sleeping habits and consumption of foods consumed in the process of being awake late at night, except meat and meat derivatives. Significant relationships were found between exercise habits, accommodation type and chocolate consumption.

Conclusion: Due to the circumstances of the research, only girl students were involved. The non-significant differences in parameters were associated with the fact that almost all of the participants were not overweight or obese, the study only conducted by female students, and the group have no bad eating or sleeping habits to cause obesity. It is anticipated that similar studies to be conducted in the future may lead to different outcomes if applied to a larger population, taking both sexes into account.

Keywords: Sleep, Sleep Patterns, Eating Habits, Food Frequencies

Introduction

Considering that communication is moving to the virtual environments and that individuals' habits of socializing based on physical activities are gradually perishing, it can be seen that a generation is being raised spending hours looking at computer screens and/or other electronic devices. Due to several reasons, including the screen time, sleep has become an ignorable option for people (1). Unfavorable changes in sleep and eating patterns are now increasing in incidence in all age groups. Factors such as gender, race, socio-economic status, and age may prove differences in people's exposure to obesity

(2). Disrupted eating habits and reduced physical activity profiles lead people into obesity which is the primary reason of a number of metabolic disorders in the long term (3,4).

Changing sleep patterns and decreased sleep duration is closely associated with obesity. It was found that the body mass index (BMI) of people from all ages who sleep less than 7.7 hours was higher than the ones who sleep more than 7.7 hours a day on an average (5). Cuypers et al. reported that a very insufficient sleep duration (less than 5 hours) will be required in order to associate sleep deprivation and obesity (6). Another study conducted on young people suggested a reciprocal relationship between obesity and sleep duration. Factors such as lower sleep quality, delayed sleep phase are separately associated with the obesity estimations (7).

Most of the studies available in the literature compare the obesity in children or adults with their sleep patterns. Reilly et al., in a study on children at the age of 3, found that the obesity risk of children who sleep less than normal pose the increased risk of obesity by 45 % when they are 7 (8).

However, the literature offers limited amount of studies on the age group which can be defined as young people. University students are found to be an attractive population to study in terms of the relationship between their sleep and nutrition patterns given their changing lifestyle and their academic responsibilities.

This study was conducted taking into account the accommodation conditions, availability of food, and sleep durations of university students. As the accommodation preferences of students coming from other cities change significantly, their eating habits tend to differ from their previous lifestyles.

In the light of all these assessments, the question if the changing lifestyle of university students increases their disposition to obesity has become an interesting subject to study. It was believed that to build this study on a comparison of students currently at different stages of their academic years is the best option in order to understand if such changes are more obvious with the increased adaptation to the conditions as the students proceed in their academic lives.

Materials and Methods

Inclusion and Exclusion Criteria

This study was conducted on a total number of 104 female students, ages ranging between 18 and 25, who currently study in the 1st, 2nd, and 3rd grade of the Faculty of Health Sciences, Department of Nutrition and Dietetics of Yeditepe University. A literature review aimed at exploring sleep patterns, nutrition and night eating habits showed that there is limited amount of research focusing on young adults, university students, which was the motivation behind the population selection of this study. As the number of male students enrolled in this department is limited (n=13) the population was limited to female students in order to avoid any possible problems in the distribution of the results.

The 4th grade students of the department were not included to the study. The reason behind the exclusion of 4th grade students was that they are working as interns three days of the week which make it difficult to qualify them as students, and that they go through a change in their eating and sleep habits due to their changing lifestyle; in addition, it was harder to reach out to these students.

Anthropometric Measurements

Body mass index, fat mass and waist circumference values are some of the valid detectors of obesity (9). Thus, BMI (Weight (kg)/ Height^2 (m^2)), body fat mass and waist circumferences of the participants were measured as part of the analysis. The height measurements for BMI scoring were taken using a stadiometer. Measurements were taken barefoot when participants' heels were in contact with the device, aligning the apparatus with the top of their heads. BMI of the participants was then calculated after using a body composition analysis device which weight measurements taken. The same InBody 230 body composition analysis device was used to measure body fat mass in kilograms. In order to cause any deviation, participants' waist circumference measurements were taken by the same researcher using inflexible tape measure suitable for medical purposes.

Questionnaire

The sleep pattern and eating behavior research part of the study was performed using a questionnaire developed building on a literature review. In order to ensure that necessary information was inquired, researchers developed new survey questions inspired by available questionnaires. In this questionnaire, all possible accommodation statuses were inquired using a classification involving "Family/Relative's Home", "Student Shared Flat", "Dormitory (Campus, State and Private)". Sleep patterns are explored in two groups, namely, weekdays and weekends.

The participants were then asked to classify themselves under one of the items: "Go to bed late and wake up early", "Go to bed early and wake up early", "Go to bed early and wake up late", and "Go to bed late and wake up late" developed taking the example of a previous study in order to investigate how long the participants sleep on weekdays and weekends, and if they have a habit of sleeping in daytime (10).

Participants were asked to specify their breakfast habits, and how many snacks and how many main meals they consume in a day as part of the inquiry about their eating habits. Building on a previous study, participants were asked to specify their frequency: "Never/Less than once in a month", "1-2 times in a month", "Once a week", "2-4 times a week", "5-6 times a week", and "Every night" of consumption of some specific food items between the dinner time and bedtime (4). As the participants are students, a number of convenient food items commonly preferred by students were included in the assessment. Also considering the possibility of different accommodation styles may affect the choice of food items, the food items investigated were not limited with "ready-to-eat" food.

Moreover, alcohol consumption of the participants was also investigated. The frequency scale used in the inquiry about their eating behaviors was used also in this section and commonly available types of alcoholic beverages were included. Exercise habits of the participants were inquired based on the fulfillment of the criteria of "At least 3 days a week and at least for 30 minutes" (11).

Ethics Committee Approval

In order to conduct this study and to confirm its ethical status, ethics committee approval for Observational Research was obtained from Bahçeşehir University Clinic Research Ethics Committee by the number of 2016-04/09 and the date of 18th May 2016.

Statistical Analysis

Number Cruncher Statistical System (NCSS) (Kaysville, Utah, USA) software was used for statistical analysis. Complementary statistics were expressed in numbers and percentages for categorical variables and in averages, standard deviation, minimum and maximum values for numerical variables. As the numerical variables do not meet the normal distribution condition, Mann Whitney U Test was used in comparison of two independent groups, while Kruskal Wallis test was used in the case of comparison of more than three groups. Subgroup analysis was performed using Mann Whitney U test and was interpreted using Bonferroni correction. Correlations between numerical variables were explored using Pearson Chi Square Analysis and Fisher-Freeman-Halton Exact test. Statistical alpha significance level was taken as $p < 0.05$.

Results

This study was conducted on a total number of 104 female students who study in the 1st, 2nd, and 3rd grades of the Faculty of Health Sciences, Department of Nutrition and Dietetics of Yeditepe University. It was defined that most of the participants are accommodated in dormitories. According to the survey, it was found that 40.2 % of the participants regularly exercise while 59.8 % do not exercise. A statistically significant difference was found in the BMI averages of the students across grades ($p=0.006$; $p < 0.05$) (Table 1). A statistically significant difference was found in the waist circumference averages of the students across grades ($p=0.005$; $p < 0.05$) (Table 1).

The BMI of 1st grade students were significantly lower than that of 2nd grade and 3rd grade students (1st-2nd grade: $p=0.024$; 1st-3rd grade: $p=0.024$; $p < 0.05$). There was no statistically significant difference between 2nd and 3rd grade students2 BMI levels ($p > 0.05$) (Table 2). A statistically significant difference was found in the waist circumference averages of the students across grades ($p=0.005$; $p < 0.05$) (Table 1). The waist circumference of 1st grade students was significantly lower than that of 2nd grade and 3rd grade students (1st-2nd grades: $p=0.012$; 1st-3rd grades: $p=0.038$; $p < 0.05$). There was no statistically significant difference between 2nd and 3rd grade students' waist circumferences ($p > 0.05$) (Table 2). A statistically significant difference was found in the fat mass averages of the students across grades ($p=0.011$; $p < 0.05$) (Table 1). The fat mass averages of 1st grade students were significantly lower than that of 2nd grade and 3rd grade students (1st-2nd: $p=0.040$; 1st-3rd: $p=0.043$; $p < 0.05$). There was no statistically significant difference between 2nd and 3rd grade students' fat mass averages ($p > 0.05$) (Table 2). There was no statistically significant difference between BMI, waist circumference and fat mass averages of the groups with regards to their accommodation types and exercise habits ($p > 0.05$).

Sleep Patterns

It was observed that majority of the participants have reported that they are in the group which "goes to bed late and wakes up late" and that they did not sleep in daytime (75.5 %, 81.4 %). There was no statistically significant relationship between the participants' sleep duration on weekends and their BMI, waist circumference and fat mass levels ($p=0.262$ $p=0.531$ $p=0.185$, respectively). There was no statistically significant difference in the BMI, waist circumference and fat mass averages

İlayda Öztürk

Tab. 1: Evaluation of BMI, Waist Circumference, Fat Mass Measurements According to General Features

		BMI (kg/m²)		Waist Circumference (cm)		Fat Mass (kg)	
	n	Mean±SD	Median	Mean±SD	Median	Mean±SD	Median
Grade 1st Grade	43	19.5±2.1	19.3	63.5±4.9	63	13.1±4.6	12.4
2nd Grade	14	21.3±2.1	20.8	68.4±6.2	67.5	16.6±4.5	16.2
3rd Grade	45	21.1±3.0	20.7	66.7±6.8	65	16.2±6.7	14.4
bp		0.006**		0.005**		0.011*	
Accommodation Family/Relative's home	32	20.6±2.4	20.3	65.7±5.8	64	15.6±6.0	14.3
Student shared flat	43	19.9±2.1	19.6	64.5±5.7	64	13.3±4.4	13
Dormitory	27	21.2±3.4	20.9	67.4±7.1	65	16.7±6.9	15.2
bp		0.275		0.191		0.079	
Exercise Yes	41	20.4±2.1	20	65.8±5.3	66	14.2±5.3	12.3
No	61	20.5±3.0	20	65.5±6.8	64	15.4±6.1	14.1
ap		0.700		0.356		0.299	

aMann Whitney U Test,   bKruskal Wallis Test,   *p<0.05,   **p<0.01

Tab. 2: Subgroup Analyses

	BMI (kg/m²)	Waist Circumference (cm)	Fat Mass (kg)
	p	p	p
1st Grade-2nd Grade	0.024*	0.012*	0.040*
1st Grade-3rd Grade	0.024*	0.038*	0.043*
2nd Grade-3rd Grade	1.000	0.756	1.000

*Bonferroni Dunn Test, *p<0.05*

of the students who sleep in daytime during weekends and who do not and those who go to bed early and wake up late (p=0.627 p=0.382 p=0.986 p=0.648 p=0.751 p=0.309, respectively). It was found that the highest BMI, waist circumference and fat mass scores are obtained from the participants classified under the group which "goes to bed late and wakes up early" on weekends. Nevertheless, it was observed that individuals who do not sleep in daytime on weekends have higher fat mass when compared to those who sleep in daytime on weekends.

Eating Patterns

It was observed that 69.6 % of the participants have the habit of having breakfast on weekdays. A statistically significant relationship was found between the numbers of snacks have on weekdays and BMI averages. (p=0.025; p<0.05) (Table 3). It was found that BMI scores of the participants who have 2 snacks were significantly higher than the participants who have 0-1 snack and 3 snacks (0-1 snack: p=0.032; 3 snacks: p=0.021; p<0.05). There was no statistically significant difference between the 0-1 snack and 3 snacks groups (p=0.687; p>0.05). A statistically significant relationship was found between the numbers of snacks have on weekdays and waist circumference averages (p=0.025; p<0.05). It was found that waist circumferences of the participants who have 2 snacks were significantly higher than the participants who have 0-1 snack and 3 snacks (0-1 snack: p=0.017; 3 snacks: p=0.042; p<0.05) (Table 3). There was no statistically significant difference between the 0-1 snack and 3 snacks groups (p=0.961; p>0.05). A statistically significant relationship was found between the numbers of snacks have on weekdays and fat mass averages (p=0.040; p<0.05). It was found that fat mass averages of the participants who have 2 snacks were significantly higher than the participants who have 3 or more snacks (p=0.018; p<0.05) (Table 3). There was no statistically significant difference between the 0-1 snack, 2 snacks and 3 or more snacks groups (0-1 snack: p=0.097; 2 snacks: p=0.393; 3 snacks: p>0.05).

Tab. 3: Relationship Between Eating Habits on Weekdays and BMI, Waist Circumference, Fat Mass

	n	BMI (kg/m²) †rho	p	Waist Circumference (cm) †rho	p	Fat Mass (kg) †rho	p
Number of meals on weekdays	102	0.149	0.134	0.033	0.741	0.059	0.558
Number of snacks on weekdays	102	0.015	0.878	0.059	0.555	-0.037	0.711

	n	BMI Mean±SD	Median	WC Mean±SD	Median	Fat Mass Mean±SD	Median
Number of meals on weekdays							
0-1 meal	•2	22.0±6.2	22	69.5±7.8	69.5	20.0±12.9	19.9
2 meals	38	19.8±2.1	19.4	64.5±4.1	64	13.9±4.3	13.5
≥3 meals	62	20.8±2.8	20.5	66.2±7.1	64	15.4±6.3	14
ᵃp		0.108		0.656		0.443	
Number of snacks on weekdays							
0-1 meal	32	19.9±2.4	19.5	64.1±4.9	63	14.1±4.9	12.9
2 meals	49	21.1±2.7	20.7	67.5±7.0	66	16.3±6.2	14.8
≥3 meals	21	19.6±2.6	19	63.6±4.8	64	13.1±5.6	11.8
ᵇp		0.025*		0.025*		0.040*	
Habit of having breakfast on weekdays							
Yes		20.7±2.7	20.2	66.1±6.8	64	15.4±6.0	14.4
No		19.8±2.4	19.2	64.5±4.4	64	13.8±5.2	12.5
ᵃp		0.054		0.557		0.171	

*Due to the small number of people in the group, it was not included in statistical evaluation, *p<0.05, †r: Spearman's Correlation Coefficient, ᵃMann Whitney U Test, ᵇKruskal Wallis Test

There was no statistically significant relationship between meal and snack numbers and BMI, waist circumference and fat mass averages of the students (p>0.05). There was no statistically significant difference in the BMI, waist circumference and fat mass averages of the students who have or have not the habit of having breakfast on weekdays (p>0.05).

Food Frequencies

In the section of this study which explored the frequency of the participants to consume a number of specific food items, it was found that 48 % of the participants consume fruits 2-4 times a week; 31.4 % of the participants consume nuts once a week; 53.9 % of the participants never consume potato chips; 29.4 % of the participants consume chocolate 2-4 times a week; 25.5 % of the participants consume biscuits and derivatives once a week; 47.1 % of the participants never consume popcorn; 26.5 % of the participants consume milk and dairy products 2-4 times a week; 55.9 % of the participants never consume meat and meat derivatives; 47.1 % of the participants never consume vegetables and vegetable derivatives; and 61.8 % of the participants never consume carbonated beverages. As reported by the participants, it was found that the consumption of milk and dairy products was the highest by 12.7 % while the consumption of meat and meat derivatives was the lowest by 1 %.

There was no statistically significant difference of BMI, waist circumference and fat mass measurements according to the frequency of students' consumption of fruits, nuts, chips, chocolate, biscuits and derivatives, popcorn, milk and derivatives, bread and derivatives, vegetables, carbonated beverages (p>0.05). A statistically significant difference was found in the BMI averages in the meat and meat derivatives consumption frequency groups (p=0.030; p<0.05). It was found that BMI average of the participants who consume meat and meat derivatives 5-6 Times a Week was significantly higher than that of those consume meat and meat derivatives 1-2 Time a Week (p=0.030; p<0.05). There was not statistically difference found other groups BMI values (p>0.05) and not statistically difference between meat and meat derivatives consumption, waist circumference and fat mass averages. (p>0.05) (Table 4).

Alcohol Consumption Frequencies

A statistically significant difference was not found in the BMI, waist circumference, fat mass averages in the alcohol consumption frequency groups for weekdays. According to the data obtained, the frequency of alcohol consumption on weekends was not more than "2-4 Times a Week" on weekdays. It was

Tab. 4: BMI, Waist Circumference, Fat Mass in Food Frequency Groups

		n	BMI (kg/m²) Mean±SD	Median	Waist Circumference (cm) Mean±SD	Median	Fat Mass (kg) Mean±SD	Median
Fruit	Never	•4	19.7±1.9	20	62.5±0.6	62.5	11.7±4.3	11.1
	1-2 times a month	8	19.6±3.1	19	63.0±6.3	62.5	13.8±6.9	11.5
	Once a week	23	20.3±1.9	20	64.5±3.5	64	14.5±4.3	14.2
	2-4 times a week	49	20.4±2.5	20	66.0±6.4	64	14.8±5.3	14.1
	5-6 times a week	18	21.3±3.7	20.5	67.8±8.2	65.5	17.1±8.1	14.6
	[b]p		0.561		0.350		0.526	
Nuts	Never	10	21.2±2.9	20.4	67.6±5.9	64	16.5±6.4	14.5
	1-2 times a month	22	20.8±3.4	19.9	66.1±7.7	65	15.5±7.1	14.5
	Once a week	32	20.0±2.2	20.2	65.0±5.9	63	14.2±4.7	13.4
	2-4 times a week	29	20.4±2.6	19.6	65.8±6.1	64	15.0±6.1	13
	5-6 times a week	9	20.4±2.0	21	63.9±3.4	64	14.1±4.9	14.8
	[b]p		0.828		0.606		0.890	
Potato Chips	Never	55	20.7±2.4	20.7	65.6±6.6	64	15.3±5.7	14.3
	1-2 times a month	39	20.0±2.8	19.3	65.6±6.1	64	14.4±5.9	12.4
	Once a week	•4	22.3±2.8	21.4	69.0±4.1	67.5	18.5±7.2	15.8
	2-4 times a week	•3	18.8±2.6	17.9	62.3±2.5	62	11.7±3.5	12.9
	5-6 times a week	•1	18.9	18.9	64	64	8.7	8.7
	[a]p		0.052		0.794		0.218	

Chocolate	Never	13	20.4±1.7	20.7	66.9±6.9	64	15.3±5.3	14.8
	1-2 times a month	24	19.9±2.0	19.7	63.9±3.8	63	13.1±4.8	12.3
	Once a week	18	20.2±1.8	19.9	64.5±6.3	63.5	14.6±3.5	14.9
	2-4 times a week	30	21.5±3.5	20.9	68.0±7.2	67	17.3±7.4	14.7
	5-6 times a week	17	19.5±2.5	18.9	63.9±5.5	63.5	13.4±5.1	12.9
	[b]p	0.180			0.064		0.127
Biscuits and derivatives	Never	23	20.3±2.4	20	65.1±6.6	63	14.0±6.0	12.4
	1-2 times a month	25	20.2±1.8	20	65.4±4.5	64	14.3±4.6	13.6
	Once a week	26	20.8±3.3	20.4	66.0±8.1	65.5	15.9±6.7	15.5
	2-4 times a week	21	20.6±2.8	20.7	65.5±4.8	64	15.7±5.9	14.2
	5-6 times a week	7	19.9±2.9	19.2	66.6±7.0	64	14.1±5.5	12.5
	[b]p	0.882			0.924		0.584
Popcorn	Never	48	20.6±2.4	20	65.9±6.2	64	15.1±5.7	14
	1-2 times a month	41	20.2±2.8	19.7	65.3±6.2	64	14.0±5.7	12.4
	Once a week	8	21.1±2.7	20.5	65.3±5.9	64	17.0±6.0	16
	2-4 times a week	5	20.4±3.9	18.4	66.6±8.6	63	16.9±7.3	12.9
	[b]p	0.605			0.938		0.315
Milk and Milk Derivatives	Never	12	20.3±2.5	19.9	64.9±6.5	63.3	14.5±6.1	12.4
	1-2 times a month	11	20.6±2.4	20.7	65.7±4.4	64	14.5±6.1	13.2
	Once a week	14	20.7±2.1	20.4	65.7±4.3	66	15.4±4.5	14.4
	2-4 times a week	27	19.6±2.4	19.2	64.7±6.2	64	13.6±4.9	12.4
	5-6 times a week	38	21.0±3.0	20.8	66.4±7.3	64.5	15.9±6.6	14.7
	[b]p	0.264			0.766		0.513

(continued on next page)

Tab. 4: Continued

		BMI (kg/m²)		Waist Circumference (cm)		Fat Mass (kg)	
	n	Mean±SD	Median	Mean±SD	Median	Mean±SD	Median
Meat and Meat Derivatives							
Never	57	20.6±2.3	20	65.1±4.9	64	15.1±5.4	13.6
1-2 times a month	7	18.3±1.2	17.9	63.6±3.3	64	11.5±3.3	11.9
Once a week	4	19.0±2.7	19.5	63.0±6.1	65.5	12.9±5.4	12.7
2-4 times a week	20	20.4±3.6	19.8	67.1±9.8	63	15.4±7.5	14.5
5-6 times a week	14	21.4±2.7	21.2	67.2±5.4	65.5	16.0±5.5	15.2
ᵇp		0.030*		0.366		0.257	
Bread and Bread Derivatives							
Never	45	20.5±2.2	20	65.3±4.8	64	14.9±5.3	13
1-2 times a month	12	20.0±2.7	19.2	64.5±5.2	63	13.4±6.2	11.5
Once a week	9	21.4±1.8	21.4	68.0±6.8	66	17.4±3.5	17
2-4 times a week	15	19.0±2.0	19.1	62.5±3.8	63	12.8±3.4	14.4
5-6 times a week	21	21.1±3.7	20.8	68.1±9.1	65	16.3±8.0	15.2
ᵇp		0.090		0.183		0.146	
Vegetables							
Never	48	20.5±2.4	19.9	64.9±4.8	63.8	15.0±5.7	13.1
1-2 times a month	9	20.0±1.5	20.4	64.9±6.4	63	14.0±3.9	13.6
Once a week	11	20.1±2.4	20	65.5±3.3	66	15.1±4.2	15.2
2-4 times a week	21	20.4±2.3	20	66.0±6.8	64	14.2±4.9	14
5-6 times a week	13	20.8±4.4	19.2	68.3±10.4	65	16.4±9.3	14.5
ᵇp		0.988		0.836		0.960	

	Never	63	20.4±2.3	20.2	65.1±5.1	64	14.8±5.3	13.8
	1-2 times a month	20	20.2±2.5	19.4	66.5±6.9	64.5	14.5±5.1	13.3
Carbonated	Once a week	6	23.1±4.5	21	70.5±11.6	66.5	19.9±9.6	16.4
Beverages	2-4 times a week	10	20.0±3.5	19.4	65.3±7.0	64	14.6±7.0	13
	5-6 times a week	•3	18.5±1.3	17.9	60.7±2.9	59	12.1±4.6	10.8
	^{b}p		0.207		0.609		0.320

^{a}Mann Whitney U Test, ^{b}Kruskal Wallis Test

*Due to the small number of people in the group, it was not included in statistical evaluation

Tab. 5: Relationship between Alcohol Consumption, BMI, Waist Circumference and Fat Mass on Weekends

	BMI (kg/m²)		Waist Circumference (cm)		Fat Mass (kg)	
	†rho	p	†rho	p	†rho	p
Beer	-0.028	0.776	0.026	0.799	-0.021	0.838
Wine	-0.200	0.044*	-0.164	0.099	-0.162	0.104
Vodka	0.016	0.874	0.046	0.647	-0.031	0.754
Vodka (with juice or energy drink)	0.014	0.892	0.089	0.375	-0.018	0.858
Raki	0.071	0.477	0.017	0.863	0.054	0.593
Whisky	0.158	0.113	0.026	0.793	0.088	0.382
Tequila	-0.091	0.362	-0.036	0.716	-0.127	0.204
Gin	0.073	0.466	0.157	0.116	0.034	0.732

† r: Spearman's Correlation Coefficient, *p<0.05

found that beer was the most commonly preferred alcoholic beverage on weekends by 2.9 %. A statistically significant and negative correlation was found in the BMI averages in the wine consumption frequency groups (p=0.044). There was no statistically significant relationship between the participants' other alcoholic beverage consumption frequencies and their BMI, waist circumference and fat mass levels (Table 5). There was no significant difference between alcohol consumption frequencies on weekdays and the students' grades. A statistically significant difference was found in the tequila consumption frequency on weekends and the participants' grade (r=0.200; p=0.010). It was found that tequila consumption frequency of 1st grade students is higher. There was no significant difference between the other alcoholic beverage consumption frequencies on weekdays and the students' grades.

Food Frequencies and Accommodation

A statistically significant difference was found in the chocolate consumption frequency and the participants' accommodation type. The frequency of chocolate consumption of those who live in a dormitory was higher than the others (p=0.004; p<0.05). There was no significant difference between the other food consumption frequencies and the students' accommodation type (Table 6). There was no significant difference between alcohol consumption frequencies on weekdays and/or weekends and the students' accommodation type.

Tab. 6: Evaluation of Food Frequencies According to Accommodation

		Family/ Relative's Home		Student Shared Flat		Dormitory		p
		n	%	n	%	n	%	
Fruits	Never	1	3.1	1	2.3	2	7.4	ᶜ0.631
	1-2 times a month	2	6.3	3	7.0	3	11.1	
	Once a week	9	28.1	9	20.9	5	18.5	
	2-4 times a week	14	43.8	25	58.1	10	37.0	
	5-6 times a week	6	18.8	5	11.6	7	25.9	
Nuts	Never	4	12.5	3	7.0	3	11.1	ᶜ0.904
	1-2 times a month	4	12.5	11	25.6	7	25.9	
	Once a week	11	34.4	12	27.9	9	33.3	
	2-4 times a week	10	31.3	13	30.2	6	22.2	
	5-6 times a week	3	9.4	4	9.3	2	7.4	
Potato Chips	Never	16	50.0	26	60.5	13	48.1	ᶜ0.256
	1-2 times a month	15	46.9	14	32.6	10	37.0	
	Once a week	1	3.1	0	0.0	3	11.1	
	2-4 times a week	0	0.0	2	4.7	1	3.7	
	5-6 times a week	0	0.0	1	2.3	0	0.0	
Chocolate	Never	10	31.3	3	7.0	0	0.0	ᶜ0.004**
	1-2 times a month	8	25.0	11	25.6	5	18.5	
	Once a week	3	9.4	10	23.3	5	18.5	
	2-4 times a week	4	12.5	13	30.2	13	48.1	
	5-6 times a week	7	21.9	6	14.0	4	14.8	
Biscuits and biscuits derivatives	Never	9	28.1	10	23.3	4	14.8	ᵈ0.515
	1-2 times a month	6	18.8	13	30.2	6	22.2	
	Once a week	7	21.9	13	30.2	6	22.2	
	2-4 times a week	7	21.9	6	14.0	8	29.6	
	5-6 times a week	3	9.4	1	2.3	3	11.1	
Popcorn	Never	15	46.9	23	53.5	10	37.0	ᶜ0.288
	1-2 times a month	14	43.8	16	37.2	11	40.7	
	Once a week	3	9.4	3	7.0	2	7.4	
	2-4 times a week	0	0.0	1	2.3	4	14.8	

(continued on next page)

Tab. 6: Continued

		Family/ Relative's Home		Student Shared Flat		Dormitory		p
		n	%	n	%	n	%	
Milk and milk derivatives	Never	7	21.9	3	7.0	2	7.4	ᶜ0.332
	1-2 times a month	3	9.4	5	11.6	3	11.1	
	Once a week	5	15.6	3	7.0	6	22.2	
	2-4 times a week	7	21.9	15	34.9	5	18.5	
	5-6 times a week	10	31.3	17	39.5	11	40.7	
Meat and meat derivatives	Never	23	71.9	21	48.8	13	48.1	ᶜ0.569
	1-2 times a month	1	3.1	3	7.0	3	11.1	
	Once a week	0	0.0	2	4.7	2	7.4	
	2-4 times a week	5	15.6	10	23.3	5	18.5	
	5-6 times a week	3	9.4	7	16.3	4	14.8	
Bread and bread derivatives	Never	17	53.1	16	37.2	12	44.4	ᶜ0.462
	1-2 times a month	4	12.5	6	14.0	2	7.4	
	Once a week	3	9.4	2	4.7	4	14.8	
	2-4 times a week	3	9.4	10	23.3	2	7.4	
	5-6 times a week	5	15.6	9	20.9	7	25.9	
Vegetables	Never	19	59.4	17	39.5	12	44.4	ᶜ0.518
	1-2 times a month	3	9.4	4	9.3	2	7.4	
	Once a week	1	3.1	5	11.6	5	18.5	
	2-4 times a week	7	21.9	10	23.3	4	14.8	
	5-6 times a week	2	6.3	7	16.3	4	14.8	
Carbonated drinks	Never	21	65.6	27	62.8	15	55.6	ᶜ0.071
	1-2 times a month	9	28.1	7	16.3	4	14.8	
	Once a week	0	0.0	1	2.3	5	18.5	
	2-4 times a week	2	6.3	5	11.6	3	11.1	
	5-6 times a week	0	0.0	3	7.0	0	0.0	

ᶜ*Fisher Freeman Halton Exact Test,* ᵈ*Pearson Chi-Square Test,* ***p<0.01*

Food Frequencies and Exercise

A statistically significant difference was found in the exercise groups and the participants' food consumption frequency. The chocolate consumption frequency of those who do not exercise was significantly higher (p=0.006; p<0.05). Considering the equal consumption frequencies of the participants who do not exercise, it was observed that they tend to consume more of almost every food item (Table 7).

Alcohol Consumption Frequencies and Exercise

There was no significant difference between alcohol consumption frequencies on weekdays and/or weekends and the students' exercise habits. Considering the equal alcohol consumption frequencies of the participants who do not exercise in each alcoholic beverage category, it was observed that they tend to consume more of almost every alcoholic beverage.

Discussion

The main purpose of this study is to explore the effects of the food items consumed between dinner time and bedtime, sleep duration and sleep timing on the increased obesity risk. Previous studies investigated the impact of night eating on the obesity risk for individuals from every age group (5,7,12,13). Many studies in the literature on sleep duration, sleep timing and night eating habits focused on adult, children, and elderly participants. The limited number of studies found in relation to young adults was one of the main reasons behind the selection of the population for this study, university students. In addition, the population consists of the students of the Department of Nutrition and Dietetics. The reason behind this specific selection was that they are better able to control their diets in the light of the education they receive when compared to students from other departments. It was attempted to observe if the individuals who receive information about eating healthy were good at applying this information in their daily lives. As students are exposed to difficult exam sessions, and the stress of delivering projects and homework within deadlines, it was believed that this age group might experience irregularities in their sleep and eating patterns (14). As daily lifestyle may be subject to change especially during exam sessions, it was assumed that the consumption of convenient and ready-made food later at night would increase accordingly. In order to underline this effect, the survey included in this study was conducted during the exam session.

Tab. 7: Exercise Habits and Food Frequencies

		Exercise		No Exercise		p
		n	%	n	%	
Fruits	Never	1	2.4	3	4.9	^c0.341
	1-2 times a month	4	9.8	4	6.6	
	Once a week	12	29.3	11	18.0	
	2-4 times a week	20	48.8	29	47.5	
	5-6 times a week	4	9.8	14	23.0	
Nuts	Never	7	17.1	3	4.9	^d0.328
	1-2 times a month	7	17.1	15	24.6	
	Once a week	12	29.3	20	32.8	
	2-4 times a week	12	29.3	17	27.9	
	5-6 times a week	3	7.3	6	9.8	
Potato Chips	Never	20	48.8	35	57.4	^c0.377
	1-2 times a month	19	46.3	20	32.8	
	Once a week	2	4.9	2	3.3	
	2-4 times a week	0	0.0	3	4.9	
	5-6 times a week	0	0.0	1	1.6	
Chocolate	Never	10	24.4	3	4.9	^d0.006**
	1-2 times a month	12	29.3	12	19.7	
	Once a week	4	9.8	14	23.0	
	2-4 times a week	12	29.3	18	29.5	
	5-6 times a week	3	7.3	14	23.0	
Biscuits and biscuit derivatives	Never	12	29.3	11	18.0	^d0.493
	1-2 times a month	10	24.4	15	24.6	
	Once a week	10	24.4	16	26.2	
	2-4 times a week	8	19.5	13	21.3	
	5-6 times a week	1	2.4	6	9.8	
Popcorn	Never	21	51.2	27	44.3	^c0.638
	1-2 times a month	17	41.5	24	39.3	
	Once a week	2	4.9	6	9.8	
	2-4 times a week	1	2.4	4	6.6	
Milk and milk derivatives	Never	8	19.5	4	6.6	^d0.293
	1-2 times a month	5	12.2	6	9.8	
	Once a week	4	9.8	10	16.4	
	2-4 times a week	9	22.0	18	29.5	
	5-6 times a week	15	36.6	23	37.7	

Tab. 7:   Continued

		Exercise		No Exercise		p
		n	**%**	**n**	**%**	
Meat and meat derivatives	Never	24	58.5	33	54.1	ᶜ0.727
	1-2 times a month	4	9.8	3	4.9	
	Once a week	2	4.9	2	3.3	
	2-4 times a week	7	17.1	13	21.3	
	5-6 times a week	4	9.8	10	16.4	
Bread and bread derivatives	Never	21	51.2	24	39.3	ᵈ0.403
	1-2 times a month	6	14.6	6	9.8	
	Once a week	3	7.3	6	9.8	
	2-4 times a week	3	7.3	12	19.7	
	5-6 times a week	8	19.5	13	21.3	
Vegetables	Never	19	46.3	29	47.5	ᵈ0.554
	1-2 times a month	4	9.8	5	8.2	
	Once a week	4	9.8	7	11.5	
	2-4 times a week	11	26.8	10	16.4	
	5-6 times a week	3	7.3	10	16.4	
Carbonated Drinks	Never	25	61.0	38	62.3	ᶜ0.577
	1-2 times a month	8	19.5	12	19.7	
	Once a week	1	2.4	5	8.2	
	2-4 times a week	6	14.6	4	6.6	
	5-6 times a week	1	2.4	2	3.3	

ᶜFisher Freeman Halton Exact Test, ᵈPearson Chi-Square Test, **p<0.01

The curriculum used in the Department of Nutrition and Dietetics has a difficulty level gradually gets harder from the 1st grade to the 3rd grade, for that reason participants were enrolled from each one of these grades with the purpose to see how the increased information level shapes their sleep and eating habits. An assessment of the intergrade differences showed that BMIs, waist circumference and fat mass measurements are significantly lower than that of 2nd and 3rd grade students. The reasons behind this finding were believed to be the fact that the Department of Nutrition and Dietetics has recently received increased attention, that it is commonly preferred by female students with the aspiration to have a healthy and fit body, that the students of Yeditepe University tend to place importance on their appearance due to their general socioeconomic backgrounds, and that students tend to disregard their eating and sleep routines with harder curriculum and increased responsibility. Increased information level in accordance with the instructions on nutrition does not seem to improve the level of adoption of this information in one's lifestyle.

Yeditepe University has a high number of students coming from other cities. Thus, students have a number of different accommodation options. Changing accommodation type may have a direct impact on students' sleep habits, while changing the availability and convenience of food. It was also predicted that the responsibility levels will change among the students who live alone in the dormitory, who live alone in an apartment or who share the apartment with another student. Therefore, this study was also designed to inquire the accommodation types of the students.

Although the findings were not statistically significant, it was found that students who live in school dormitory have higher BMI, waist circumference and fat mass scores when compared to other accommodation types. Students who live alone, who share an apartment and who live with family have better chances to access healthy food options. In private dormitories, on the other hand, students are often provided with a shared kitchen facility. As the campus dormitory does not offer such facilities, students commonly prefer ready-made and high-calorie food as an alternative to healthy food served at the cafeteria. Thus, it is believed that this is the reason behind higher scores obtained from students living in campus dormitory. Nevertheless, the fact that students living in the campus do not make an extra effort to go to classes was also considered as another reason for the higher scores.

This study also investigates the physical activity statues as it can be a factor in reducing the obesity risk or prevalence of obesity. Studies in this field do not consider an exercise pattern of less than 3 days a week and less than 30 minutes a session as a physical activity (11). Therefore, this study inquires the level of physical activity of the participants based on these levels. According to the results obtained from the survey, there was no significant difference between participants who exercise and who do not. This is explained by the fact that BMI, waist circumference and fat mass scores of all the participants are in a normal range and that they pursue a rather active lifestyle as required by their age group.

It is assumed that insufficient sleep and sleeping late at night are risk factors of obesity. Thus, this study explored the sleep duration of the participants and their sleep timing under four sleep start and end conditions. Previous studies have also used similar subgroup inquiries (7).

According to the results obtained, it was found that sleep duration on weekdays, sleeping late or early and waking up late or early and daytime sleep were not significantly correlated with their BMIs, waist circumference and fat mass. This finding may be explained with the fact that although the participants had different patterns of sleep start and end, the average duration of sleep was 7.1 hours which is not significantly below the duration recognized as insufficient (5,15). Young adult participants often wake up early in order to maintain successful results at school. It was found that changes in the sleep pattern on weekends do not result in a significant difference in the measurements of BMI, waist circumference and fat mass. This can be explained with the increased social activity accompanying increased sleep duration (9 hours at an average) which translates into increased physical activity. Previous studies suggest that increased sleep duration on weekends does not improve the relationship between sleep and obesity risk (16). Another aspect which differs depending on the sleep habits is the frequency of meals. Eating habits may change depending on the sleep pattern of the student. For example, it is found that students who prefer to increase their sleep duration tend to skip breakfast or to go for ready-made high-calorie food. As the population of this study involves female students only, it was predicted that they would rather take their time in the morning to get ready for school, and skip breakfast in favor of convenient food. Although there was no significant difference in the data obtained from this study, it was found that BMI, waist circumference and fat mass measurements gave higher results in students who have breakfast on weekdays when compared to those skip breakfast. This result changed with almost all the participants having breakfast on weekends. Although their number is rather low, BMIs, waist circumference, and fat mass measurements of those who did not have breakfast on weekends were higher than those who have breakfast on weekends. It was predicted that there will be differences in the frequency of snacks and meals on weekdays and weekends due to changing social activity level and bedtime. However, the results of this study did not give any significant difference between the number of meals and snacks both on weekdays and weekends. This can be explained with the fact that participants who are engaged in school on weekdays are engaged in social activities on weekends which result in the same pattern for the time spent with meals.

Consumption of a number of specific foods is investigated in order to find a correlation between the participants' possible eating habits after dinner or night eating habits and obesity. Previous research also investigated specific foods and their consumption after 8 pm in connection with night eating and its effects on obesity (4,10,12,17). Even the consumption of food which is commonly deemed healthy may lead to obesity when they are consumed at late hours resulting in increased calorie intake. This can be explained with the changes in circadian rhythm and hormone activity (18-21).

According to the data obtained, "Meat and Meat Derivatives" consumption were found to have statistically significant impact on BMI scores. A review of the food preferences with respect to accommodation showed that students living in the campus dormitory consume significantly more chocolate than the others. There was also significant difference between the food consumption frequencies and exercise habits of the students. Students who exercise tend to consume significantly less amount of chocolate than who do not exercise according the study criteria. Having snacks also had significant effects on BMI, waist circumference and fat mass. Students who had 0-1 snack and 3 snacks on weekdays have significantly lower BMI, waist circumference and fat mass when compared to students who had 2 snacks on weekdays. As this study focuses on university students, alcohol consumption was considered as another possible factor which may lead to obesity. Given the fact that consumption frequency may differ from weekdays to weekends, consumption of different alcoholic beverages was investigated for both timeframes. According to the data obtained, tequila consumption of 1st grade students is significantly higher than the other grades. Considering it is a beverage commonly preferred in nightclubs, it could be explained with the 1st grade students' enthusiasm about new university life. There was a negative but statistically significant relationship between wine consumption on weekends and BMI for all participants. There was no statistically significant relationship between students' alcohol consumption on weekdays and their BMI, waist circumference and fat mass measurements. This can be explained with reduced alcohol consumption on weekdays. There was no statistically significant relationship between the accommodation type and exercise habits off the students and their alcohol consumption both on weekdays and weekends.

In short, this study focuses on young adults which makes it distinguished from the previous research. When the data obtained is considered in general, there was no significant correlation between the sleep and eating habits of university students and their BMI, waist circumference and fat mass measurements. Among the reasons behind this finding are the possibility of having a high basal metabolism rate due to physiologic features (22), increased physical activity level as a requirement of social and academic lifestyle, having the necessary information level especially in healthy eating as students of the Department of Nutrition and Dietetics, and increased attention to healthy living in connection with the aspiration to have a specific body image as the participants were all female students. Moreover, a previous study on the same age group was only able to establish a statistically significant relationship between sleep duration, night eating and BMI in male participants. This study shows that there is no correlation between BMI, sleep duration and night eating in the light of studies conducted on female participants (7).

Conclusion

It was observed that consuming potato chips after dinner and consuming meat and meat derivatives 5-6 times a week has a negative but significant relationship with BMI. A statistically significant and negative correlation was found between BMI and wine consumed on weekends. When compared with other grades, BMIs, waist circumference and fat mass measurements of the 1st grade students are to be significantly lower. Students who consume 3 snacks on weekdays tend to have significantly lower BMI, waist circumference and fat mass than who consume 2 snacks. It was also observed that exercise habits do not result in a significant difference in the parameters explored. It was found that changes in the accommodation type do not result in a significant difference in the measurements of BMI, waist circumference and fat mass. Students living in campus dormitory tend to consume more chocolate than others. As reported by the previous research, increasing responsibility level of the students and having a more routine lifestyle may lead to a negative impact on the parameters used in this study in terms of sleep duration, sleep timing and night eating habits. In order to have better results in future research, it will be a good idea to increase the number of participants included. In addition, a comparison of more than one department may lead to different results. Nevertheless, it may be possible to define a statistically significant relationship between BMI and sleep and eating patterns with a comparison of the two genders. When the data obtained is considered, there is no significant correlation between the sleep and night eating habits of university students with ages ranging between 18 and 24 and their BMI, waist circumference and fat mass measurements. More studies are needed in this field if it is to establish the correlation between sleep and night eating habits and obesity in this age group.

References

1. Mitchell, J. A., Rodriguez, D., Schmitz, K. H., Audrain-McGovern, J. (2013). Greater screen time is associated with adolescent obesity: A longitudinal study of the BMI distribution from Ages 14 to 18. *Obesity*, *21*(3), 572-575. doi:10.1002/oby.20157

2. Pisa, P. T., Pedro, T. M., Kahn, K., Tollman, S. M., Pettifor, J. M., & Norris, S. A. (2015). Nutrient patterns and their association with socio-demographic, lifestyle factors and obesity risk in rural South African adolescents. *Nutrients, 7*(5), 3464-3482. doi:10.3390/nu7053464

3. Eng, S., Wagstaff, D. A., & Kranz, S. (2009). Eating late in the evening is associated with childhood obesity in some age groups but not in all children: The relationship between time of consumption and body weight status in U.S. children. *International Journal of Behavioral Nutrition and Physical Activity, 6*, 27. doi:10.1186/1479-5868-6-27

4. Sun, W., Huang, Y., Wang, Z., Yu, Y., Lau, A., Ali, G. . . . Shan, G. (2015). Sleep duration associated with body mass index among Chinese adults. *Sleep Medicine, 16*(5), 612-616. doi:10.1016/j.sleep.2014.12.011

5. Taheri, S., Lin, L., Young, T., & Mignot, E. (2004). Short sleep duration is associated with reduced leptin, elevated ghrelin, and increased body mass index. *PLoS Medicine, 1*(3), e62. doi:10.1371/journal.pmed.0010062

6. Cuypers, K., Kvaløy, K., Bratberg, G., Midthjell, K., Holmen, J., & Holmen, T. L. (2012). Being normal weight but feeling overweight in adolescence may affect weight development into young adulthood-an 11-year followup: The HUNT study. Norway. *Journal of Obesity.* doi:10.1155/2012/601872

7. Roberts, R. E., & Duong, H. T. (2015). Is there an association between adolescent sleep restriction and obesity. *Journal of Psychosomatic Research, 79*(6), 651-656. doi:10.1016/j.jpsychores.2015.05.012

8. Reilly, J. J., Armstrong, J., Dorosty, A. R., Emmett, P. M., Ness, A., Rogers, I., . . . Sherriff, A. (2005). Early life risk factors for obesity in childhood: Cohort study. *BMJ, 330*(7504), 1357. doi:10.1136/bmj.38470.670903.E0

9. Karakas, P., & Bozkir, M. G. (2012). Anthropometric indices in relation to overweight and obesity among Turkish medical students. *Archives of Medical Science, 9;8*(2), 209-213. doi:10.5114/aoms.2012.28546

10. Olds, T. S., Maher, C. A., & Matricciani, L. (2011). Sleep duration or bedtime? Exploring the relationship between sleep habits and weight status and activity patterns. *Sleep, 34*(10), 1299-1307. doi:10.5665/SLEEP.1266

11. Peitis, C. L., Taylor, N. F., & Shields, N. (2013). Patients receiving inpatient rehabilitation for lower limb orthopaedic conditions do much less physical activity than recommended in guidelines for healthy older adults: An observational study. *Journal of Physiotherapy, 59*(1), 39-44. doi:10.1016/S1836-9553(13)70145-0

12. Baron, K. G., Reid, K. J., Kern, A. S., & Zee, P. C. (2011). Role of sleep timing in caloric intake and BMI. *Obesity, 19*(7), 1374-1381. doi:10.1038/oby.2011.100

13. Spaeth, A., Dinges, D. F., & Goel, N. (2013). Effects of experimental sleep restriction on weight gain, caloric intake, and meal timing in healthy adults. *Sleep, 36*(7), 981-990. doi:10.5665/sleep.2792

14. Tajik, E., Zulkefli, N. A. M., Baharom, A., Minhat, H. S., & Latiff, L. A. (2014). Contributing factors of obesity among stressed adolescents. *Electron Physician, 6*(1), 771-778. doi:10.14661/2014.771-778

15. Cleator, J., Abbott, J., Judd, P., Sutton, C., & Wilding, J. P. H. (2012). Night eating syndrome: Implications for severe obesity. *Nutrition and Diabetes, 2*(9), e44. doi:10.1038/nutd.2012.16

16. Meyer, K. A., Wall, M. M., Larson, N. I., Laska, M. N., & Neumark-Sztainer, D. (2012). Sleep duration and BMI in a sample of young adults. *Obesity, 20*(6), 1279-1287. doi:10.1038/oby.2011.381

17. Gunes, F. E., Bekiroglu, N., Imeryuz, N., & Agirbasli, M. (2012). Relation between eating habits and a high body mass index among freshman students: A cross-sectional study. *Journal of the American College of Nutrition, 31*(3), 167-174. doi:10.1080/07315724.2012.10720024

18. Golley, R. K., Maher, C. A., Maricciani, L., & Olds, T. S. (2013). Sleep duration or bedtime? Exploring the association between sleep timing behavior, diet and BMI in children and adolescent. *International Journal of Obesity, 37*(4), 546-551. doi:10.1038/ijo.2012.212

19. Sancar, A., Lindsey-Boltz, L. A., Kang, T. H., Reardon, J. T., Lee, J. H., & Ozturk, N. (2010). Circadian clock control of the cellular response to DNA damage. *FEBS Letters, 584*(12), 2618-2625. doi:10.1016/j.febslet.2010.03.017

20. Crnko, S., Cour, M., Van Laake, L. W., & Lecour, S. (2018). Vasculature on the clock: Circadian rhythm and vascular dysfunction. *Vascular Pharmacology, 108*, 1-7. doi:10.1016/j.vph.2018.05.003

21. Utpal, B., Thakkar, N., Das, P., & Bhadra, M. P. (2017). Evolution of circadian rhythms: From bacteria to human. *Sleep Medicine, 35*, 49-61. doi:10.1016/j.sleep.2017.04.008

22. Ferreira-Figueiredo, M., Detrano, F., Oliveria-Coelho, G. M., Barros, M. E., Lanzillotti R. S., Neto J. F. N., ... Soares, E. de A. (2014). Body composition and basal metabolic rate in women with type 2 diabetes mellitus. *Journal of Nutrition and Metabolism*, 574057. doi:10.1155/2014/574057

Yonca Sevim

Recreational Athletes' Food Choices

Abstract

Objective: There are many factors that affect a person's food choices. Recreational athletes (Rec), which are a special group, do sports for different purposes and in environment than professional athletes do. The aim of this study is to determine the factors affecting the food choices of this group, considering the different conditions and physical and individual differences than professional athletes.

Materials and Methods: This study was conducted on a total of 184 volunteer rec-athletes, 94 men and 90 women, aged 18-56, who do sports in private fitness centers. A questionnaire containing sociodemographic information, recreational objectives, pre-post training and general food preferences, and Food Choice Questionnaire (FCQ) were administered to the participants.

Results: In this study, it was found that the most motivational participation in sports of recreational athletes was to relieve stress and then to increase body muscle mass and the feeling of well-being. Rec-athletes stated that they preferred foods rich in carbohydrates before exercise (p<0.01), while they preferred foods rich in protein and water content after exercise (p<0.01). The first 3 items with the highest average in the FCQ scoring were found as "Keeps me healthy" (mean 3.34±0.87), "Contains a lot of vitamins and minerals" (mean 3.16±0.95) and "Tastes good" (mean 3.12±0.97). Rec-athletes gave importance to health, natural content, and convenience factor in their food choices, respectively. When the participants were asked about their food choice, apart from FCQ, the order changed in terms of taste, health, and nutritional content, respectively.

Conclusion: In this study, it has been determined that the factors affecting the food choices of rec-athletes may be different from those of professional/elite athletes and general consumers. In understanding food choices, rec-athletes should be evaluated separately from other populations and more studies are needed.

Keywords: Recreational, Athlete, Food Choice Questionnaire, Fitness, Nutrition, FCQ

Introduction

The number of food-related decisions of an individual's made been estimated as more than 220 decisions per day and these decisions influenced by both external and internal factors (1,2).

There is a complex interaction between sensory factors, such as appearance, taste, odor and texture characteristics, and non-sensory factors such as expectations and attitudes toward food, health claims, price, ethical concerns, mood and familiarity in food preferences. (3,4). In addition, it is known that cultural and religious beliefs (5,6), subculture and ethnic characteristics (7), access to food and food safety (8), individual level of knowledge about food and nutrition (9) as well as personal and family beliefs (10) also affect food choices.

Despite numerous studies with general populations, a small number of studies has been carried out with athletes. The majority of the studies have indicated that performance related factors affect the food choice of athletes from different sports and countries. (11,12). These items include stage of competitive season, intensity of training, weight modification and gastrointestinal issues (13). Also, coaches, the behaviors and practices of other athletes and the culture within sport have influence on athletes (14-16). Both athletes and general population report that food choices are often influenced by food choice of teammates or peers in social place where meals are eaten with together (10,17). Similar with the general population, factors such as price, sensory appeal, familiarity, and hunger have influence on athletes (11,13). However, most of these researchers have focused on specific sports, single countries, and genders rather than examining food choice in athletes on a wide scale (13).

A recreational athlete (rec-athlete) can be defined as a person who is physically active but who does not train for competition at the same level of intensity and focus as a competitive athlete (18). The expression "recreationally active" is also used as physical activity at least 3 times a week and lasting at least 30 minutes (19). Since sport participants can range from the recreational (leisure or amateur sport) to the elite (compete at the national or international level), factors affecting the food choice may vary according to the priorities of the athlete (20). A recreational athlete can spend time in a very different physical condition and environment than an elite athlete. Recreative sports are outdoor sports, team sports, individual sports, water sports, air sports, motor sports, combat sports, racket sports, recreational activities in parks, folk dances and dances, exercise in fitness centers (21,22). In so many countries around the world, publicly founded and private recreational facilities are existing. Studies on food alternatives in these facilities are very insufficient. In a systematic review, it was shown that unhealthy foods are more dominant in the accessible food environment in sports environments (23). Publicly funded sport complexes providing access to affordable physical activities have been also identified as a community setting with substantial potential to improve public health, but which, by virtue of unhealthy food environments, may be paradoxically contributing to obesity risk (24). In addition, it has been reported that unhealthy food brands contribute to obesity by increasing brand awareness and sponsor product preference while reaching large masses with sports sponsorship (25).

Other priorities that differ recreational athletes from elite athletes are the gains from these activities. Participation in leisure activities has also been reported to increase reported happiness (26) and reduce the effects of stress (27) and provide individual and social benefits including physical and mental health and academic success (28). Studies have also shown that participation in recreational sports reduces work stress, and the more participation increases, the more decreases in stress (29-31). Similarly, the main purpose of activities in recreational sports is to increase the level of physical fitness and participation including entertainment and socialization (32).

One of the goals in improving fitness level may be the fact that physical inactivity is one of the biggest Public Health problems of the 21st century (33). Physical inactivity is responsible for 6 % of deaths in the world and has been identified as the fourth risk leading factor for global mortality. This follows high blood pressure (13 %), tobacco use (9 %) and high blood glucose (6 %). Overweight and obesity are responsible for 5 % of global mortality (34). Inactivity is responsible for more than 5.3 % of the 57 million deaths that occurred worldwide in 2008. By eliminating physical inactivity, life expectancy of the world's population is estimated to increase by 0.68 (0.41-0.95) years (35). The health benefits of physical activity and exercise are certain; in fact, everyone can benefit from becoming more physically active (36). Recreation and sport settings are increasingly identified as ideal settings for promoting overall health through creation of environments that support positive health behaviors and increasing number of these settings typically support health through physical activity promotion. However, the food environment within them is often not reflective of nutrition guidelines (24). Professional athletes think that their food choices have a positive effect on performance, fitness level and health, and therefore it is known that this awareness affects their food choices (37). Evidence also showed that many health-related decisions are often made very quickly with little conscious. Thus, although many individuals express an intention to eat healthy, in practice they more commonly select unhealthy foods for immediate reasons such as taste and convenience (38,39).

It is important to detect factors affect food choices and numerous approaches have been studied on this area (13). One of the most widely used quantitative tools to examine these factors that are important in individual food choice is the Food Choice Questionnaire (FCQ) developed by Steptoe and Wardle in 1995 (40). This questionnaire has been used to understand the food choice factors of various populations, including consumers from around the world, adolescents, dental students and the factors behind organic food choices, however, it has not been used on athlete populations (4,41-43).

The FCQ contains 36 items grouped into nine dimensions, measuring the importance of food choice factors: "health", "mood", "convenience", "sensory appeal", "natural content", "price", "weight control", "familiarity" and "ethical concern" (40). Each subscale consists of 3-6 items. In the FCQ, questions starting with "on a typical day" related to the food choices are asked to participants and it is requested that they evaluate them on a four-point scale (1=not at all important to 4=very important) (44). The scale has been translated into more than 20 languages and used as a tool in over 40 countries (45). Dikmen and et al tested the validity and reliability of the food choice questionnaire (FCQ) for Turkish consumers and they showed that the Turkish validation of FCQ appears to be a reliable research instrument.

With a recent study, Truchet and Pelly (46) developed a new version of FCQ as Athlete Food Choice Questionnaire (AFCQ) to determine the key factors influencing food choice in an international cohort of athletes. This questionnaire contains 84 items on a 5-point scale and the dimensions in the special version for athletes are "nutritional attributes of the food", "emotional influences", "food and health awareness", "influence of others", "usual eating practices", "weight control", "food values and beliefs", "sensory appeal" and "performance". This new version has a very convenient scale potential for athlete populations, as it also includes factors specific to athletic performance and sports environment. To be able to use this version in our country, Turkish validation of AFCQ is needed.

Studies investigating food choices specific to rec-athletes are much less numerous. Since the environment where recreational sports are performed and the purposes of participating in these sports differ, it is very important to have information about the food choices of these athletes. For all these reasons, in this study, it was aimed to evaluate the food choices of rec-athletes with the FCQ tool. In this sense, this study will make an important contribution to the literature.

Materials and Methods

Participants

This study was conducted on a total of 184 volunteers, 94 males and 90 females, between the ages of 18-56, who do exercise in various fitness centers in İstanbul, Turkey. Data were collected between February and March 2020. Four hundred people were informed about the survey, 20 people refused to participate in the study, 180 people who wanted to participate in the study were not rec-athletes (19), and 16 people were excluded from the study, and the study data were evaluated with 184 people. Food choice behavior is a complex process and mainly influenced by taste, convenience, cost of the food items and health status of the individuals (47). Since receiving medical treatment and having chronic diseases may affect the decision process in food choice, people without medical treatment or chronic diseases were included in the study. Volunteer participants did not receive any incentives to participate.

Questionnaire

The questionnaire form used in the study was developed by the researcher after the relevant literature review. The questionnaire form consists of questions about sociodemographic characteristics such as gender, age, marital status, income and education, sports participation goals, and food preferences. The FCQ is the last part of the questionnaire.

The FCQ comprised 36 items in 9 dimensions (health, mood, convenience, sensory appeal, natural content, price, weight control, familiarity, and ethical concern (40). Some researchers have used 5-point or 7-point Likert scales in recent studies (48-51). The FCQ scale was scored as originally with a 4-point Likert scale (1=not at all important to 4=very important) in this current study. The Turkish validation and adaptation studies were conducted by Dikmen et al. FCQ was concluded to be a suitable tool for use in our population (44). Questions starting with "on a typical day" related to the food choices are asked to participants and it was requested that they evaluate them on a four-point scale (1=not at all important to 4=very important). Participants filled in the questionnaire and the FQC themselves. Permission was obtained from Dikmen et al. for the use of the Turkish validated version of the FCQ in this study.

Statistical Analysis

Statistical Package for Social Sciences (SPSS) version 20.0 was used to statistically evaluate the data obtained from the study. Continuous variables were presented with mean and standard deviation. Categorical variables were presented with number and percentage values. Between men and women, continuous variables showing normal distribution were evaluated by the Significance Test of the Difference Between Two Means and categorical variables were evaluated by the Chi-Square. Chi-square test (McNemar) was applied to dependent groups for food choice comparisons before and after exercise. The relationships between sub-dimensions and sociodemographic levels of the study group were made by ANOVA analysis. The statistical significance level in the analyzes was taken as p<0.05.

Results

The demographic and general characteristics of the participants are shown in Table 1. The average age of the participants was found to be 28 (±9.7) years. The average age of women participating in the study was found to be significantly higher than men (29.4±10.7 and 26.3±8.5, respectively, p<0.05). 80.4 % of the participants are single, 84.8 % have undergraduate and postgraduate education. The mean body mass index value has a significant difference between men (24.8±3.2 kg/m^2) and women (22.5±3.7 kg/m^2) (p<0.05).

Participants stated that they mostly engaged in recreational sports to relieve stress (53.3 %), to increase body muscle mass (51.1 %), and to feel well-being

Tab. 1: General Characteristics of Participants

	Male n=94		Female n=90		
	Mean±SD		Mean±SD		*p*
Age (year)	26.3±8.5		29.4±10.7		*0.033**
Weight (kg)	80.3±13.3		61.2±11.4		*0.000**
Height (cm)	179.7±7.6		164.5±6.3		*0.000**
BMI (kg/m^2)	24.8±3.2		22.5±3.7		*0.000**
	n	%	n	%	
Marital Status					
Single	80	85.1	68	75.6	*0.103***
Married	14	14.9	22	24.4	
Education					
Primary Education	1	1.1	2	2.2	
High School	13	13.8	12	13.3	*0.823***
License Degree	80	85.1	76	84.4	
Income Statue					
Income>Expense	35	37.2	32	35.6	
Income=Expense	40	42.2	48	53.3	*0.168***
Income<Expense	19	20.2	10	11.1	

*Independent Samples test was used, ** Chi-Square Tests was used
BMI: Body Mass Index

(50.5 %) (Table 2). The number of people who do sports to gain weight and socialize has been found very few.

Table 3 shows the factors affecting the food choices of the participants, which were asked in the questionnaire as an additional part beside FCQ. Participants stated that they mostly give importance to "Taste", then "Health Benefit" and "Nutritional Content" food choice.

The food choices of rec-athletes before and after exercise were questioned based on the content of macronutrients and the results are shown in Table 4. While the choice of foods rich in protein and water increased after exercise (p=0.001), the choice of foods rich in carbohydrate decreased (p=0.001). The number of people who did not pay attention to any macronutrient content before exercise decreased after exercise (p=0.013). Fat content of foods to be consumed after exercise was not a factor affecting food choices.

Tab. 2: Goals of Participation in Recreational Sports

Goals	n	%
Well-being	93	50.5
Boosting immunity	37	20.1
Improving general health	81	44.0
Weight loss / fat burning	79	42.9
Increase body muscle mass	94	51.1
Weight gain	17	9.2
Weight maintenance	46	25.0
Stress relief, relaxing	98	53.3
Socializing	24	13.0

Tab. 3: Factors Affecting Food Choice of Participants

Factors	n	%
Taste	132	71.7
Health benefit	121	65.8
Nutritional Content	109	59.2
Freshness	88	47.8
Cost	53	28.8
The package appearance	20	10.9
Social environment	11	6.0
Brand	10	5.4

Tab. 4: Comparison of Participants' Pre- and Post-exercise Food Preferences

Foods	Before n	Before %	After n	After %	p
	Exercise				
	Before		After		
Rich in carbohydrate	95	51.6	46	25.0	*0.001**
Rich in protein	83	45.1	135	73.4	*0.001**
Rich in fat	10	5.4	10	5.4	1.000*
Rich in water	49	26.6	79	42.9	*0.001**
Rich in fiber	28	15.2	30	16.3	0.871*
Not paying attention	21	11.4	10	5.4	*0.013**

* Chi-square test (McNemar) was applied to dependent groups.

Food choice item scores of the participants according to the FCQ are shown in Table 5. According to the FCQ results, the three items with the highest score were found as 29th item "keeps me healthy" (mean 3.34±0.87), the 22nd item being "contains a lot of vitamins and minerals" (mean 3.16±0.95) and the 4th item "tastes good" (mean 3.12±0.97). Item 27 "is high in protein", item 10 "is nutritious", and item 12 "is good value for money" scored 3 and above. When the sub-dimensions of the FCQ are examined, the "Health" dimension has a higher average (mean 2.94±0.63) than the other dimensions, the dimension with the lowest mean is "ethical concerns" (2.10±0.86).

When the dimensions were evaluated according to the gender difference, it was found that men and women made similar preferences, and men only give more importance to the price factor than women (p<0.05) (Table 6).

Correlations between dimensions of the FCQ are shown in Table 7. There are weak correlations between the sub-dimensions at 0.05 significance level (between 0.151 and 0.184) and 0.001 significance level (between 0.209 and 0.496). Among the factors affecting food choice, a moderate correlation was found between "mood" and "sensory appeal" (0.560), "natural content" and "health" (0.515) at a significance level of 0.001.

When the relationship between educational status and dimensions was examined, it was seen that the factors of "health" and "mood" (p=0.01 and p=0.048, respectively) were affected by the education level. The education level that made this difference has been high school and postgraduate education.

Considering the effect of marital status on food choices, it was found that married individuals gave more importance to the factors of "health", "sensory appeal", "natural content", "familiarity" and "ethical concern" (p=0.008, p=0.030, p=0.000, p=0.009, p=0.000, respectively).

Tab. 5: Mean and Standard Deviation (SD) of FCQ Items and Dimensions

Dimensions		Items	Mean±SD
Health	9	Is high in fiber and roughage	2.33±1.01
	10	Is nutritious	3.00±0.96
	22	Contains a lot of vitamins and minerals	3.16±0.95
	27	Is high in protein	3.05±0.98
	29	Keeps me healthy	3.34±0.87
	30	Is good for my skin/teeth/hair/nails etc.	2.76±1.05
		Mean score of the dimension	2.94±0.63
Mood	13	Cheers me up	2.75±1.08
	16	Helps me cope with stress	2.31±1.12
	24	Keeps me awake/alert	2.65±1.05
	26	Helps me relax	2.63±1.04
	31	Makes me feel good	2.97±1.00
	34	Helps me cope with life	2.35±1.05
		Mean score of the dimension	2.61±0.75
Convenience	1	Is easy to prepare	2.77±1.01
	11	Is easily available in shops and supermarkets	2.79±0.93
	15	Can be cooked very simply	2.54±1.05
	28	Takes no time to prepare	2.80±0.96
	35	Can be bought in shops close to where I live or work	2.78±0.94
		Mean score of the dimension	2.74±0.70
Sensory Appeal	4	Tastes good	3.12±0.97
	14	Smells nice	2.62±1.07
	18	Has a pleasant texture	2.36±1.03
	25	Looks nice	2.54±1.06
		Mean score of the dimension	2.66±0.72
Natural Content	2	Contains no additives	2.86±1.06
	5	Contains natural ingredients	2.95±0.95
	23	Contains no artificial ingredients	2.73±1.10
		Mean score of the dimension	2.84±0.84
Price	6	Is not expensive	2.55±0.96
	12	Is good value for money	3.01±1.02
	36	Is cheap	2.44±0.95
		Mean score of the dimension	2.67±077

(continued on next page)

Tab. 5: Continued

Dimensions		Items	Mean±SD
Weight Control	3	Is low in calories	2.61±1.08
	7	Is low in fat	2.81±0.97
	17	Helps me control my weight	2.86±0.96
		Mean score of the dimension	2.76±0.74
Familiarity	8	Is familiar	2.90±0.92
	21	Is like the food I ate when I was a child	1.78±1.00
	33	Is what I usually eat	2.56±0.97
		Mean score of the dimension	2.42±0.68
Ethical Concern	19	Is packaged in an environmentally friendly way	2.23±1.08
	20	Comes from countries I approve of politically	1.84±1.03
	32	Has the country of origin clearly marked	2.22±1.06
		Mean score of the dimension	2.10±0.86

Tab. 6: Comparison of FCQ Dimensions According to Gender

Dimensions	Male n=94 Mean±SD	Female n=90 Mean±SD	p*
Health	2.96±0.6	2.92±0.69	*0.652*
Mood	2.54±0.75	2.69±0.73	*0.170*
Convenience	2.75±0.75	2.74±0.66	*0.914*
Sensory Appeal	2.62±0.75	2.71±0.70	*0.380*
Natural Content	2.82±0.84	2.87±0.85	*0.681*
Price	2.79±0.77	2.55±0.76	*0.036*
Weight Control	2.67±0.75	2.87±0.72	*0.066*
Familiarity	2.40±0.68	2.44±0.68	*0.665*
Ethical Concern	2.02±0.83	2.19±0.88	*0.177*

*Independent Samples test was used

Discussion

This is the first study conducted to determine the motives for food choice of recreational athletes by using the FCQ. FCQ was used for the first time in Turkey by Derya et al for a Turkish validation study with the general population. In both studies, participants' characteristics such as body mass index and marital status were similar.

Tab. 7: Correlation matrix of the FCQ Dimensions (s=184)

	Health	Mood	Convenience	Sensory Appeal	Natural Content	Price	Weight Control	Familiarity
Mood	0.488**							
Convenience	0.229**	0.271**						
Sensory Appeal	0.256**	0.560**	0.273**					
Natural Content	0.515**	0.295**	0.111	0.125				
Price	0.125	0.191**	0.496**	0.151*	-0.050			
Weight Control	0.411**	0.278**	0.279**	0.139	0.366**	0.195**		
Familiarity	0.283**	0.356**	0.222**	0.407**	0.120	0.167*	0.184*	
Ethical Concern	0.386**	0.412**	0.106	0.362**	0.474**	0.138	0.209**	0.414**

* Correlation is significant at the 0.05 level (2-tailed.) ** Correlation is significant at the 0.001 level (2-tailed).

FCQ has not been applied to any athlete group before. It was applied to students, children, adolescents, older, households and mostly consumers. Considering the characteristics that distinguish the recreational athlete from the professional athlete, it would be more accurate to compare the results of this study with both athletes and general population groups. Steptoe et al. (40) reported the sensory appeal, health, convenience, and price are the most important factors in the original FCQ. In FCQ studies conducted in Balkans, northern and southern Europe showed that price and sensory appeal were the most important food choice motives, and the second important motives were health and convenience (45). In this study, sensory appeal ranks seventh. According to the results of Dikmen et al. (44) study in Turkey, sensory appeal, price, natural content, and health are the important food choice motives and results are similar to European studies (49-51). When we look at the rank of importance of sensory appeal, it is seen that recreational athletes have different priorities than the general population.

In this current study, health, natural content, and convenience were the most important food choice motives of rec-athletes, respectively. When the participants were asked about their food choice, apart from FCQ, the order changed in terms of taste, health, and nutritional content, respectively. Health has been found to be an important factor with both methods. Participants in this study do rec-sports voluntarily and goals of participation on sports are relieving stress / relaxing, increasing muscle mass and wellness. In addition, the education level of almost all participants is undergraduate degree. The reason behind health motivation as an important factor may be their educational level and goal in sports participation. The health-conscious consumers often give more importance on exercise, nutrition, and weight control (52). Consumers who give greater importance on health and nutrition, often include more females, older adults and those with higher incomes and education levels (53,54). In this current study, as a result of the post-hoc analysis, those with high school and above education level gave more importance to the "health" and "mood" factors.

Cognitive dietary restriction is referred to as the conscious restriction of food intake in order to control body weight (55). Data shows that weight is an important factor in food choice, especially for those concerned with body shape and size (40). Cognitive dietary restraint is defined as the conscious restriction of food intake to control body weight. (56). These behaviors may include two basics "diet rules" such as choosing products low in fat and calories or restricting selected food groups. (57,58). Dietary restraint has been examined broadly in non-athlete populations, in terms of weight loss, dieting and disordered eating (55,58-60). Besides, dietary restraint has been explored in relation to disordered eating, bone health and ovulatory disturbances in athlete populations. (61,62). Many athletes try to adjust body weight and composition believing this will improve performance (63). Also, many athletes feel pressure to change body composition to have a lean, athletic look (64). Body mass and physique have been shown to influence sport performance (65,66), physique goals may have effect on the food choices of athletes. In this study, it was determined that rec-athletes give importance to the selection of foods with low energy and fat content as in the general population aiming for weight control. The scores of FCQ's items in the weight control dimension were found to be higher than the results of the study of Dikmen et al. (44). It has been observed that recreational athletes may give more importance on weight control than the general population, but further studies are needed for a firm statement.

There are other reasons why people participate in sport, such as friendship, stress release and personal satisfaction. These individuals have different characteristic such as age, fitness levels and personal backgrounds and their motives for food choice may differ to an international level elite athlete (67,68). Motives for participating in sport may have an effect on food choice as individual goals may differ from an athlete with physique goals to non-athlete who eat whatever they desire and enjoys of this freedom (20,67). The motivation to participate in sport may be depends on a lifestyle that affect food choice. In this study, it was determined that the motivation of rec-athletes to participate in sports is to relieve stress the most, then to increase the body muscle mass and the feeling of wellness.

Historically, hunger was thought to be the primary factor influencing individual food choice (69). In fact, hunger is a factor that can motivate individual food choice (70) and may take place on preference (71) and price (70) especially in food deprivation. Research showed that the immediate availability of food is more important than taste to the food deprived individual (71). Exercise may elevate the appetite of athletes and, for this reason they may have a bigger impulse to eat (72). In this current study, convenience is among the top three dimensions and have more importance than the factors that trigger hunger such as taste and appetite. The fact that the convenience factor is important may be due to the metropole city life and the fact that sports can be done in the time remaining from business life and traffic. Similarly, in this study the score of the taste item was found lower than the general Turkish population (44).

Exercise induced anorexia is a temporary suppression of appetite may occur after having moderate to intense exercise, shown in a large study with non-athletes (both active and sedentary) (73-75). However, appetite suppression is not always evident with differences cause by variations in study designs, in respects of the intensity, duration and type of exercise (75,76). Also, the effect of exercise on appetite suppression may differ by sex and environmental conditions (77,78). Athletes may eat despite a loss of appetite (79) or may ignore hunger cues and restrict intake in order to reach weight goals (80). These behaviors show a conflict with the appetite suppressive effects of exercise and suggest hunger may not be a primary factor influencing individual food choice. Considering only hunger as an indicator of an athlete's energy needs may not be proper when working with this population (81). Considering the differences between the athletes and non-athletes groups, as well as the differences within the athletes themselves, the improvement of the FCQ, which does not contain an item on appetite, will be very important for future studies and help to understand what the athlete actually feels and does with regard to appetite.

It has been suggested that homeostatic mechanisms related with macronutrient balance help regulate eating behavior and energy balance (82). Imbalances in carbohydrate or protein (i.e. low carbohydrate, low protein, or low-calorie diets) may stimulate regulatory signals that direct to eat in order to restore macronutrient balance (81,83). In the presence of low carbohydrates, glycogen stores are reduced, which can lead to more eating until the stores are restored (84,85). Similarly, a low-protein diet (below the recommended daily protein requirement) can serve as a signal for increased energy intake to maintain nitrogen balance (81,86,87). The nutrients used as an energy source during exercise vary according to the physiological and physical characteristics of the athlete, the sport branch, the frequency, duration and intensity of the exercise, energy stores, appropriate diet, environmental temperature, etc. (88). Therefore, the complex relationship between exercise and appetite can affect athletes' pre- and post-exercise/training food preferences (46). Athletes may turn to carbohydrate or protein-based foods as a body impulse, or they may display an attitude different from their impulses (80). In this study, it was determined that rec-athletes give importance to foods rich in carbohydrates before exercise and foods rich in protein and water after exercise. Fat content of the foods to be consumed after exercise has not been a factor affecting food preferences. However, it was concluded that they give importance to the low-fat content of the food on the FCQ. According to this result, the general food preferences of the athletes during the day and the food preferences during the exercise/training time may be different. In further studies, it will be important to investigate the food choice differences depending on exercise and general habits.

When the relationships among the dimensions of the FCQ were examined, the most significant correlations were found between sensory appeal and mood, health and natural content, price, and convenience. In two separate studies conducted by Thurecht and Pelly in athletes (46) and Dikmen et al. (44) in the general population, a significant correlation was found between "weight control" and "nutritional content" factors. Similarly, in this study, a correlation was found in natural content and health dimensions. It is a fact that the professional athlete's performance is affected by weight and nutritional intake, and athletes may try to manipulate their diet to improve their performance (17,89).

Conclusion

Rec-athletes differ from professional athletes and general consumers. However, it has been found that they may have common features with these two groups in their food preferences. The difference of sports participation goals and health goals, lack of seasonal and weight differences or lack of competitive features in recreational sports are the main differences that differentiate them from professional athletes and thus affect their food preferences. Different methods have been used to investigate the food choices of individuals, the FCQ is the most widely used of these methods. However, the FCQ has not been used in athletes before. Given that athletes also show different food preferences as professional, elite, and recreational, it will be beneficial to develop restructured food choice questionnaire specific to these groups. General health and nutritional awareness of recreational athletes may differ from general consumers. However, the existence of nutritional environments that meet these needs of the athletes in recreational facilities is doubtful and one of the most important factors affecting food choices is the availability of food. It would be better understanding to evaluate rec-athletes food choices separately from other populations.

References

1. Wansink, B., & Sobal, J. (2007). Mindless eating: The 200 daily food decisions we overlook. *Environment and Behavior, 39*(1), 106-123. doi:10.1177/0013916506295573

2. Sobal, J., & Bisogni, C. A. (2009). Constructing food choice decisions. *Annals of Behavioral Medicine, 38*(Suppl 1), 37-46. doi:10.1007/s12160-009-9124-5

3. Honkanen, P., & Frewer, L. (2009). Russian consumers' motives for food choice. *Appetite, 52*(2), 363-371. doi:10.1016/j.appet.2008.11.009

4. Prescott, J., Young, O., O'neill, L., Yau, N. J. N., & Stevens, R. (2002). Motives for food choice: A comparison of consumers from Japan, Taiwan, Malaysia and New Zealand. *Food Quality and Preference, 13*(7-8), 489-495. doi:10.1016/S0950-3293(02)00010-1

5. Parraga, I. M. (1990). Determinants of food consumption. *Journal of the American Dietetic Association, 90*(5), 661-663.

6. Rozin, P., Fischler, C., Imada, S., Sarubin, A., & Wrezesniewski, A. (1999). Attitudes to food and the role of food in life in the U.S.A., Japan, Flemish Belgium and France: possible implications for the diet-health debate. *Appetite, 33*(2), 163-180. doi:10.1006/appe.1999.0244

7. Sobal, J., Bisogni, C. A., Devine, C. M., & Jastran, M. (2006). A conceptual model of food choice process over the life course. In R. Shepherd & M. Raats (Eds.), *The psychology of food choice* (pp. 1-18). Wallingford: CABI. doi:10.1079/9780851990323.0001

8. Mello, J. A., Gans, K. M., Risica, P. M., Kirtania, U., Strolla, L. O., Fournier, L. (2010). How is food insecurity associated with dietary behaviors? An analysis with low-income, ethnically diverse participants in a nutrition intervention study. *Journal of the American Dietetic Association, 110*(12), 1906-1911. doi:10.1016/j.jada.2010.09.011

9. Worsley, A. (2002). Nutrition knowledge and food consumption: Can nutrition knowledge change food behaviour? *Asia Pacific Journal of Clinical Nutrition, 11*(3), 579-585. doi:10.1046/j.1440-6047.11.supp3.7.x

10. Contento, I. R., Williams, S. S., Michela, J. L., & Franklin, A. B. (2006). Understanding the food choice process of adolescents in the context of family and friends. *The Journal of Adolescent Health, 38*(5), 575-582. doi:10.1016/j.jadohealth.2005.05.025

11. Pelly, F., Burkhart, S., & Dunn, P. (2018). Factors influencing food choice of athletes at international competition events. *Appetite, 121*, 173-178. doi:10.1016/j.appet.2017.11.086

12. Pelly, F., King, T., & O'connor H. (2006). *Factors influencing food choice of elite athletes at an international competition dining hall*. Paper presented at the Proceedings of the 2nd Australian Association for Exercise and Sports Science Conference.

13. Birkenhead, K., & Slater, G. (2015). A review of factors influencing athletes' food choices. *Sports Medicine, 45*(11), 1511-1522. doi:10.1007/s40279-015-0372-1

14. Rodriguez, N. R., Di Marco, N. M., & Langley, S. (2009). American college of sports medicine position stand. Nutrition and athletic performance. *Medicine and Science in Sports and Exercise, 41*(3), 709-731. doi:10.1249/MSS.0b013e31890eb86

15. Robins, A., & Hetherington, M. M. (2005). A comparison of pre-competition eating patterns in a group of non-elite triathletes. *International Journal of Sport Nutrition and Exercise Metabolism, 15*(4), 442-457. doi:10.1123/ijsnem.15.4.442

16. Ono, M., Kennedy, E., Reeves S., & Cronin, L. (2012). Nutrition and culture in professional football. A mixed method approach. *Appetite, 58*(1), 98-104. doi:10.1016/j.appet.2011.10.007

17. Smart, L. R., & Bisogni, C. A. (2001). Personal food systems of male college hockey players. *Appetite, 37*(1), 57-70. doi:10.1006/appe.2001.0408

18. Blake, J. (2008). *Nutrition and you.* San Francisco: Pearson Benjamin Cummings Publishing Company.

19. Baggaley, M., Noehren, B., Clasey, J. L., Shapiro, R., & Pohl, M. B. (2015). Frontal plane kinematics of the hip during running: Are they related to hip anatomy and strength? *Gait & Posture, 42*(4), 505-510. doi:10.1016/j.gaitpost.2015.07.064

20. Lamont, M., & Kennelly, M. (2011). I can't do everything! competing priorities as constraints in triathlon event travel careers. *Tourism Review International, 14*(2), 85-97. doi:10.3727/154427211X13044361606333

21. Khasnabis, C., Heinicke Motsch, K., & Achu, K. (2010). *Community-based rehabilitation. CBR guidelines.* Geneva: World Health Organization.

22. Ardahan, F. (2013). Investigation of recreational exercise motivation scale according to recreative sports type: Antalya example. *Igdir University, Journal of Social Sciences, 4*, 95-108.

23. Carter, M. A., Edwards, R., Signal, L., & Hoek, J. (2012). Availability and marketing of food and beverages to children through sports settings: A systematic review. *Public Health Nutrition, 15*(8), 1373-1379. doi:10.1017/S136898001100320X

24. Mclsaac, J. L. D., Jarvis, S., Olstad, D. L., Naylor, P. J., Rehman, L., & Kirk, S. F. L. (2018). Voluntary nutrition guidelines to support healthy eating in recreation and sports settings are ineffective: Findings from a prospective study. *AIMS Public Health, 5*(4), 411-420. doi:10.3934/publichealth.2018.4.411

25. Dixon, H., Lee, A., & Scully, M. (2019). Sports sponsorship as a cause of obesity. *Current Obesity Reports, 8*(4), 480-494. doi:10.1007/s13679-019-00363-z

26. Godbey, G. C. (1999). *Leisure in your life: An exploration.* State College, PA: Venture Publishing.

27. Coleman, D. (1993). Leisure based social support, leisure dispositions and health. *Journal of Leisure Research, 25*(4), 350-361. doi:10.1080/00222216.1993

28. Rasberry, C. N., Lee, S. M., Robin, L., Laris, B. A., Russell, L. A., Coyle, K. K., & Nihiser, A. J. (2011). The association between school-based physical activity, including physical education, and academic performance: A systematic review of the literature. *Preventive Medicine, 52*(Suppl 1), 10-20. doi:10.1016/j.ypmed.2011.01.027

29. Kuo, C. T. (2013). The effect of recreational sport involvement on work stress and quality of life in central Taiwan. *Social Behavior and Personality, 41*(10), 1705-1716. doi:10.2224/sbp.2013.41.10.1705

30. Kerr, J. H., & Vlaswinkel, E. H. (1995). Sports participation at work: An aid to stress management? *International Journal of Stress Management, 2,* 87-96. doi:10.1007/BF01566164

31. Oshio, T., Tsutsumi, A., & Inoue, A. (2016). The association between job stress and leisure-time physical inactivity adjusted for individual attributes: Evidence from a Japanese occupational cohort survey. *Scandinavian Journal of Work, Environment & Health, 42*(3), 228-236. doi:10.5271/sjweh.3555

32. Hoffman, J. R., Kang, J., Faigenbaum, A. D., & Ratamess, N. A. (2005). Recreational sports participation is associated with enhanced physical fitness in children. *Research in Sports Medicine, 13*(2), 149-161. doi:10.1080/15438620590956179

33. Faude, O., Zahner, L., & Donath, L. (2015). Exercise guidelines for health oriented recreational sports. *Therapeutische Umschau, 72*(5), 327-334. doi:10.1024/0040-5930/a000683

34. World Health Organization. (2009). *Global health risks: Mortality and burden of disease attributable to selected major risks.* Geneva: World Health Organization.

35. Lee, I. M., Shiroma, E. J., Lobelo, F., Puska, P., Blair, S. N., & Katzmarzyk, P. T. (2012). Effect of physical inactivity on major non-communicable diseases worldwide: An analysis of burden of disease and life expectancy. *Lancet, 380*(9838), 219-229. doi:10.1016/S0140-6736(12)61031-9

36. Warburton, D. E. R., & Bredin, S. S. D. (2017). Health benefits of physical activity: A systematic review of current systematic reviews. *Current Opinion in Cardiology, 32*(5), 541-556. doi:10.1097/HCO.0000000000000437

37. Maughan, R., Depiesse, F., & Geyer, H. (2007). The use of dietary supplements by athletes. *Journal of Sports Sciences, 25*(Suppl 1), 103-113. doi:10.1080/02640410701607395

38. Cohen, D., & Farley, T. A. (2008). Eating as an automatic behavior. *Preventing Chronic Disease, 5*(1), A23.

39. Marteau, T. M., Hollands, G. J., & Fletcher, P. C. (2012). Changing human behavior to prevent disease: The importance of targeting automatic processes. *Science, 337*(6101), 1492-1495. doi:10.1126/science.1226918

40. Steptoe, A., Pollard, T. M., & Wardle, J. (1995). Development of a measure of the motives underlying the selection of food: The food choice questionnaire. *Appetite, 25*(3), 267-284. doi:10.1006/appe.1995.0061

41. Honkanen, P., & Frewer, L. (2009). Russian consumers' motives for food choice. *Appetite, 52*(2), 363-371. doi:10.1016/j.appet.2008.11.009

42. Share, M., & Stewart-Knox, B. (2012). Determinants of food choice in Irish adolescents. *Food Quality and Preference, 25*(1), 57-62. doi:10.1016/j.foodqual.2011.12.005

43. Lockie, S., Lyons, K., Lawrence, G., & Mummery, K. (2002). Eating 'green': Motivations behind organic food consumption in Australia. *Sociologia Ruralis, 42*(1), 23-40. doi:10.1111/1467-9523.00200

44. Dikmen, D., Inan Eroğlu, E., Göktas, Z., Barut-Uyar, B., & Karabulut, E. (2016). Validation of a Turkish version of the food choice questionnaire. *Food Quality and Preference, 52*, 81-86. doi:10.1016/j.foodqual.2016.03.016

45. Cunha, L. M., Cabral, D., Mourab, A. P., & Vaz De Almeida, M. D. (2018). Application of the food choice questionnaire across cultures: Systematic review of cross-cultural and single country studies. *Food Quality and Preference, 64*, 21-36. doi:10.1016/j.foodqual.2017.10.007

46. Thurecht, R. L., & Pelly, F. E. (2019). Development of a new tool for managing performance nutrition: The athlete food choice questionnaire. *International Journal of Sport Nutrition and Exercise Metabolism, 29*(6), 620-627. doi:10.1123/ijsnem.2018-0386.

47. Shepherd, R. (1990). The psychology of food choice. *Nutrition & Food Science, 90*(3), 2-4. doi:10.1079/9780851990323.0001

48. Dowd, K., & Burke, K. J. (2013). The influence of ethical values and food choice motivations on intentions to purchase sustainably sourced foods. *Appetite, 69*, 137-144. doi:10.1016/j.appet.2013.05.024

49. Markovina, J., Stewart-Knox, B. J., Rankin, A., Gibney, M., Almeida, M. D. V., Fischer, . . . Frewer, L. J. (2015). Food4Me study: Validity and reliability of food choice questionnaire in 9 european countries. *Food Quality and Preference*, *45*, 26-32. doi:10.1016/j.foodqual.2015.05.002

50. Milosevic, J., Zezelj, I., Gorton, M., & Barjolle, D. (2012). Understanding the motives for food choice in western balkan countries. *Appetite*, *58*(1), 205–214. doi:10.1016/j.appet.2011.09.012

51. Pieniak, Z., Verbeke, W., Vanhonacker, F., Guerrero, L., & Hersleth, M. (2009). Association between traditional food consumption and motives for food choice in six european countries. *Appetite*, *53*(1), 101-108. doi:10.1016/j.appet.2009.05.019

52. Glanz, K., Basil, M., Maibach, E., Goldberg, J., & Snyder, D. (1998). Why Americans eat what they do: Taste, nutrition, cost, convenience, and weight control concerns as influences on food consumption. *Journal of American Dietetic Association*, *98*(10), 1118-1126. doi:10.1016/S0002-8223(98)00260-0

53. Wardle, J., Haase, A. M., Steptoe, A., Nillapun, M., Jonwuties, K., & Bellisle, F. (2004). Gender differences in food choice: The contribution of health beliefs and dieting. *Annals of Behavioral Medicine*, *27*(2), 107-116. doi:10.1207/s15324796abm2702_5

54. Steptoe, A., & Wardle, J. (1999). Motivational factors as mediators of socioeconomic variations in dietary intake patterns. *Psychology and Health*, *14*(3), 391-402. doi:10.1080/08870449908407336

55. Vartanian, L. R., Wharton, C. M., & Green, E. B. (2012). Appearance vs. health motives for exercise and for weight loss. *Psychology of Sport and Exercise*, *13*(3), 251-256. doi:10.1016/j.psychsport.2011.12.005

56. Stunkard, A. J., & Messick, S. (1985). The three-factor eating questionnaire to measure dietary restraint, disinhibition, and hunger. *Journal of Psychosomatic Research*, *29*(1), 71-83. doi:10.1016/0022-3999(85)90010-8

57. Ward, A., & Mann, T. (2000). Don't mind if I do: Disinhibited eating under cognitive load. *Journal of Personality and Social Psychology*, *78*(4), 753-763. doi:10.1037//0022-3514.78.4.753

58. Forestell, C. A., Spaeth, A. M., & Kane, S. A. (2012). To eat or not to eat red meat. A closer look at the relationship between restrained eating and vegetarianism in college females. *Appetite*, *58*(1), 319-325. doi:10.1016/j.appet.2011.10.015

59. Meule, A., Westenhöfer, J., & Kübler, A. (2011). Food cravings mediate the relationship between rigid, but not flexible control of eating behavior and dieting success. *Appetite*, *57*(3), 582-584. doi:10.1016/j.appet.2011.07.013

60. Timko, C. A., & Perone, J. (2006). Rigid and flexible control of eating behavior and their relationship to dieting status. *Eating and Weight Disorders, 11*(3), 90-95. doi:10.1007/BF03327564

61. Williams, N., Leidy, H., Flecker, K., & Galucci, A. (2006). Food attitudes in female athletes: Association with menstrual cycle length. *Journal of Sports Sciences, 24*(9), 979-986. doi:10.1080/02640410500456986

62. Barrack, M. T., Rauh, M. J., Barkai, H. S., & Nichols, J. F. (2008). Dietary restraint and low bone mass in female adolescent endurance runners. *The American Journal of Clinical Nutrition, 87*(1), 36-43. doi:10.1093/ajcn/87.1.36

63. O'Connor, H., Olds, T., & Maughan, R. J. (2007). Physique and performance for track and field events. *Journal of Sports Sciences, 25*(Suppl 1), 49-60. doi:10.1080/02640410701607296

64. Smart, L. R., & Bisogni, C. A. (2001). Personal food systems of male college hockey players. *Appetite, 37*(1), 57-70. doi:10.1006/appe.2001.0408

65. Knechtle, B., Wirth, A., Baumann, B., Knechtle, P., & Rosemann, T. (2010). Personal best time, percent body fat, and training are differently associated with race time for male and female ironman triathletes. *Research Quarterly for Exercise Sport, 81*(1), 62-68. doi:10.1080/02701367.2010.10599628

66. Landers, G. J., Blanksby, B. A., Ackland, T. R., & Smith, D. (2000). Morphology and performance of world championship triathletes. *Annals of Human Biology, 27*(4), 387-400. doi:10.1080/03014460050044865

67. Lamont, M., & Kennelly, M. (2012). A qualitative exploration of participant motives among committed amateur triathletes. *Leisure Sciences, 34*(3), 236-255. doi:10.1080/01490400.2012.669685

68. Brown, T. D., O'Connor, J. P., & Barkatsas, A. N. (2009). Instrumentation and motivations for organised cycling: The development of the cyclist motivation instrument (CMI). *Journal of Sports Science & Medicine, 8*(2), 211-218.

69. Lowe, M. R., & Butryn, M. L. (2007). Hedonic hunger: A new dimension of appetite? *Physiology & Behavior, 91*(4), 432-439. doi:10.1016/j.physbeh.2007.04.006.

70. Furst, T., Connors, M., Bisogni, C. A., Sobal, J., & Falk, L. W. (1996). Food choice: A conceptual model of the process. *Appetite, 26*(3), 247-265. doi:10.1006/appe.1996.0019

71. Hoefling, A., & Strack, F. (2010). Hunger induced changes in food choice. When beggars cannot be choosers even if they are allowed to choose. *Appetite, 54*(3), 603-606. doi:10.1016/j.appet.2010.02.016

72. Long, D., Perry, C., Unruh, S. A., Lewis, N., & Stanek-Krogstrand, K. (2011). Personal food systems of male collegiate football players: A grounded theory investigation. *Journal of Athletic Training*, 46(6), 688-695. doi:10.4085/1062-6050-46.6.688

73. King, N. A., Burley, V. J., & Blundell, J. E. (1994). Exercise-induced suppression of appetite: Effects on food intake and implications for energy balance. *European Journal of Clinical Nutrition*, 48(10), 715-724.

74. Deighton, K., Zahra, J. C., & Stensel, D. J. (2012). Appetite, energy intake and resting metabolic responses to 60min treadmill running performed in a fasted versus a postprandial state. *Appetite*, 58(3), 946-954. doi:10.1016/j.appet.2012.02.041

75. Broom, D. R., Batterham, R. L., King, J. A., & Stensel, D. J. (2009). Influence of resistance and aerobic exercise on hunger, circulating levels of acylated ghrelin, and peptide YY in healthy males. *American Journal of Physiology. Regulatory, Integrative and Comparative Physiology*, 296(1), R29-35. doi:10.1152/ajpregu.90706.2008

76. Deighton, K., Barry, R., Connon, C. E., & Stensel, D. J. (2013). Appetite, gut hormone and energy intake responses to low volume sprint interval and traditional endurance exercise. *European Journal of Applied Physiology*, 113(5), 1147-1156. doi:10.1007/s00421-012-2535-1

77. Aeberli, I., Erb, A., Spliethoff, K., Meier, D., Götze, O., Frühauf, H., ... Lutz, T. A. (2013). Disturbed eating at high altitude: Influence of food preferences, acute mountain sickness and satiation hormones. *European Journal of Nutrition*, 52(2), 625-635. doi:10.1007/s00394-012-0366-9

78. Hagobian, T. A., Sharoff, C. G., Stephens, B. R., Wade, G. N., Silva, J. E., Chipkin, S. R., & Braun, B. (2009). Effects of exercise on energy-regulating hormones and appetite in men and women. *American Journal of Physiology. Regulatory, Integrative and Comparative Physiology*, 296(2), R233-242. doi:10.1152/ajpregu.90671.2008

79. Robins, A., & Hetherington, M. M. (2012). A comparison of pre-competition eating patterns in a group of non-elite triathletes. *International Journal of Sport Nutrition Exercise Metabolism*, 15(4), 442-457. doi:10.1123/ijsnem.15.4.442

80. Pettersson, S., Pipping Ekström, M., & Berg, C. M. (2012). The food and weight combat. A problematic fight for the elite combat sports athlete. *Appetite*, 59(2), 234-242. doi:10.1016/j.appet.2012.05.007

81. Loucks, A. B. (2004). Energy balance and body composition in sports and exercise. *Journal of Sports Science*, 22(1), 1-14. doi:10.1080/0264041031000140518

82. Flatt, J. P. (1987). Dietary fat, carbohydrate balance, and weight maintenance: Effects of exercise. *The American Journal of Clinical Nutrition, 45*(1 Suppl), 296-306. doi:10.1093/ajcn/45.1.296

83. Flatt, J. P. (1987). The difference in the storage capacities for carbohydrate and for fat, and its implications in the regulation of body weight. *Annals of the New York Academy of Science, 499*, 104-123. doi:10.1111/j.1749-6632.1987.tb36202.x

84. Hopkins, M., Jeukendrup, A., King, N. A., & Blundell, J. E. (2011). The relationship between substrate metabolism, exercise and appetite control does glycogen availability influence the motivation to eat, energy intake or food choice? *Sports Medicine, 41*(6), 507-521. doi:10.2165/11588780-000000000-00000

85. Flatt, J. P. (1996). Glycogen levels and obesity. *International Journal of Obesity and Related Metabolic Disorders, 20*(Suppl 2), 1-11.

86. Gosby, A. K., Conigrave, A. D., Lau, N. S., Iglesias, M. A., Hall, R. M., Jebb, S. A., . . . Sipmpson, S. J. (2011). Testing protein leverage in lean humans: A randomised controlled experimental study. *Public Library of Science One, 6*(10), e25929. doi:10.1371/journal.pone.0025929

87. Martens, E. A., Lemmens, S. G., & Westerterp-Plantenga, M. S. (2013). Protein leverage affects energy intake of high-protein diets in humans. *The American Journal of Clinical Nutrition, 97*(1), 86-93. doi:10.3945/ajcn.112.046540

88. Potgieter, S. (2013). Sport nutrition: A review of the latest guidelines for exercise and sport nutrition from the American college of sport nutrition, the international olympic committee and the international society for sports nutrition. *South African Journal of Clinical Nutrition, 26*(1), 6-16. doi:10.1080/16070658.2013.11734434

89. O'Connor, H., Olds, T., & Maughan, R. J. (2007). Physique and performance for track and field events. *Journal of Sports Science, 25*(Suppl 1), 49-60. doi:10.1080/02640410701607296

Kardelen Besen, Dilara Güler, Mirsad Alkan, and Dilber
Karagözoğlu Coşkunsu

Acute Effects of Myofascial Release Technique Applied with Foam Roller on Posterior Plane Muscles in Patients with Mechanical Neck Pain

Abstract

Objective: This study aimed to investigate the acute effects of myofascial release with foam roller on hamstring and gastrocnemius muscles to patients with mechanical neck pain (MNP) on parameters that cervical range of motion, pain and muscle strength on cervical region.

Materials and Methods: The research consisted of pre-test and post-test evaluation phases. Forty-one participants (mean age: 22.1±2.3 years; mean height: 160±8 cm, mean weight: 65.2±16 kg) with MNP who scored 45 points in New York Posture Rating Chart were involved. To the hamstring and gastrocnemius muscles of participants on both extremities, the foam roller myofascial release technique was applied for a total duration of 12 minutes, consisting of 3 recurrences of 1-minute treatments. The evaluations were made prior to, and after the application. Pain intensity was assessed with Visual Analogue Scale. Cervical flexion, extension, lateral flexion, and rotation was measured by cervical range of motion device (C-ROM®). Muscle strength was measured by microFET2® hand dynamometer. The gathered datasets were analyzed via a non-parametric test.

Results: Upon comparing the pre-test and post-test datasets, statistically significant improvements were observed in the measurements of pain intensity level, cervical range of motion and muscle strength throughout the spectrum (for all evaluations p<0.001).

Conclusion: A one-time session that involved the foam roller myofascial release technique was observed to have positive impacts on cervical range of motion, pain, and muscle strength of patients with mechanical neck pain.

Keywords: Neck, Pain, Myofascial, Myofascial Release, Foam Roller

Introduction

Mechanical neck pain (MNP); is a result of degenerative alterations at cervical region muscle tissues, stemming from small traumas and postural defections, instead of systemic and/or neurologic problems (1). Such discomforts could be observed in unilateral or bilateral forms and are fundamentally biomechanical defections, limiting the cervical motional capabilities consequently (2). Likewise, decreased muscular activation during cervical movements, muscular strength loss, increase in tonus and spasm occurrence levels are amongst other probable issues (3). It is commonly considered that the decreased flexibility of the fascia tissue is the root cause of such non-specific pains. Furthermore, the indications of several experiments conducted on both humans and animals were that chronical MNP was accompanied with limited motional capabilities of the fascial tissue (4).

Fascia is a closely packed band tissue, structurally similar to tendons and ligaments. It covers organs, muscles, blood vessels and nerves, connecting tissues and enabling motion via creating a mechanism of tissues sliding amongst themselves (5). Physical actions applied to an area of the body, and/or forces that the body is exposed to, is conducted via the entire fascial structure (6). This structure (packed with collagen and elastic fibers) of independent sheets packed on top of each other in horizontal, vertical, and oblique formations, enveloping muscle tissues for reinforcing structural integrity. The fascia also has roles such as local suspension, protection, separation, shock absorption, reduced pressure and preserving stability. Its innervation comes from the autonomous nervous system. The sensory receptors of fascia tissues are 10 times that of a regular muscle tissue. Moreover, it is sensitive to alterations in hormones as well as movement (7). Like all connective tissues, the fascia has numerous Golgi receptors, Pacini corpuscles and Ruffini corpuscles. The tissues of muscles and fascia form the myofascial system and a functional deprivation at the fascia could directly result in muscular strength loss and inefficient power production (8). From a systematic point of view, the myofascial system is responsible for pain conductivity, maintaining posture, fascia chain conduction, coordination, and load distribution (7). Bad posture, trauma, gynecologic problems, surgical scars, adhesions, inflammations, stress and erroneous movement could disrupt the force distribution on the facia and consequently, short-term loss of flexibility and loss of stability could be accompanied by long-term pain and dysfunctionality (8).

Amongst the fascial chains defined by Myers, the Superficial Back Line (SBL) is a fascial band stretching from the toes all the way to the supraorbital foramen. Plantar begins with the fascia connecting to the Achilles tendon, while the upper tips of the gastrocnemius muscle are connected with the lower tips of the hamstring tendons. The structure proceeds to the sacrotuberous ligament and connects with the erector spinals. After covering the occipital edge, the SBL ends at the supraorbital foramen (9). There are two SBL's, at the right-hand side and at the left-hand side. Because two structures interact, any irregularities must be observed and compensated. Some of the medical postural conditions associated with SBL are ankle dorsiflexion limitation, knee hypertension, hamstring shortness, anterior pelvic tilt, sacral nutation, irregular muscle elongation due to thoracic flexion, upper cervical hyperextension inducing suboccipital limitation, the forward shifting or rotation of the occiput on the atlas, and eye-spinal cord connection issues (10).

A self-myofascial release (SMR) technique, the utilization of a foam roller (FR*) to increase the cervical range of motion consists of applying a dense FR* in a rolling motion across the neck, in proportion with the body weight. During the rolling process, because the soft tissue is treated with a sweeping pressure, the fascial structure is assumed to be contracted, consequently increasing the cervical are range of motion (11,12).

In this investigation, in order to evaluate the interactions amongst available interactive components, the FR* SMR technique was applied to the hamstring and gastrocnemius muscles of patients who suffer from MNP. The acute effects of such treatment to cervical range of motion, pain and muscle strength was analyzed.

Materials and Methods

Study Design

Study is designed as pretest–posttest. This study was performed in accordance with the Declaration of Helsinki in the Physiotherapy Laboratory of Bahçeşehir University Faculty of Health Sciences Physiotherapy and Rehabilitation Department from February 2019 to May 2019. Study protocol was approved by the Bahçeşehir University Clinical Research Ethics Committee (Decision date: 2019-06/02). Informed consents of the participants who attend to study had been taken before the study.

Forty-one participants attending in the study were treated with FR and SMR applications and, evaluations were made before and after the treatment. Treatment and the evaluations were performed by the same persons (Treatment: K.B, evaluations: D.G.).

Participants

Forty-one participants were involved in the study who are determined based on criteria of being compatible with the study.

Criteria for being involved in the study:

- Being 18-40 years old,
- Having MNP (Pains caused by minor traumas and posture disorders that give rise to changes in neck muscle and connective tissues (9), not caused by systemically or neurologic problems),

- Being minimally active according to the International Physical Activity Questionnaire (13),
- Getting 45 points or lower from the New York Posture Chart (14),
- Being volunteer to get involved in the study.

Criteria for being excluded from the study:

- Having neurological disorder (hemiplegia, Parkinson's disease, multiple sclerosis etc.),
- Lacking cognitive function to let them attend actively,
- Having severe psychiatric disorder, disc herniation, severe neck anterior tilt,
- Taking Medical Supports,
- History of neck trauma or surgery in the last 1 year,
- Having diagnosed with osteoporosis,
- Having diagnosed with cancer.

Treatment

Participants were treated with FR° and SMR just after the first evaluation.

Self-Myofascial Release (SMR) Treatment with Foam Roller (FR°): The treatment was performed on SBL which is limiting the trunk flexion or causing trunk extension according to functional disfunction. SBL is affecting the posture in sagittal plane primarily. Application was performed on hamstring and gastrocnemius muscles of lower extremities from proximal to distal. Treatment was performed to myofascia of both muscles for one minute and three repetitions for a total of 12 minutes (15). The pressure that FR° applies to the soft tissue stretches the tissue. This movement causes fascia to warm up. This dissolves fibrous adhesions between fascia layers and restores soft tissue extensibility (16). Participants were positioned on the floor with FR° under their extremities and their hands beside the body. It was asked participants to apply the greatest force they can between the FR° and the muscle (17).

Assessments

The VAS of the participants before and after the application was evaluated with C-ROM° and microFET2°.

Visual Analogue Scale (VAS): VAS was used in order to convert the participants' level of pain into numerical values. Two opposite definitions of the parameters that would be evaluated were put on both ends of a line of 100 mm (0: No pain at all, 10: Very severe pain). The patients were asked to mark their own level of pain on this line (18).

Cervical Range of Motion Assessment: Range of motion of patients with MNP was evaluated by C-ROM® device (19,20). Test-retest reliability of the measurements made by C-ROM (ICC, 0.89-0.98) (19) and the reliability between practitioners for patients with MNP are shown (20).

After a brief explanation of the evaluation process, the participants were asked to sit on a chair in an upright position and to relax their shoulders with their feet flat on the floor and their arms touching their body. Before taking the measurements, a trial was made in each cervical movement direction so that the individuals could get used to the procedure. For flexion, extension, and lateral flexion, the corresponding inclinometer was read and recorded (starting position). At the end of each movement, the inclinometer was read again (ending position), and the value was recorded. For rotation, the dial of the magnetic inclinometer was manually set to zero before movement so that the end position value would directly reflect the amount of movement. If a participant has not followed the instructions of the testing machine correctly in any of the cervical movements, the measurement was not taken, and both the instructions and the movement were repeated. After each measurement, the test machine was reset to the starting position before proceeding to the next measurement. The order and the direction of the measurements were picked randomly. Three measurements were taken for each cervical movement and their average was taken.

Special instructions given for the flexion movement were, "first move your chin close to your chest, then move your head forwards and downwards as much as possible until your movements are limited by tension or discomfort." Special instructions for extension were, "first lift your chin, then move your head backwards and look away until your movements are limited by tension or discomfort." Additional instructions were given in order to prevent the movement of the chest, which were "do not move your shoulders or change the amount of pressure applied at the back of your chair." During these movements, manual balance was not made; only verbal instructions were given.

Special instructions for each direction of lateral flexion performance were, "look straight and tilt your neck to the sideways towards your ears as much as possible, until your movements are limited by tension or discomfort." In order to avoid thoracic and shoulder girdle movements, the individual was told not to move their shoulders and not to change the amount of pressure applied to the back of the chair. In addition to this, the test machine was manually balanced while the individual was performing the movements.

Special instructions for the rotation movement were "turn your head as much as possible as if you are looking at an imaginary horizontal line on the wall, until your movement is limited by tension or discomfort." In order to avoid thoracic and shoulder girdle movements, the individual was told not to move their shoulders and not to change the amount of pressure applied to the back of the chair. Furthermore, while the participant was performing the movement, the contralateral shoulder was manually stabilized by placing the hand on the distal clavicle and acromion.

Dynamometer Measurements: MicroFET2® dynamometer was used to take the neck extension, flexion, right lateral flexion, left lateral flexion muscle strength measurements of the participants, both before and after the study. The muscle strength measurements were taken while the participant was sitting and the microFET2 dynamometer was placed by an applicator (21,22).

Cervical muscle strength was measured in neutral head posture, in four contraction directions (flexion, extension, right-left lateral flexion) by using manual dynamometer. All of the measurements were taken while the individual was sitting in an upright position on a chair with thoracic stabilization, back supported, hip and knee flexion at 90 degrees, feet fully flat on the ground and hands on the lap. All of the contractions were made by keeping a time of three seconds with the dynamometer and with 15 seconds of resting time between each trial. Each measurement was repeated for three times and the average was recorded (23).

Statistical Analysis

SPSS (Statistical Package for the Social Sciences) version 20.0 was used for the statistical analysis. Shapiro Wilk test was performed to determine whether data was compatible with normal distribution. As the data was not compatible with normal distribution, non-parametric tests were used. The difference within the group was evaluated with 95 % confidence interval. In all of the analyses, $p<0.05$ values were considered statistically significant. The effect size of the change between before and after the process was calculated by using the formula "$r=z/\sqrt{(nx2)}$." Effect size was defined as small ($r\leq0.1$), medium ($r=0.30$) and large ($r\geq0.5$) (24).

Results

Forty-one participants (mean age: 22.1±2.3 years; mean height: 160±8 cm, mean weight: 65.2±16 kg) were completed the study. A statistically significant difference in pain, cervical range of motion and muscle strength measurements was seen after the FR® application ($p<0.001$ in all parameters). Considering the effect size values, the FR® application was found to be moderately effective in right rotation ROM and right rotation strength and largely effective in all other parameters (Table 1).

Tab. 1: Changes Before and After Application

	Before Application		After Application		Results of Analysis	
	Min.-Max.	Mean-S.D.	Min.-Max.	Mean-S.D.	p	E.S. (d)
VAS (0-10)	2.0-7.0	4.0±1.7	0.0-6.0	1.6±1.7	p<0.001	1.40
C-ROM L.F. Right (°)	30.0-53.0	38.8±6.1	33.0-64.0	44.8±6.8	p<0.001	0.98
C-ROM L.F. Left (°)	25.0-55.0	40.7±6.5	31.0-63.0	46.0±6.9	p<0.001	0.81
C-ROM Ext. (°)	43.5-81.0	63.3±9.1	48.0-85.0	66.8±7.4	p<0.001	0.38
C-ROM Flex. (°)	5.0-71.0	51.1±12.5	37.0-78.0	59.1±9.7	p<0.001	0.64
C-ROM R. Right (N)	5.0-81.0	61.0±12.5	5.0-81.0	65.9±12.5	p<0.001	0.39
C-ROM R. Left (N)	5.0-80.0	61.7±11.0	55.0-83.0	67.6±6.1	p<0.001	0.53
Dynam. L.F. Right (N)	6.1-23.4	12.2±4.2	7.1-25.7	13.6±4.5	p<0.001	0.33
Dynam. L.F. Left (N)	5.8-26.8	12.1±4.1	6.4-28.7	13.8±4.9	p<0.001	0.41
Dynam. Ext. (N)	5.6-31.5	14.4±5.5	7.0-34.5	16.3±6.4	p<0.001	0.34
Dynam. Flex. (N)	6.0-20.4	11.2±3.8	5.6-21.6	12.4±4.3	p<0.001	0.31

VAS: Visual analogue scale, C-ROM: Cervical Active Range of Motion, LF: lateral flexion, R: rotation

Discussion

As a result of pretest- posttest study, one-time session that involved the FR° SMR technique applied on hamstring and gastrocnemius muscles was observed to have positive impacts on cervical range of motion, and muscle strength which is connected to the SBL of patients with MNP. This impact was moderate on the right cervical rotation ROM and right cervical rotation strength; however, the impact was large on the other parameters.

Overuse and overstress of the soft tissue causes abnormal cross bonds and scar tissue on fascia (16). In use of FR°, it causes frictional force and creates pressure on the soft tissue and stretches the tissue. Friction warms up the fascia. Warmth and stretching disrupts the adhesions between fascia layer and bring back the flexibility of the soft tissue.

Muscle and fascia form the myofascial system and the fascia is whole on its own. In addition, the force, which is applied on fascial chain, so the stimuli are conducted over the SBL. Thus, it is thought that this results in a friction which increases the cervical range of motion.

In a conducted study, FR° SMR technique was applied on hamstring muscles for 5 and 10 seconds with one and two sets. It was concluded that not significant increase in muscle strength was found. Moreover, if it was applied for a longer time of period, there will be significant impact on range of motion (25).

In our study, a significant difference was observed in cervical range of motion and strength when SMR was applied for 3 minutes for each hamstring and gastrocnemius muscles.

In a review which was searching for acute effects of myofascial releasing techniques; it was found that the applications increase the flexibility and decrease the muscle pain. However, no impact on athletic performance was observed (26). It observed that SMR had a recovery effect on both sportsmen and on general population. In previous studies, it was found that FR° and SMR technique recover parameters related to performance, pain, and some of the circulation system (27-30).

In the study SMR was used by applying pressure on the soft tissue of participants' own body weight. At the end of the study, results supported the hypothesis that the myofascia is a complete structure. Moreover, increases in muscle strength and range of motion of participants was found while decrease in pain score was determined. In a systematic review (31) which examines the effect of FR and roll massage myofascial release techniques on ROM, muscle strength and performance, FR a roll massage which were applied before activity was found to whether increasing the muscle performance or having no impact. However, it was illustrated that it affects the fatigue. In our study, the results which meet the criteria of the current literature with the hypothesis of FR and SMR have an impact on mechanical neck pain. In recent studies, it was noticed that the whole active components of the motion system were connected to each other in a chain with a fibrosis connective tissue and the result of our study had supporting the findings of these results.

Conclusion

In this study, the acute effect of FR® SMR technique on cervical range of motion, pain, and muscle strength in individuals with MNP was investigated with application on gastrocnemius and hamstring muscles in order to evaluate the interaction between active components. The term acute in this study refers to the period immediately after FR® application. As a result of our study, an increase was observed in the cervical range of motion in the measurements performed after FR® application. Dynamometer measurements supported our hypothesis in terms of the effects of FR® SMR technique on muscle strength, and an increase in muscle strength was observed after application. In the treatment of MNP, our hypothesis was supported in terms of the effects of FR SMG technique on pain with an observation of decrease in VAS scores after the application. In this study, it was observed that FR applied to lower extremity muscles had beneficial effects on the cervical region in the acute period, supporting the evidence that myofascia is a whole.

References

1. Türk Nöroşirurji Derneği. (2020). Boyun ağrısı. Retrieved from https://www.turknorosirurji.org.tr/menu/74/boyun-agrisi

2. Ahn, N. U., Ahn, U. M., Ipsen, B., & An, H. S. (2007). Mechanical neck pain and cervicogenic headache. *Neurosurgery, 60* (1 Suppl 1), S21-7. doi:10.1227/01.neu.0000249258.94041.C6

3. Falla, D., O'Leary, S., Farina, D., & Jull, G. (2011). Association between intensity of pain and impairment in onset and activation of the deep cervical flexors in patients with persistent neck pain. *The Clinical Journal of Pain, 27*(4), 309-314. doi:10.1097/AJP.0b013e31820212cf

4. Langevin, H. M., Bishop, J., Maple, R., Badger, G. J., & Fox, J. R. (2018). Effect of stretching on thoracolumbar fascia injury and movement restriction in a porcine model. *American Journal of Physical Medicine & Rehabilitation, 97*(3), 187-191. doi:10.1097/PHM.0000000000000824

5. Chaitow, L. (2009). Understanding soft-tissue injuries. In W. W. Lowe (Ed.), *Orthopedic massage e-book: Theory and technique.* United States: Elsevier.

6. Lindsay, M., & Robertson, C. (2008). *Fascia: Clinical applications for health and human performance.* New York: Delmar Pub.

7. Acarkan, T., & Nazlıkul, H. (2017). Fasya fonksiyonları, işlevsel görevleri ve nöralterapi yaklaşımı. *Bilimsel Tamamlayıcı Tıp Regülasyon ve Nöral Terapi Dergisi, 11*(3), 9-15.

8. Poletti, S. (2006). *The fasciae: Anatomy, dysfunction, and treatment.* Seattle: Eastland Press.

9. Myers, T. W. (2006). Anatomy trains early dissective evidence. Retrieved from http://bti.edu/pdfs/Myers_Anatomy-Trains-Early-Evidence.pdf

10. Myers, T. W. (2001). *Anatomy trains: Myofascial meridians.* London: Elsevier Churchill Livingstone.

11. Healey, K. C., Hatfield, D. L., Blanpied, P., Dorfman, L. R., & Riebe, D. (2014). The effects of myofascial release with foam rolling on performance. *The Journal of Strength & Conditioning Research, 28*(1), 61-68. doi:10.1519/JSC.0b013e3182956569

12. Kelly, S., & Beardsley, C. (2016). Specific and cross-over effects of foam rolling on ankle dorsiflexion range of motion. *International Journal of Sports Physical Therapy, 11*(4), 544-551.

13. Craig, C. L., Marshall, A. L., Sjöström, M., Bauman, A. E., Booth, M. L., Ainsworth, B. E., ... Oja, P. (2003). International physical activity questionnaire: 12-country reliability and validity. *Medicine & Science in Sports & Exercise, 35*(8), 1381–1395. doi:10.1249/01.MSS.0000078924.61453.FB

14. Magee, D. J. (1987). *Orthopedic physical assessment.* Gait assessment (pp. 362-376). Toronto: W.B. Saunders Company.

15. Cheatham, S. W. (2019). Roller massage: A descriptive survey of allied health professionals. *Journal of Sport Rehabilitation, 28*(6), 640-649. doi:10.1123/jsr.2017-0366

16. Sefton, J. (2004). Myofascial release for athletic trainers, part I: Theory and session guidelines. *International Journal of Athletic Therapy and Training, 9*(1), 48-49. doi:10.1123/att.9.1.48

17. Aune, A. A., Bishop, C., Turner, A. N., Papadopoulos, K., Budd, S., Richardson, M., & Maloney, S. J. (2019). Acute and chronic effects of foam rolling vs eccentric exercise on ROM and force output of the plantar flexors. *Journal of Sports Sciences, 37*(2), 138-145. doi:10.1080/02640414.2018.1486000.

18. Hayes, M. H. (1921). Experimental development of the graphics rating method. *Psychological Bulletin, 18,* 98-99.

19. Audette, I., Dumas, J. P., Côté, J. N., & De Serres, S. J. (2010). Validity and between-day reliability of the cervical range of motion (CROM)

device. *Journal of Orthopaedic & Sports Physical Therapy, 40*(5), 318-323. doi:10.2519/jospt.2010.3180

20. Fletcher, J. P., & Bandy, W. D. (2008). Intrarater reliability of CROM measurement of cervical spine active range of motion in persons with and without neck pain. *Journal of Orthopaedic & Sports Physical Therapy, 38*(10), 640-645. doi:10.2519/jospt.2008.2680

21. Krause, D. A., Hansen, K. A., Hastreiter, M. J., Kuhn, T. N., Peichel, M. L., & Hollman, J. H. (2019). A comparison of various cervical muscle strength testing methods using a handheld dynamometer. *Sports Health, 11*(1), 59-63. doi:10.1177/1941738118812767

22. Buckinx, F., Croisier, J. L., Reginster, J. Y., Dardenne, N., Beaudart, C., Slomian, J., . . . Bruyère, O. (2017). Reliability of muscle strength measures obtained with a hand-held dynamometer in an elderly population. *Clinical Physiology and Functional Imaging, 37*(3), 332-340. doi:10.1111/cpf.12300

23. Fiebert, I. M., Roach, K. E., Yang, S. S., Dierking, L. D., &Hart, F. E. (1999). Cervical range of motion and strength during resting and neutral head postures in healthy young adults. *Journal of Back and Musculoskeletal Rehabilitation, 12*(3), 165-178. doi:10.3233/BMR-1999-12304

24. Rosenthal, R. (1994). Parametric measures of effect size. In H. Cooper & L. V. Hedges (Eds.), *The handbook of research synthesis* (pp. 231-244). New York: Russell Sage Foundation.

25. Sullivan, K. M., Silvey, D. B., Button, D. C., & Behm, D. G. (2013). Roller-massager application to the hamstrings increases sit-and-reach range of motion within five to ten seconds without performance impairments. *International Journal of Sports Physical Therapy, 8*(3), 228-236.

26. Beardsley, C., & Škarabot, J. (2015). Effects of self-myofascial release: A systematic review. *Journal of Bodywork and Movement Therapies, 19*(4), 747-758. doi:10.1016/j.jbmt.2015.08.007

27. Castiglione, A. (2008). Self myofascial release therapy and athletes. *Australian Institute of Self Myofascial Release Therapy.*

28. MacDonald, G. Z., Penney, M. D., Mullaley, M. E., Cuconato, A. L., Drake, C. D., Behm, D. G., & Button, D. C. (2013). An acute bout of self-myofascial release increases range of motion without a subsequent decrease in muscle activation or force. *The Journal of Strength & Conditioning Research, 27*(3), 812-821. doi:10.1519/JSC.0b013e31825c2bc1

29. Okamoto, T., Masuhara, M., & Ikuta, K. (2014). Acute effects of self-myofascial release using a foam roller on arterial function. *The Journal of Strength & Conditioning Research, 28*(1), 69-73. doi:10.1519/JSC.0b013e31829480f5

30. Renan-Ordine, R., Alburquerque-Sendín, F., Rodrigues De Souza, D. P., Cleland, J. A., & Fernández-de-las-Peñas, C. (2011). Effectiveness of myofascial trigger point manual therapy combined with a self-stretching protocol for the management of plantar heel pain: A randomized controlled trial. *Journal of Orthopaedic & Sports Physical Therapy, 41*(2), 43-50. doi:10.2519/jospt.2011.3504

31. Cheatham, S. W., Kolber, M. J., Cain, M., & Lee, M. (2015). The effects of self-myofascial release using a foam roll or roller massager on joint range of motion, muscle recovery, and performance: A systematic review. *International Journal of Sports Physical Therapy, 10*(6), 827-838.

Hazal Genç, Esra Atılgan, and Beyza İnce

Comparison of Muscle Activation Level, Pain, Posture, Disability, and Balance in Individuals with and without Temporomandibular Joint Dysfunction

Abstract

Objective: Temporomandibular dysfunction is a common condition seen in 60-70 % of the population and can affect all age groups. The aim of this cross-sectional study is to compare muscle activation level, pain, posture, disability, and balance between individuals with temporomandibular dysfunction and healthy individuals.

Materials and Methods: Total 44 participants, 21 with temporomandibular joint dysfunction and 23 healthy individuals, were included in the study. Demographic data of the two groups were obtained. Superficial electromyography was applied to Masseter Muscle to evaluate muscle activation level. Pain was evaluated with an algometer. New York Posture Analysis, Neck Pain and Disability Index and Biodex Balance System were used to compare overall body health between the two groups.

Results: No significant differences found for demographic data between groups (p≥0.05). Right-left masseter muscle activation level was found higher in the healthy group compared to the Temporomandibular Joint Dysfunction group (p≤0.05). According to the algometer results, pain level both sides masseter muscle; both sides temporalis muscle was higher in Temporomandibular Joint Dysfunction group (p≤0.05). Posture of healthy individuals was better than Temporomandibular Joint Dysfunction group (p≤0.05). Most of the static and dynamic balance measurements performed on single and double legs were found significantly better (p≤0.05) in the healthy group except static double legs (p=0.12) and dynamic left legs (p=0.08). No significant difference was found between groups in Neck Pain and Disability Index (p≥0.05).

Conclusion: Pain and muscle activation level were found higher in individuals with temporomandibular joint dysfunction compared to healthy individuals. Balance parameters were found better in healthy individuals than temporomandibular joint dysfunction group. Posture score was decreased in temporomandibular joint dysfunction group compared to healthy individuals and there was no significant difference in the level of disability between two groups.

Keywords: Musculoskeletal Pain, Balance, Posture, Temporomandibular Joint Dysfunction

Introduction

Temporomandibular joint dysfunction (TMJD) is a term related to pain and dysfunction of masticatory muscles and temporomandibular joint, seen in approximately 60-70 % of the population (1,2). Jaw pain, muscle pain, mal-occlusion of the temporomandibular joint and snicking with jaw motions are common symptoms (2). Mostly seen in adults between the ages of 20-40, it is seen 4 times more in women than in men (3). Etiology of TMJD is unknown but TMJD is affected by anatomical, pathophysiological, and psychosocial factors. Normal range of motion of the jaw is 35-45 mm, lower degrees signalizes dysfunction (2).

In individuals with TMJD, it is thought that there is a decrease in muscle thickness and length as a result of the decrease in postural activity, stretching and relaxation in the masticatory muscles. Having proper muscle activity of masticatory muscles will reduce parafunctional force effects (4). It is thought that the decrease in muscle strength can lead to insufficient range of motion and cause pain.

Increased muscle tone in the cervical region leads to the formation of compensatory mechanisms at the spinal level for the correct posture (5). Also, direct relationship between temporomandibular joint and cervical region, effects lower segments of the spine. Cervical movements and mandibular movements are related to body posture through postural synergies (6).

Balance may be affected when the capacity to compensate for pathological changes in the body is exceeded (6,7). This situation may lead to disability in individuals. But between temporomandibular dysfunction and body posture, there is not sufficient evidence, and it is still under debate.

After researching literature, we aimed to compare muscle activation level, pain, body posture, disability, and body balance between individuals with temporomandibular joint dysfunction and healthy individuals.

Materials and Methods

This study conducted with Bahçeşehir University personnel and students on 2018 December-2019 June. A total of 44 individuals, 21 individuals with temporomandibular joint dysfunction and 23 healthy individuals were included in the study.

The including criteria were as follows: aged between 18 and 45, 5 or more points according to the Helkimo Index, being Bahçeşehir University employee or student. In the Helkimo Index, evaluation is made on 5 parameters (0 points,

3 points, 5 points) including range of motion, mandibular deviation, dysfunction, joint pain, and muscle pain. Minimum score is 0, maximum score is 25. High score indicates more serious illness (8).

The excluding criteria were as follows: who have had surgery in the mandibular region, displacement of the temporomandibular joint disc with/without reduction, have a history of trigeminal neuralgia, receiving orthodontic dental treatment, individuals with orthopedic and/or neurological problems. All participants were evaluated with Biodex Balance System, EMG-BF, Algometer, Neck Pain Disability Questionnaire, New York Posture Scale.

The sample size was calculated using the G*Power package program (G*Power, Ver. 3.1.9.2, Axel Buchner, Kiel University, Germany). With Type 1 error 0.05 (α=0.05), Type 2 error 0.10 (=0.1), the total number of cases at 90 % power was found to be at least 44.

Ethics committee approval was obtained from İstanbul Medipol University Non-Interventional Clinical Research Ethics Committee, dated 21/12/2018, number 10840098-604.01.01-E.53718. Study was organized in accordance with the Helsinki Declaration principles and the consent of the individuals was obtained with the "Voluntary Information Form".

Balance was evaluated with Biodex Balance System SD, USA. According to the amount of deviation of the individual from 49 axes as anterior-posterior (AP) and medial-lateral (ML); Anterior-posterior index (API), medial-lateral index (MLI), total (OAI) deviation amounts are calculated. Tests were applied with both feet on the ground and eyes open on one leg. All individuals were tested on the same platform level on hard ground.

EMG-BF (Intelect Advanced Color Combo+ EMG, Chattanooga Group, TN, USA) was used to evaluate the muscle activation level. Graphic visual feedback on the screen was used as auditory feedback, and the signal sound that increased or decreased with changing muscle activity. The average muscle activation level was determined with the "set target" option on the device. The participant was asked to have maximum contraction for 10 seconds and then minimal relaxation. Only the average muscle activation level was recorded. The obtained findings are shown in microvolt (μV) units above the bar graph, at the top of the screen. Dura-Stick II 1.25 inch (3 cm) round 2 active electrodes were placed in the masseter muscle at one cm intervals and in the same direction with the muscle fibers, and one reference electrode was placed in the same direction with the active electrodes.

Digital algometer (Wagner FDX 25 Forge Gage, USA) was used for pain assessment. The masseter muscle body, anterior part of the temporalis muscle and temporomandibular joint were measured three times and averaged.

Posture was evaluated using the New York Posture Analysis. New York Posture Analysis is a cheap, easy, and fast applicable subjective assessment method that is widely used for clinical postural assessment. Thirteen regions of the body posteriorly; (head-A, shoulder levels-B, vertebral column-C, hip levels-D, medio-lateral position of feet-E, foot arches-F), anteriorly; (head-G, thorax-H, shoulders-I, upper back-J, trunk-K, abdomen-L, lower back-waist-M) and laterally scored on the form by monitoring. According to this, if the position of the examined area is correct, five points are given, if it is moderately impaired, three points, if seriously impaired, one point is given. Total score is maximum 65 and minimum 13. Accordingly, the score is classified as "very good" if it is "45", "good" if it is between 40 and 44, "medium" if it is 30-39, weak if it is 20-29, and "bad" if it is 19 (9). High score signifies good posture.

Disability was evaluated by Neck Pain and Disability Index (NPDI) (10). Each item consists of five items and is scored between 0 and 4 points. High scores indicate an increase in limitation in activities.

Statistical Analysis

All analyses were performed with the SPSS (version 22.0) statistical package program. Kolmogorov-Smirnov method was used for evaluation of normal distribution. It was observed that the data did not conform to normal distribution. Independent Sample T-Test was used for evaluating the demographic data. The level of significance was set at $p<0.05$. Mann Whitney U test was used for the other variables. All the p values related to this variable and less than 0.05 was considered significant.

Results

Participants were examined in terms of age, height, body weight and body mass index. There was no difference in demographic data (age, height, body weight and body mass index) between two groups ($p\geq0.05$) (Table 1).

According to the data obtained as a result of the study, a statistically significant difference was found between healthy individuals and individuals with temporomandibular joint dysfunction in balance parameters ($p\leq0.05$). There was no statistically significant difference in static double legs mediolateral and dynamic right legs mediolateral measurements ($p\geq0.05$) (Table 2).

According to EMG muscle activation measurement performed on the masseter muscle, the level of muscle activation was found significantly higher in individuals with temporomandibular joint dysfunction compared to healthy individuals ($p\leq0.05$).

Tab. 1: Comparison of Demographic Data

	Healthy	TMJD		
	Mean±SD	Mean±SD	Z	P
Age (year)	23.00±0.47	23.95±0.77	-0.61	0.54*
Height (cm)	170.04±2.05	167.62±1.90	-0.92	0.36*
Body Weight (kg)	63.13±2.37	60.95±2.22	-0.49	0.62*
Body Mass Index (kg/m²)	21.65±0.43	21.56±0.48	-0.15	0.88*

Independent Samples T test, cm: centimeter, kg: kilogram, m: meter

Tab. 2: Comparison of Balance Parameters of Healthy Individuals and Individuals with Temporomandibular Dysfunction

	Healthy	TMJD		
	Mean±SD	Mean±SD	Z	P
Static Double Legs OA	0.34±0.04	0.57±0.10	-2.26	**0.02***
Static Double Legs AP	0.30±0.04	0.48±0.09	-2.01	**0.04***
Static Double Legs ML	0.21±0.02	0.33±0.07	-1.56	0.12*
Static Right Legs OA	0.59±0.08	1.46±0.18	-3.83	**0.00***
Static Right Legs AP	0.44±0.05	1.02±0.14	-3.60	**0.00***
Static Right Legs ML	0.41±0.04	1.10±0.20	-3.11	**0.00***
Static Left Legs OA	0.62±0.13	1.51±0.21	-3.70	**0.00***
Static Left Legs AP	0.55±0.09	1.05±0.16	-2.68	**0.01***
Static Left Legs ML	0.62±0.10	0.98±0.15	-2.07	**0.04***
Dynamic Double Legs OA	0.61±0.07	0.94±0.11	-2.69	**0.01***
Dynamic Double Legs AP	0.47±0.06	1.00±0.27	-2.42	**0.02***
Dynamic Double Legs ML	0.38±0.05	0.67±0.13	-2.00	**0.04***
Dynamic Right Legs OA	0.84±0.09	1.49±0.19	-2.66	**0.01***
Dynamic Right Legs AP	0.58±0.07	1.00±0.14	-2.14	**0.03***
Dynamic Right Legs ML	0.56±0.07	1.07±0.18	-2.16	**0.03***
Dynamic Left Legs OA	1.03±0.15	1.52±0.19	-2.12	**0.03***
Dynamic Left Legs AP	0.67±0.12	1.11±0.15	-2.61	**0.01***
Dynamic Left Legs ML	0.83±0.16	1.26±0.21	-1.77	0.08*

Mann Whitney-U, OA: overall, AP: anterior-posterior, ML: medio-lateral

138   Hazal Genç, Esra Atılgan, and Beyza İnce

Tab. 3: Comparison of EMG, Algometer and Posture Parameters of Healthy Individuals and Individuals with Temporomandibular Dysfunction

	Healthy	TMJD		
	Mean±SD	Mean±SD	Z	P
EMG Right	127.26±8.50	163.29±8.87	-2.58	**0.01***
EMG Left	116.73±7.48	160.33±10.47	-3.09	**0.00***
M. Masseter Right	2.44±0.16	1.66±0.12	-3.49	**0.00***
M. Masseter Left	2.40±0.17	1.72±0.10	-2.86	**0.00***
M. Temporalis Right	2.44±0.17	1.71±0.10	-3.21	**0.00***
M. Temporalis Left	2.52±0.18	1.71±0.93	-3.35	**0.00***
TMJ Right	2.52±0.16	1.69±0.09	-3.61	**0.00***
TMJ Left	2.58±0.17	1.94±0.13	-2.56	**0.01***
NYPA	59.39±0.62	55.33±1.13	-3.67	**0.00***
NPDI	17.43±2.13	24.57±3.07	-1.68	0.09*

*Mann Whitney-U, NPDI: Neck Pain Disability Index
NYPA: New York Posture Analysis

The level of pain evaluated on the masseter, temporalis and temporomandibular joints was found significantly higher in individuals with temporomandibular joint dysfunction compared to healthy individuals ($p \leq 0.05$).

The posture score was found significantly higher in healthy individuals than in individuals with temporomandibular joint dysfunction ($p \leq 0.05$). However, there was no significant difference between the two groups on disability level ($p \geq 0.05$) (Table 3).

Discussion

We emphasize that in our study, muscle activation level, pain, posture, disability, and balance parameters were compared between individuals with temporomandibular joint dysfunction and healthy individuals.

Evaluation should be made to include especially muscular structures in individuals with temporomandibular joint dysfunction can be useful in planning multidimensional therapy (11). In our study, we examined the masseter muscle with superficial EMG for this purpose. It was observed that individuals with TMJD were more affected in muscle activation values than in healthy individuals.

Stiesch-Scholz et al. found a significant correlation between chewing and sensitivity in palpation of neck muscles TMJD group in their study. These results pointed out that cervical region problems and TMJD may have a common etiology or that one of the diseases may have an etiological role in the other (12). They suggested conducting more specific treatment studies for these problems in order to clarify the issue. Barbosa et al. found similar results in individuals with cervicobrachial symptoms. (4). Tümen et al. stated that it is important to examine the masseter muscle with EMG in individuals with temporomandibular joint dysphonia (13).

There is functional closeness of the temporomandibular joint system and the cervical spine. Visscher et al. reported that individuals with craniomandibular pain have more cervical spinal pain regardless of whether this pain is due to muscle or joint (14). Pain and dysfunction in the cervical region can be caused by changes in head posture. This may cause dysfunction in the chewing system (15). Neurophysiologically, altered central neural plasticity can be responsible for this situation, together with a deviated and continuous afferent input on the trigeminal nucleus (16).

In addition, in order for the mandibular region to perform an optimal chewing activity, the cervical region that carries this region and works in coordination with this region must also show appropriate muscle activity (17). In another research, it was reported that limited mouth opening often occurs due to masseter muscle spasm (18).

Silveria et al. examined individuals with TMJD in their study. They compared pain sensitivity of masticatory muscles and cervical region muscles in 20 healthy women with 20 TMJD. The results showed that the pain sensitivity of the cervical region muscles was lower in the group with temporomandibular joint problems compared to the healthy group (19).

Ardıç et al. examined pain and posture disorders in temporomandibular joint problems in their study. As a result of the study, they found that various posture disorders such as head-anterior posture and shoulder drop were observed (20). In our study, it was found that the posture was more affected in individuals with temporomandibular joint dysfunction according to the findings obtained as a result of the study and evaluated by New York Posture Analysis.

In a systematic review by Bevilaqua-Grossi et al, they emphasized that the methodological quality of many studies is low and the relationship between TMJD and head-neck posture is still unclear (21).

While there are studies investigating cervical region dysfunctions in cases with TMJD in the literature, there are very few studies investigating the symptoms of temporomandibular joint in cases with cervical pathology in isolation.

The fact that most of the studies conducted on this subject are not controlled and single-blind studies makes it difficult to compare the results of the studies.

In the data obtained at the results of our study, no statistically significant relationship was found in the neck disability index of individuals with TMJD.

In the study conducted individuals with or without temporomandibular joint dysfunction whose average age was 65 years, balance was evaluated in elderly by Oltramari-Navarro et al in 2017. However, temporomandibular joint dysfunction was not associated with balance in this population (22).

These results are different from our study. We think that this difference is due to the fact that the selected population is older than our study group and therefore it is more likely to have balance disorder

The most important symptoms of the functional disorders of the masticatory muscles are pain and dysfunction. Subaşı et al. examined the frequency of temporomandibular joint dysfunction in patients with cervical disc herniation. According to the results, temporomandibular dysfunction is more common in individuals with cervical problems compared to individuals without cervical problems (23).

Conclusion

As a result of the study, we concluded that individuals with temporomandibular joint dysfunction were negatively affected in terms of balance, pain, muscle activation level, pain tolerance and posture. However, no significant relationship was found in the level of neck disability. In our study, patient evaluation was not completed, and it is predicted to obtain new results by updating the data in the future.

References

1. Roda, R. P., Fernández, J. M. D., Bazán, S. H., Soriano, Y. J., Margaix, M., & Sarrión, G. (2008). A review of temporomandibular joint disease (TMJD). Part II: Clinical and radiological semiology. Morbidity processes. *Medicina Oral Patologia Oral Cirugia Bucal, 13*(2), 102-109.
2. Lomas, J. (2018). Temporomandibular dysfunction. *Australian Journal of General Practice, 47*(4), 212-215. doi:10.31128/AFP-10-17-4375
3. Sharma, S., Gupta, D. S., Pal, U. S., & Jurel, S. K. (2011). Etiological factors of temporomandibular joint disorders. *National Journal of Maxillofacial Surgery, 2*(2), 116-119. doi:10.4103/0975-5950.94463
4. Barbosa, M. A., Tahara, A. K., Ferierre, I. C., Intelango, L., & Barbosa, A. C. (2019). Effects of 8 weeks of masticatory muscles focused endurance

exercises on women with oro-facial pain and temporomandibular disorders: A placebo randomised controlled trial. *Journal of Oral Rehabilitation, 46*(10), 885-894. doi:10.1111/joor.12823

5. Miernik, M., Wieckiewicz, M., Paradowska, A., & Wieckiewicz, W. (2012). Massage therapy in myofascial TMD pain management. *Advances in Clinical and Experimental Medicine. 21*(5), 681-685.

6. Ries, L. G. K., & Bérzin, F. (2008). Analysis of the postural stability in individuals with or without signs and symptoms of temporomandibular disorder. *Brazilian Oral Research, 22*(4), 378-381. doi:10.1590/s1806-8324200800040001

7. Wiesinger, B., Malker, H., Englund, E., & Wänman, A. (2009). Does a dose-response relation exist between spinal pain and temporomandibular disorders?. *BMC Musculoskeletal Disorders, 10*(1), 23-28. doi:10.1186/1471-2474-10-28

8. Rani, S., Pawah, S., Gola, S., & Bakshi, M. (2017). Analysis of Helkimo index for temporomandibular disorder diagnosis in the dental students of Faridabad city: A cross-sectional study. *The Journal of the Indian Prosthodontic Society, 17*(1), 48-52. doi:10.4103/0972-4052.194941

9. McRoberts, L. B., Cloud, R. M., & Black, C. M. (2013). Evaluation of the New York posture rating chart for assessing changes in postural alignment in a garment study. *Clothing and Textiles Research Journal, 31*(2), 81-85. doi:10.1177/0887302X13480558

10. Bicer, A., Yazici, A., Camdeviren, H., & Erdogan, C. (2004). Assessment of pain and disability in patients with chronic neck pain: Reliability and construct validity of the Turkish version of the neck pain and disability scale. *Disability and Rehabilitation, 26*(16), 959-962. doi:10.1080/09638280410001696755

11. Carlson, C. R., Bertrand, P. M., Ehrlich, A. D., Maxwell, A. W., & Burton, R. G. (2001). Physical self-regulation training for the management of temporomandibular disorders. *Journal of Orofacial Pain, 15* (1), 47-55.

12. Stiesch-Scholz, M., Fink, M., & Tschernitschek, H. (2003). Comorbidity of internal derangement of the temporomandibular joint and silent dysfunction of the cervical spine. *Journal of Oral Rehabilitation, 30*(4), 386-391. doi:10.1046/j.1365-2842.2003.01034

13. Tümen, D. S., & Arslan, S. G. (2007). Çiğneme kas aktivitesi ve ölçüm yöntemleri. *Dicle Tıp Dergisi, 34*(4), 316-322.

14. Visscher, C. M., Lobbezoo, F., De Boer, W., Van Der Zaag, J., & Naeije, M. (2001). Prevalence of cervical spinal pain in craniomandibular pain patients. *European Journal of Oral Sciences, 109*(2), 76-80. doi:10.1034/j.1600-0722.2001.00996.x

142   Hazal Genç, Esra Atılgan, and Beyza İnce

15. Armijo-Olivo, S., Silvestre, R. A., Fuentes, J. P., da Costa, B. R., Major, P. W., Warren, ... Magee, D. J. (2012). Patients with temporomandibular disorders have increased fatigability of the cervical extensor muscles. *The Clinical Journal of Pain, 28*(1), 55-64. doi:10.1097/AJP.0b013e31822019f2

16. La Touche, R., Alba, P. A., Harry von, P., Mannheimer, J. S., Fernández-Carnero, J., & Rocabado, M. (2011). The influence of craniocervical posture on maximal mouth opening and pressure pain threshold in patients with myofascial temporomandibular pain disorders. *The Clinical Journal of Pain, 27*(1), 48-55. doi:10.1097/AJP.0b013e3181edc157

17. Ries, L. G. K., & Bérzin, F. (2008). Analysis of the postural stability in individuals with or without signs and symptoms of temporomandibular disorder. *Brazilian Oral Research, 22*(4), 378-383. doi:10.1590/s1806-83242008000400016

18. Souza, J. A., Pasinato, F., Corrêa, E. C., & da Silva, A. M. T. (2014). Global body posture and plantar pressure distribution in individuals with and without temporomandibular disorder: A preliminary study. *Journal of Manipulative and Physiological Therapeutics, 37*(6), 407-414. doi:10.1016/j.jmpt.2014.04.003

19. Silveira, A., Gadotti, I. C., Armijo-Olivo, S., Biasotto-Gonzalez, D. A., & Magee, D. (2015). Jaw dysfunction is associated with neck disability and muscle tenderness in subjects with and without chronic temporomandibular disorders. *BioMed Research International,* (3), 512792 doi:10.1155/2015/512792

20. Ardıç, F., Yılmaz, M., Palulu, N., Okumuş, M., Yorgancıoğlu, Z. R., & Güner, S. (2005). Temporomandibuler sistemdeki miyofasyal ağrı bozukluğunda postürün değerlendirilmesi. *Archives of Rheumatology, 20*(3), 7-11.

21. Bevilaqua-Grossi, D., Chaves, T. C., & Oliveira, A. S. D. (2007). Cervical spine signs and symptoms: Perpetuating rather than predisposing factors for temporomandibular disorders in women. *Journal of Applied Oral Science, 15*(4), 259-264. doi:10.1590/s1678-77572007000400004

22. Oltramari-Navarro, P. V. P., Yoshie, M. T., Silva, R. A. D., Conti, A. C. D. C. F., Navarro, R. D. L., Marchiori, L. L. D. M., & Fernandes, K. B. P. (2017). Influence of the presence of Temporomandibular Disorders on postural balance in the elderly. *Communication Sciences and Disorders and Associated, 29*(2), e20160070 doi:10.1590/2317-1782/20172016070

23. Subaşı, S. S., Gelecek, N., İlçin, N., & Çeliker, Ö. (2012). Servikal disk hernili hastalarda temporomandibular eklem disfonksiyonu görülme sıklığı. *Türk Plastik Rekonstrüktif ve Estetik Cerrahi Dergisi, 19*(3), 125-130.

İlkay Öztürk, Mirsad Alkan, and Hasan Kerem Alptekin

Evaluation of the Relationship Between Physical Activity and Fatigue with Presenteeism

Abstract

Objective: This research aims that, evaluate the relationship between Socio-demographic characteristics, body mass index, physical activity, and fatigue with presenteeism.

Materials and Methods: In this study, 53 individuals selected as the sample from academic and administrative staff of Bahçeşehir university whose ages between 18 and 65 with their job description requires working at least 5 days a week and an average of 8 hours a day. Demographic data form (DDF), fatigue severity scale (FSS), international physical activity scale (IPAQ) and Stanford presenteeism scale (SPS) were used with quantitative research method. Statistical analysis was done with SPSS 25.0 package program.

Results: Thirty-five women and 18 men whose SPS score were 21.11±4.68, FSS score were 3.80±1.27, energy expenditure according to IPAQ were 1966.20±1767.78 (METs) and BMI were 24.79±4.96 kg/m² participated in this study. There were negative significant weak correlation between SPS with FSS (p=0.03, p<0.05; r=-0.29; 0.2<r<0.4) and positive significant weak correlation between SPS with BMI (p=0.00, p<0.05; r=0.39, 0.2<r<0.4). There was not any significant correlation between IPAQ with SPS, FSS, BMI (p>0.05).

Conclusion: At the end of this study, it was seen that insufficient or irregular physical activities did not affect presenteeism. Researchers recommended that healthy living programs must be planned individually by the professional health expertise to protect employees from presenteeism. Addition that, these must be include regular physical activity components, which careful about the fatigue and protection from risk of injuries, to control of health-related risk factors.

Keywords: Presenteeism, Physical Activity, Fatigue, Body Mass Index

Introduction

"Presenteeism" is the state of being (not being) in the workplace despite being sick or unwell. In the other words, this is being physically at work but spiritually not and performance loss as a result of medical conditions (1). We should underline that the concept of presenteeism is understood with different expressions. In previous studies, presenteeism was mostly defined as coming to work while sick. However, diseases are not the only cause of presenteeism. Sometimes people come to work even if they do not feel well and they show poor performance due to different reasons other than the disease. Chapman has described presenteeism as the measurable extent to which physical or psycho-social symptoms, conditions and diseases adversely affect the work productivity of individuals who choose to remain at work (2). Presenteeism is a medical problem that need to be diagnosed and treated. For all reasons of presenteeism, generally arise in response to overworking and stress from workplace (3). Presenteeism incidence is highest in education sectors. Education is one of the sectors where presenteeism is highest (4). Employee Assistance Programs (EAP) has been used in EU and USA for years. EAP includes relaxation techniques, biofeedback mechanisms and sensation skills and it was reported that EAP helps employees to reducing stress related symptoms. Employee Assistance Programs (EAP) has been used in EU and USA for years. EAP includes relaxation techniques, biofeedback mechanisms, sensation skills. Addition that, it was reported the EAP helps employees to reducing stress related symptoms (5). However, such support programs have not yet become widespread in our country. On the other hand, sedentary lifestyle is one of the biggest risk factors for all diseases. Addition that, a great part of the daily sedentary habit is together with time spent during desk work (6). Physical activity guideline of World Health Organization (WHO) recommends to minimum 150-minute moderate intensity aerobic or 75 minutes vigorous intensity aerobic activities for adults aged 18-65 years (7). This research evaluated the relationship between Socio-demographic characteristics, body mass index, physical activity, and fatigue with presenteeism.

Materials and Methods

Fifty-three individuals between 18 and 65 ages, whose job descriptions required to work at least 5 days in a week and an average of 8 hours in a day from academic and administrative staff of Bahçeşehir University included in this study. The research was carried out between dates of March 15, 2019 and July 15, 2019 with the permissions of the Bahçeşehir University Scientific Research and Publication Ethics Board and the Rectorate of Bahçeşehir University. Initially, an online survey invitation was sent to Bahçeşehir University employees via e-mail. The "Google Forms" system was used for the online surveys. An informed consent declaration was presented to volunteers before the survey begins and 53 individuals who declared to their acceptance included in this study. Individuals answered forms that "International Physical Activity Questionnaire-Short Form (IPAQ)", "Fatigue Severity Scale (FSS)", "Stanford Presenteeism Scale (SPS)" and "Demographic Data Form (DDF)".

Physical activity questionnaires are inexpensive and can be answered easily. (8). IPAQ is a standardized instrument developed by many researchers from different countries with the encouragement of the World Health Organization and the Centers for Disease Control to assess physical activities. (9). Physical activity can be assessed with using the two different self-administered short (7-item) and long (27-item) forms of the IPAQ. Both of them asks to listed activities and request estimates of durations and frequencies for each activity did in last week. As a result of the validity and reliability study for Turkish language of both IPAQ forms, it was reported that they are suitable for use in Turkish language (10).

Fatigue levels of participants were assessed with FSS. Krupp et al. Developed and reported that FSS is suitable for both of patients with multiple sclerosis and healthy people (11). FSS includes 9 Likert type questions and each question includes 7 items where 1 indicates strongly disagree to 7 indicates agree. When scoring FSS, indicating numbers of all answers summons and score of above 36 indicates significant fatigue and maximum score is 63. Also, it has been reported as a result of Turkish validity and reliability study of FSS that Turkish version is suitable (12).

The Stanford Presenteeism Scale was developed by the Stanford University School of Medicine with the support of Merck & Co Inc. SPS includes 6 Likert type questions and each question includes 5 items where 1 indicates strongly disagree to 5 indicates agree. When scoring SPS, indicating numbers of all answers summons and scores between 6 to 10 indicates highest presenteeism level controversy that 26-30 indicates lowest presenteeism level (13,14). SPS showed good psychometric properties and it has been reported in a past study (15) Also it has been reported as a result of Turkish validity and reliability study of SPS that Turkish version is suitable (16).

Descriptive statistics of the data; mean, standard deviation, median, and frequency values were used. The distribution of the variables was measured with "Kolmogorov Smirnov" test and "Shapiro-Wilk Test" in 95 % confidence interval. Parametric data's correlation was analyzed with "Pearson Correlation" and non-parametric data's correlation analyzed with "Spearman Correlation". All analysis was performed with SPSS 25.0.

DDF has been used for age, gender, marital status, number of children, education level, income level and job duties information's. Each parameter included sub-parameters, and these used for creating to independent subgroups for

Tab. 1: Distribution of the Variables

	Kolmogorov-Smirnov[a]			Shapiro-Wilk		
	Statistics	df	p	Statistics	df	p
SPS	0.105	53	0.200	0.963	53	0.095
FSS	0.099	53	0.200	0.958	53	0.060
IPAQ	0.182	53	0.000*	0.881	53	0.000*
BMI	0.122	53	0.046*	0.928	53	0.003*

Significance Level p=0.05.

assess to SPS, IPAQ, FSS, BMI changes with DDF data. Subgroups did not have enough individuals for parametric tests so that the data analyzed with "Mann Whitney-U" Test which nonparametric test.

Results

The demographic characteristics of the participants were analyzed with frequency analysis. Results of characteristics data analysis listed that: genders were 35(66 %) women and 18(34 %) men; ages were 3 (5.7 %) 18-24, 25 (47.2 %) 25-34, 14 (26.4 %) 35-44, 5 (9.4 %) 45-54, 5 (9.4 %) 55-64, 1(1.9 %) over 65; martial statuses were 23 (43.4 %) single, 23 (43.4 %) married, 7 (13.2 %) divorced; number of children were 15 (23.9 %) 1 child, 5 (9 %) 2 children, 1 (1.9 %) 3 children, 32 (60.4) don't have a child; education levels were 2 (3.8 %) vocational school, 19 (35.8 %) bachelor, 16 (30.2) master of science, 15 (28.3 %) doctor of philosophy, 1 (1.9 %) post doctorate degrees; their jobs were 10 (18.9 %) teaching fellow as academic member, 8 (15.1 %) lecturer, 6 (11.3 %) research assistant, 14 (26.4 %) secretary, 9 (17.0 %) administrator without academic member, 3 (5.7 %) administrator with academic member, 3 (5.7 %) other staff; income levels were; 1 (1.9 %) lower than 1,600 Turkish Liras (TL), 10 (18.9 %) 1,601 TL to 3,000 TL, 23 (43.4 %) 3,001 TL to 6,000 TL, 11 (20.8 %) 6,001 TL to 9,000 TL, 8 (15.1 %) higher than 9,001 TL.

Participants' presenteeism level measured with SPS was 21.11±4.68, fatigue level measured with FSS is 3.80±1.27, MET's expenditure measured with IPAQ was 1966.20±1767.78, BMI questioned with DDF was 24.79±4.96 kg/m^2.

Results of distribution of the variables according to Kolmogorov Smirnov Test and Shapiro Wilk Test showed in Table 1. SPS and FSS variables were parametric (p>0.05) but IPAQ and BMI variables were non-parametric (p<0.05).

Results of analysis for assess to relation between SPS with FSS according to Pearson Correlation Test showed in Table 2. Negative significant weak

Tab. 2: Relationship Between SPS with FSS

		SPS	
	n	Pearson Correlation	p (2-tailed)
FSS	53	-0.296*	0.031

Significance Level p=0.05 (2-tailed)

Tab. 3: Relationships Between SPS and FSS with IPAQ and BMI

		IPAQ			BMI	
	n	Correlation Coefficient	Sig. (2-tailed)	n	Correlation Coefficient	Sig. (2-tailed)
SPS	53	0.052	0.712	53	0.398**	0.003
FSS	53	-0.131	0.350	53	-0.265	0.055

** Significance Level for Correlation p=0.01 (2-tailed)

correlation was shown between SPS with FSS (p=0.03, p<0.05; r=-0.29; 0.2<r<0.4).

Results of analysis for assess to relations between SPS and FSS with IPAQ and BMI according to Spearman Correlation Test showed in Table 3. Positive significant weak correlation was shown between SPS with BMI (p=0.00, p<0.05; r=-0.39; 0.2<r<0.4). There was any significant correlation between FSS with BMI, SPS with IPAQ and FSS with IPAQ (p>0.05).

Age effects researched with two subgroups which are under 34 ages and above 35 ages. Results of analysis for assess to age effects on SPS, FSS, BMI and IPAQ according to "Mann Whitney U Test" showed in Table 4. Individuals who under 34 ages showed significantly lower values for SPS and BMI (p<0.05) and significantly higher values for FSS (p<0.05). There were any significant changes for IPAQ (p>0.05).

Gender effects researched with two subgroups which are women and men. Results of analysis for assess to gender effects on SPS, FSS, BMI and IPAQ according to "Mann Whitney U Test" showed in Table 5. Women showed significantly higher values for FSS (p<0.05), and significantly lower values for BMI (p<0.05). There were any significant changes for IPAQ and SPS (p>0.05).

Marital status effects researched with two subgroups which are single and married. Results of analysis for assess to marital status effects on SPS, FSS, BMI and IPAQ according to "Mann Whitney U Test" showed in Table 6. There are divorced individuals included to single group. There were any significant changes on SPS, FSS, BMI and IPAQ values between groups (p>0.05).

Tab. 4: Age Effects on SPS, FSS, BMI and IPAQ

	n	Min.	Max.	Avg.	±SD	u	w	z	p
SPS									
Under 34	28	9	30	19.678	4.422	232.500	638.500	-2.106	0.03
Above 34	25	16	30	22.720	4.532				
FSS									
Under 34	28	1.56	5.78	4.29	1.158	179.000	504.000	-3.049	0.00
Above 34	25	1.33	5.78	3.25	1.185				
BMI									
Under 34	28	17.30	36.00	23.666	4.527	237.000	643.000	-2.013	0.04
Above 34	25	18.67	43.08	26.048	5.214				
IPAQ									
Under 34	28	0.00	6933.00	1934.321	1754.357	340.500	665.500	-0.169	0.86
Above 34	25	0.00	6318.00	2001.920	1818.239				

Descriptive Statics, Mann Whitney U Test

Educations effects researched with two subgroups which are under bachelor and above Master of Science. Results of analysis for access to education effects on SPS, FSS, BMI and IPAQ according to "Mann Whitney U Test" showed in Table 7. There were any significant changes on SPS, FSS, BMI and IPAQ values between groups (p>0.05).

Tab. 5: Gender Effects on SPS, FSS, BMI and IPAQ

	n	Min.	Max.	Avg.	±SD	u	w	z	p
SPS									
Women	35	9	30	20.428	4.779	246.500	876.500	-1.294	0.19
Men	18	17	30	22.444	4.328				
FSS									
Women	35	2.22	5.78	4.17	1.117	171.500	342.500	-2.697	0.00
Men	18	1.33	5.22	3.09	1.279				
BMI									
Women	35	17.30	43.08	23.460	5.022	129.000	759.000	-3.493	0.00
Men	18	19.37	36.00	27.376	3.767				
IPAQ									
Women	35	0.00	6318.00	1717.200	1579.818	254.500	884.500	-1.137	0.25
Men	18	0.00	6933.00	2450.388	2047.322				

Descriptive Statics, Mann Whitney U Test

Tab. 6: Marital Status Effects on SPS, FSS, BMI and IPAQ

	n	Min.	Max.	Avg.	±SD	u	w	z	p
SPS									
Single	30	9	29	20.100	4.588	260.000	725.000	-1.535	0.12
Married	23	16	30	22.434	4.580				
FSS									
Single	30	1.44	5.78	4.05	1.292	258.500	534.500	-1.554	0.12
Married	23	1.33	5.22	3.47	1.193				
BMI									
Single	30	17.30	43.08	24.023	5.315	242.000	707.000	-1.848	0.06
Married	23	17.90	36.00	25.790	4.374				
IPAQ									
Single	30	0.00	6933.00	1742.966	1624.155	296.000	761.000	-0.880	0.37
Married	23	0.00	6318.00	2257.391	1937.199				

Descriptive Statics, Mann Whitney U Test

Tab. 7: Education Effects on SPS, FSS, BMI and IPAQ

	n	Min.	Max.	Avg.	±SD	u	w	z	p
SPS									
Under B	21	13	30	20.952	4.521	322.500	553.500	-0.247	0.80
Above MSc	32	9	30	21.218	4.864				
FSS									
Under B	21	1.44	5.78	3.85	1.345	325.000	853.000	-0.200	0.84
Above MSc	32	1.33	5.78	3.77	1.242				
BMI									
Under B	21	19.37	30.45	23.949	3.256	305.500	536.500	-0.555	0.57
Above MSc	32	17.30	43.08	25.342	5.804				
IPAQ									
Under B	21	0.00	6933.00	2203.809	1956.044	295.500	823.500	-0.737	0.46
Above MSc	32	0.00	5598.00	1810.281	1646.289				

Descriptive Statics, Mann Whitney U Test, B: Bachelor, MSc: Master of Science

Tab. 8: Income Effects on SPS, FSS, BMI and IPAQ

	n	Min.	Max.	Avg.	±SD	h	df	p
SPS								
Low Income	11	13	30	21.272	5.001			
Average Income	23	9	30	20.040	4.733	2.053	2	0.35
High Income	19	16	30	22.315	4.384			
FSS								
Low Income	11	1.44	5.33	3.78	1.159			
Average Income	23	1.56	5.78	4.20	1.246	4.991	2	0.08
High Income	19	1.33	5.78	3.3275	1.25679			
BMI								
Low Income	11	17.30	30.45	22.819	4.044			
Average Income	23	19.03	43.08	25.266	5.881	3.058	2	0.21
High Income	19	17.90	33.53	25.356	4.099			
IPAQ								
Low Income	11	0.00	5394.00	1782.454	1710.714			
Average Income	23	0.00	6318.00	1679.695	1628.639	1.346	2	0.51
High Income	19	0.00	6933.00	2419.421	1953.945			

Descriptive Statics, Kruskal Wallis Test

Income effects analyzed three subgroups which are low income (under 3,000 TL), average income (3,001 TL- 6,000 TL) and high income (above 6,001 TL). Results of analysis for assess to income effects on SPS, FSS, BMI and IPAQ according to "Kruskal Wallis Test" showed in Table 8. There were any significant changes on SPS, FSS, BMI and IPAQ values between groups ($p > 0.05$).

Job duties effects analyzed two subgroups which are academic and administrative. Results of analysis for assess to job duties effects on SPS, FSS, BMI and IPAQ according to "Mann Whitney U Test" showed in Table 9. There were any significant changes on SPS, FSS, BMI and IPAQ values between groups ($p > 0.05$).

Discussion

If presenteeism is experienced due to health problems, it is one of the precautions can be taken that inform the managers about this. Periodic health checks which made by the enterprises will be helps to detect undiagnosed or misdiagnosed but revealing the existing health problems (17).

Tab. 9: Job Duties Effects on SPS, FSS, BMI and IPAQ

	n	Min.	Max.	Avg.	±SD	u	w	z	p
SPS									
Academic	28	9	30	21.428	4.887	311.000	636.000	-0.699	0.48
Administrative	25	13	30	20.760	4.530				
FSS									
Academic	28	1.33	5.78	3.77	1.296	340.500	746.500	-0.169	0.86
Administrative	25	1.44	5.78	3.83	1.270				
BMI									
Academic	28	17.30	43.08	25.183	5.448	313.000	638.000	-0.659	0.51
Administrative	25	18.99	36.00	24.350	4.426				
IPAQ									
Academic	28	0.00	6933.00	1946.500	1953.957	323.000	729.000	-0.482	0.63
Administrative	25	0.00	6318.00	1988.280	1573.165				

Descriptive Statics, Mann Whitney U Test

Individuals who included in this study showed different sociodemographic characteristics but both presenteeism and fatigue are common in the sample group. The randomly selected sample group includes many sociodemographic classes.

The result of the study showed that presenteeism and fatigue are inversely proportional, BMI is directly proportional to presenteeism, and IPAQ does not affect presenteeism.

That has been already known; FSS value affect physical activity choices and many activities does not affects BMI. So that one-off our limitation for this study that we do not have information about detailed activity analysis.

It is necessary to identify personnel who have problems with overweight, chronic pain, sleep disorders, depression, and diabetes, which are common and cause loss of productivity. Moreover, healthy living programs should be planning with the focusing on these personnel. In previous studies, it is emphasized that interventions related to stress management, improving sleep patterns, relieving muscle pain, balanced nutrition, diabetes, weight control, and improving mental health and physical activity should be carried out in health promotion programs (18).

Our results showed that SPS value did not relate to sociodemographic data such as education level, marital status, income level and duties at work. On the other side, BMI which is considered as one of the general health indicators, affects the SPS value.

It was observed in this research that younger individuals had lower SPS and BMI values but higher FSS values. According to this, it is thought that future studies are needed for research to lifestyle habits and physical activities effects on FSS and SPS in young population.

That was seen in our study that SPS and IPAQ values did not showed significant differences between genders, on the other hand women had lower BMI but higher FSS. According to this, it is thought that future studies are needed for research about specific causes of womens' presenteeism. It has been thought the causes of that put their health in second plan for compensate their decreased working level and deadlines (19).

Conclusion

Altough physical activity is a good prognostic factor, unconscious physical activity did not effect presenteeism. Furthermore enterprises should provide healthy living programs with physical activity for controlling BMI and fatique and in order to prevent presenteeism.

References

1. Çiftçi, B. (2010). İşte var ol(ama)ma sorunu ve işletmelerin uygulayabileceği çözüm önerileri. *Çalışma ve Toplum, 1*, 153-174.

2. Brown, H. E., Gilson, N. D., Burton, N. W., & Brown, W. J. (2011). Does physical activity impact on presenteeism and other indicators of workplace well-being?. *Sports Medicine, 41*(3), 249-262. doi:10.2165/11539180-000000000-00000

3. Middaugh, D. J. (2006). Presenteeism: Sick and tired at work. *Medsurg Nursing, 15*(2), 103-106.

4. Aronsson, G., Gustafsson, K., & Dallner, M. (2000). Sick but yet at work. An empirical study of sickness presenteeism. *Journal of Epidemiology & Community Health, 54*(7), 502-509. doi:10.1136/jech.54.7.502

5. Aytaç, S. (2009). *İş stresi yönetimi el kitabı iş stresi: oluşumu, nedenleri, başa çıkma yolları.* Ankara, Türkiye: Labour Ministry-CASGEM.

6. Urda, J. L., Larouere, B., Verba, S. D., & Lynn, J. S. (2017). Comparison of subjective and objective measures of office workers' sedentary time. *Preventive Medicine Reports, 8*, 163-168. doi:10.1016/j.pmedr.2017.10.004

7. Wicker, P., & Frick, B. (2017). Intensity of physical activity and subjective well-being: An empirical analysis of the WHO recommendations. *Journal of Public Health, 39*(2), e19-e26. doi:10.1093/pubmed/fdw062

8. Washburn, R. A., & Montoye, H. J. (1986). The assessment of physical activity by questionnaire. *American Journal of Epidemiology, 123*(4), 563-576. doi:10.1093/oxfordjournals.aje.a114277

9. Craig, C. L., Marshall, A. L., Sjöström, M., Bauman, A. E., Booth, M. L., Ainsworth, B. E., ... Oja, P. (2003). International physical activity questionnaire: 12-country reliability and validity. *Medicine & Science in Sports & Exercise, 35*(8), 1381-1395. doi:10.1249/01.MSS.0000078924.61453. FB

10. Saglam, M., Arikan, H., Savci, S., Inal-Ince, D., Bosnak-Guclu, M., Karabulut, E., & Tokgozoglu, L. (2010). International physical activity questionnaire: Reliability and validity of the Turkish version. *Perceptual and Motor Skills, 111*(1), 278-284. doi:10.2466/06.08.PMS.111.4.278-284

11. Krupp, L. B., Alvarez, L. A., LaRocca, N. G., & Scheinberg, L. C. (1988). Fatigue in multiple sclerosis. *Archives of Neurology, 45*(4), 435-437. doi:10.1001/archneur.1988.00520280085020

12. Armutlu, K., Korkmaz, N. C., Keser, I., Sumbuloglu, V., Akbiyik, D. I., Guney, Z., & Karabudak, R. (2007). The validity and reliability of the fatigue severity scale in Turkish multiple sclerosis patients. *International Journal of Rehabilitation Research, 30*(1), 81-85. doi:10.1097/ MRR.0b013e3280146ec4

13. Koopman, C., Pelletier, K. R., Murray, J. F., Sharda, C. E., Berger, M. L., Turpin, R. S., ... Bendel, T. (2002). Stanford presenteeism scale: Health status and employee productivity. *Journal of Occupational and Environmental Medicine, 44*(1), 14-20. doi:10.1097/00043764-200201000-00004

14. Mandıracıoğlu, A., Bölükbaş, O., Demirel, M., & Gümeli, F. (2016). Kronik hastalıklar ile absentizm ve presentizm ilişkisinin belirlenmesi. *Verimlilik Dergisi, 4*(4), 75-90.

15. Özmen, G. (2011). *Presenteeism ile örgütsel bağlılık ilişkisi: Tekstil çalışanları üzerinde bir araştırma.* (Unpublished master's thesis). Eskişehir Osmangazi University, Eskişehir, Turkey.

16. Coşkun, Ö. Y. (2012). *İki işyerinde işe devamsızlık ve kendini işe verememede etkili faktörlerin değerlendirilmesi* (Doctoral dissertation). Ankara University, Ankara, Turkey.

17. Hemp, P. (2004). Presenteeism: At work--but out of it. *Harvard Business Review, 82*(10), 49-58.

18. Şahin, D. (2019). Sağlığı geliştirme programlarının işte var olamama (presenteeism) üzerindeki etkisine yönelik alanyazın incelemesi. *Sağlık Bilimleri ve Meslekleri Dergisi, 6*(2), 427-436. doi:10.17681/hsp.457111

19. Biron, C., Brun, J. P., Ivers, H., & Cooper, C. L. (2006). At work but ill: Psychosocial work environment and well-being determinants of presenteeism propensity. *Journal of Public Mental Health*, 5(4), 26-37. doi:10.1108/17465729200600029

Pelin Pişirici and Evrim Karadağ Saygı

Investigation the Effectiveness of Low-Dose Laser Treatment in Patellofemoral Pain Syndrome-Randomized Controlled Study

Abstract

Objective: This study was conducted to investigate the effects of low-dose laser therapy (LDLT) on pain, disability, and quality of life (QoL) in patients with patellofemoral pain syndrome (PFPS).

Materials and Methods: Forty patients, 31 females and 9 males, were randomized into 2 groups of 20 people each, as laser group (LG) and control group (CG), by simple matching method. Knee extension and hip abduction muscle strength, hamstring, and iliotibial band (ITB) flexibility measurements were repeated at pretreatment and posttreatment. Patients' resting and activity pain levels are measured by visual analog scale (VAS), mental and physical disability levels are measured by pain disability index (PDI) and QoL is assessed by short form 36 (SF-36) at the pretreatment, posttreatment and 8th week. LG received hot pack, ultrasound (US), exercise, and LDLT. CG received same treatment but US and LDLT is applied placebo. LDLT is applied 10 sessions: 5 days a week for 2 weeks.

Results: The mean age of the LG and CG was 40±9.8 and 44±6 years, respectively. In LG, resting and activity VAS values showed improvement at posttreatment and 8th week. In the CG, while there was an improvement in activity and resting in VAS values at posttreatment, this decrease continued only in activity at the 8th week. In SF-36 evaluation, intragroup comparison of physical values; significant improvement was observed at posttreatment and at the 8th week in LG. In the intragroup comparison of PDI values, improvement was observed in both groups at the 8th week.

Conclusion: We recommend the use of LDLT in the treatment of PFPS for longer-term pain control and improvement in QoL.

Keywords: Anterior Knee Pain, Patellofemoral Pain Syndrome, Low Level Laser Therapy

Introduction

Patellofemoral pain syndrome (PFPS) is a painful disease of the musculoskeletal system, usually seen in active young adults. Activities that cause repetitive loading of the patellofemoral joint cause diffuse anterior or retropatellar knee pain (1). Anterior knee (retropatellar-peripatellar) pain, which increases in activities such as sitting for a long time, climbing up and down stairs, squatting even though there is no pathological condition, is defined as PFPS (2,3). The main complaint in patellofemoral joint diseases is pain in the back of the patella, in the anteromedial joint line or in the popliteal fossa. The pain increases with activity, is often bilateral and continuous, occasionally showing exacerbations (3,4).

Extensor mechanism dysfunction and associated dislocation of the patella within the femoral trochlea are considered to be the possible cause of PFPS. Decreased knee extension strength may also contribute to the formation of PFPS. The cause of pain is not the same for each patient. Although there is no valid test to diagnose PFPS, a specific combination of signs and symptoms is generally considered sufficient for diagnosis. Patients often complain of anterior knee pain associated with sitting, crouching, kneeling, climbing stairs, or running for a long time (5).

In the treatment of PFPS, firstly activity level should be reduced. Ice application is recommended. Quadriceps strengthening exercises are the most recommended treatment because the quadriceps has an important role in patellar movement. After the physical examination, strengthening exercises for weak hip muscles and stretching exercises for various muscle groups are recommended. Other treatment options include knee bands and braces, bandaging, shoe selection and arch supports (6).

Low-dose laser therapy (DDLT) is a safe physical therapy agent that has been used for years. The therapeutic laser is a non-thermic agent and does not cause any damage since it cannot transfer heat to the tissue. It is well known that laser is tolerated at all ages and does not cause pain (7). Although there are many studies on laser application in knee osteoarthritis, studies conducted with laser application in PFPS patients are limited. The aim of this study is to investigate the effect of DDLT applied to patients with anterior knee pain due to PFPS on pain, quality of life (QoL) and disability.

Materials and Methods

This study is approved by the İstanbul Number 9 Clinical Research Ethics Committee' "Ethics Committee Decision" dated 24.12.2010, numbered B.30.2.MAR.0.01.02/AEK/673. It is carried out in Marmara University Physical Medicine and Rehabilitation Department Outpatient Treatment Unit. All participants were informed about the study and their written and verbal consents were obtained.

Participants

The population of the study is the patients with anterior knee pain who live in the Anatolian side of İstanbul. This study was carried out on 40 patients between the ages of 20-50 who were diagnosed with PFPS and applied to the outpatient clinic of Marmara University Faculty of Medicine, Department of Physical Medicine and Rehabilitation. After the clinical examination of the patients by a specialist physician, general locomotor system evaluations were made by a physiotherapist.

Inclusion Criteria

- Being between the ages of 20-50
- Having anterior knee pain for at least 6 weeks
- Having pain in at least two of the activities such as sitting, kneeling, squatting, running, jumping, climbing stairs
- Having tension in patella palpation
- Having pain of at least 2 cm in the 10 cm Visual Analogue Scale (VAS) assessment during activity or at rest.
- Volunteering to participate in the study

Exclusion Criteria

- Having an advanced cardiac disease
- Having uncontrolled hypertension or diabetes mellitus
- Having a systemic, infectious, inflammatory, tumoral or major psychiatric disease
- Having a sensory defect
- Pregnancy
- Having physical therapy for the knee region in previous year
- Having major knee trauma or surgery

After signing voluntary consent forms, the patients who will participate in the study were divided into 2 groups of 20 people by simple matching method. LG received hot pack, ultrasound (US), exercise, and LDLT. Control group (CG) received same treatment but US and LDLT is applied placebo. Placebo and real applications were applied with the same procedures, only in the placebo group without turning on laser and US devices. Placebo US for 3 minutes and hot packs for 20 minutes were applied to the knee to be treated. Uni-LAZER 201 device was used in our study. Laser application was applied to 4 painful points, at right angles, in full contact, to both groups, for 30 seconds to each point and twice times. Patients who received laser therapy were included in a 10-session treatment program for 2 weeks, 5 days a week.

Exercise programs of the patients include strengthening of quadriceps, vastus medialis oblique (VMO) (0-30° terminal extension), hip flexor, abductor, and external rotator muscles, and stretching of hamstring muscles and iliotibial band (ITB). Patients applied exercise programs once during the treatment and 2 times at home (total 3 times a day) with 10 repetitions per session. Patients continued their exercises as a home program during the treatment program and until the 8th week control. No drugs other than paracetamol were allowed during the study. Those who regularly used blood pressure medication, psychiatric drugs or hormones continued their treatment.

Evaluation

Demographic Features

Patients' age, gender, body mass index, occupation, educational status, history of diseases and medications used, and activity-pain relationship were questioned. All patients' manual muscle testing, flexibility, effusion, lower extremity alignment (varus, valgus, recurvatum), patellar tilt, patellar mobility, crepitation, VMO and foot posture evaluations were performed.

Flexibility Evaluation

Modified Ober Test: This test was used to evaluate the shortness of ITB. The participant was placed on its side, with the side to be tested on top, and the lower hip and knee flexed. During the test, the pelvis is stabilized. Tested leg was gently released after being passively abducted and extended from the hip. If the leg cannot fall from the horizontal position, the test is recorded as positive. While performing the test, it is important that the hip is in slight extension position, in terms of passing the ITB over the trochanter major. Evaluation was made as "present" or "absent".

Hamstring Flexibility Test: Patients were asked to lie forward in the hamstring stretching position while the patient was sitting in the bed, and the distance between the fingertip and the foot was measured.

Manual Muscle Testing: The quadriceps and abductor muscle strength of the patients were measured by manual muscle test. All patients were evaluated by the same physiotherapist's ipsilateral hand. Muscle strength was scored between 0 and 5 according to manual muscle strength evaluation.

Quadriceps Muscle Testing: While the patient was sitting at the edge of the bed, he was asked to bring his leg to extension. When he completed the movement, he was asked to extend his leg by giving resistance towards the opposite direction of the movement.

Hip Abduction Muscle Testing: The patient is positioned with the leg to be tested above. When the patient's leg completes the abduction movement, resistance is given in the opposite direction of the movement and patient was asked to maintain his legs' position.

Foot Evaluation

Evaluation of Foot Arch: The evaluation was made in a standing position, with his feet bare and on a firm surface, transferring equal load to both feet. The longitudinal arch of the foot was evaluated by combining 3 points between the 1st metatarsal head, navicular, and calcaneus. Arch height graded as; normal arc, pes planus and pes cavus. In a normal foot, the scaphoid tubercle of the navicular bone falls on a line drawn between the medial malleolus and the center of the metatarsophalangeal joint of the thumb. This line is called the "Feiss Line". Pes planus degrees are evaluated according to the separation of the scaphoid tubercle from this line towards the ground. If the tubercle has decreased by 1/3 of the distance between the feiss line and the ground, there is 1st degree pes planus if it has decreased by 2/3, 2nd degree if it completely touches the ground, 3rd degree pes planus. If the tubercle stays above the feiss line, it is mentioned as pes cavus.

Knee Evaluation

Valgus-Varus Evaluation: Evaluation performed in standing position while patients' knees and feet were bare. Genu valgum is accepted if there is a gap of more than 2 cm between the medial malleoli, and genu varum is accepted if there is a distance of more than 2 cm between the knees. Evaluation was made as "present" or "absent".

Recurvatum Evaluation: Evaluation performed by observing the knees from the side while the patient was in a standing position, if hyperextension was detected, genu recurvatum was accepted. Evaluation was made as "present" or "absent".

Outcome Measures

The pain assessment at rest and during activity was made by VAS. Disability assessment were made using the pain disability index (PDI). Quality of life was evaluated with Short Form-36 (SF-36). The patients were evaluated at pretreatment, posttreatment and one month after the end of the treatment (8th week follow up).

Visual Analog Scale: On a line of 0-10 cm, the patient's absence of pain is indicated with 0 and unbearable pain with 10. After explaining that the pain gradually increased on the line, patients were asked to mark their pain at resting and activity. Then, the distance of the marked point to 0 was measured with a millimeter ruler.

Pain Disability Index: It evaluates the relationship of pain with 7 different functional areas. The areas addressed during the measurement are family/home responsibilities, social activity, occupation, sexual behavior, personal care, and life support activities. Responses are expressed using an 11-point Likert scale ranging from 0 points (no disability) to 10 points (complete disability). PDI developed by Tait et al. in 1990 (8) and its' Turkish validity and reliability study was conducted in 2016 by Uğurlu et al. (9).

Short Form-36: SF-36 is a scale of 36 items used in the assessment of life quality. It has 8 subgroups; physical function (10 items), social function (2 items), role limitations due to physical problems (4 items), role limitations due to emotional problems (3 items), mental health (5 items), fitness (4 items), pain 2 (item) and general health (6 items). It was developed by Rand Corporation in 1992 (10). Turkish validity and reliability study of the form was conducted in 1999 by Koçyiğit et al. (11).

Statistical Analysis

Data are expressed as mean ± standard deviation. While evaluating the study data, in addition to descriptive statistical methods, intragroup changes were analyzed using the Friedman test. Comparison of the groups with each other was analyzed using a double non-parametric test (Mann Whitney U). The cases where the "p" value is less than 0.05 are considered statistically significant. While evaluating the findings obtained in the study, SPSS (Statistical Package for Social Science) 11.5 program was used for statistical analysis.

Results

The demographic characteristics of the patients are shown in Table 1. Groups are statistically similar in terms of demographic characteristics. However, in LG, education level is higher and patellar mobility is more limited. No significant diseases other than hypertension and diabetes mellitus were found in

Tab. 1: Demographic Characteristics of the Patients

Variables		Laser Group	Control Group
Gender	Female	15	16
	Male	5	4
Occupation	Housewife	6	11
	Public server	8	4
	Worker	4	5
	Student	2	0
Education	Elementary school	5	11
	High school	4	6
	University	11	3
Modified Ober Test	Present	8	10
	Absent	12	10
Hamstring flexibility Test	Absent	11	9
	Slight	5	9
	Evident	4	2
Effusion	Present	5	6
	Absent	15	14
Patellar tilt	Lateral	9	14
	Normal	11	6
Crepitation	Present	18	19
	Absent	2	1
Patellar Mobility	Normal	4	1
	Limited	16	19
VMO	Normal	4	1
	Atrophy	16	19
Foot evaluation	Pes planus	1	3
	Pes cavus	1	2
	Normal	18	15
Age (years)		40±9.8	44±6
Body Mass Index		29±5.4	26.1±4.5

the history of the patients in either group. One patient with pes planus and pes cavus detected in LG; 3 patients with pes planus and 2 patients with pes cavus were detected in CG. Valgus was detected in 1 patient in LG. One patient with genu recurvatum detected in CG and 4 patients with genu recurvatum detected in LG.

Pain Assessment with Visual Analogue Scale

Intragroup Evaluations

Resting Pain

In the intragroup evaluation performed at posttreatment, it was found that while there was a statistically significant decrease in both groups (LG p=0.000, CG p=0.003), this decrease continued only in LG at the first month (LG p=0.005, CG p=0.119) (Table 2).

Activity Pain

In the intragroup evaluation performed at the end of the treatment, a statistically significant decrease was observed in both groups (LG p=0.000, CG p=0.001). It was observed that this decrease continued in both groups in one month after the treatment (LG p=0.000, CG p=0.003).

Intragroup Evaluations

Resting Pain

In the intergroup evaluation performed at posttreatment, no statistically significant decrease was observed in both groups (p=0.178). However, a statistically significant decrease was detected only in the LG in the one month after the end of treatment (p=0.032; p<0.05) (Table 3).

Activity Pain

No statistically significant decrease was observed in the intergroup evaluation performed in both posttreatment and one month after the end of treatment (p=0.401, p=0.150) (Table 3).

Tab. 2: Intragroup Resting and Activity VAS Assessments

	Laser Group				Control Group			
	PreT	PostT	8W	p	PreT	PostT	8W	p
Resting	2.5±1.7	0.8±0.9		0.000	3.6±3	1.9±2.3		0.003
	2.5±1.7		0.9±1.9	0.005	3.6±3		2.6±2.9	0.119
Activity	5.9±2	3.4±2.3		0.000	6±3.2	4.1±2.6		0.001
	5.9±2		2.1±2.6	0.000	6±3.2		3.7±3.3	0.003

PreT: Pretreatment, PostT: Posttreatment, 8W: One month after the end of treatment
*Friedman Test

Tab. 3: Intergroup Resting and Activity VAS Assessments

	VAS Resting			VAS Activity		
	Laser Group	Control Group	p	Laser Group	Control Group	p
PostT	0.8±0.9	1.9±2.3	0.178	3.4±2.3	4.1±2.6	0.401
8W	0.9±1.9	2.6±2.9	0.032	2.1±2.6	3.7±3.3	0.150

*PostT: Posttreatment, 8W: One month after the end of treatment *Mann Whitney U Test*

Quality of Life Assessment with Short Form-36

Intragroup Evaluations

SF-36 Mental Evaluations

In the intragroup evaluation performed at posttreatment, no statistically significant change was observed in both groups (LG p=0.070, CG p=0.117). In the evaluation made in one month after the treatment, a statistically significant decrease was found only in the LG (LG p=0.030, CG p=0.526) (Table 4).

SF-36 Physical Evaluations

In the intragroup evaluation performed at posttreatment, a statistically significant change was observed only in the LG (LG p=0.017, CG p=0.723). In the evaluation made in one month after the treatment, a statistically significant change was found only in LG (LG p=0.005, CG p=0.765) (Table 4).

Tab. 4: SF-36 Intragroup Mental and Physical Evaluations

	Laser Group				Control Group			
	PreT	PostT	8W	p	PreT	PostT	8W	p
Mental	43.3±9.5	48.8±11		0.070	45.3±9.1	44.8±11.2		0.117
	43.3±9.5		51.0±7	0.030	45.3±9.1		46.4±8.9	0.526
Physical	37.8±11	41.9±11		0.017	38.5±11	42.5±9		0.723
	37.8±11		44.5±10	0.005	38.5±11		43.5±11	0.765

PreT: Pretreatment, PostT: Posttreatment, 8W: One month after the end of treatment
Friedman Test

Intragroup Evaluations

SF-36 Mental Evaluations

There was no statistically significant decrease in the intergroup evaluation performed both at the posttreatment and in the first month follow up (p=0.330, p=0.066; p<0.05 respectively) (Table 5).

SF-36 Physical Evaluations

There was no statistically significant decrease in the intergroup evaluation performed both at the posttreatment and in the first month follow up (p=0.776, p=0.256; p<0.05 respectively) (Table 5).

Disability Assessment with Pain Disability Index

Intragroup Evaluations

In the intragroup evaluation performed in the first month follow up, a statistically significant decrease was observed in both groups (LG p=0.009, CG p=0.002; p<0.005) (Table 6).

Tab. 5: SF-36 Intergroup Mental and Physical Evaluations

| | Mental SF-36 | | | Physical SF-36 | | |
	Laser Group	Control Group	p	Laser Group	Control Group	p
PostT	48.8±11	44.8±11.2	0.330	41.9±11	42.5±9	0.776
8W	51.0±7	46.4±8.9	0.066	44.5±10	43.5±11	0.256

*PostT: Posttreatment, 8W: One month after the end of treatment *Mann Whitney U Test*

Tab. 6: PDI Intragroup Evaluations

| | Laser Group | | | Control Group | | |
	PostT	8W	p	PostT	8W	p
PDI	16.6±15	10.5±10	0.009	18.7±11	15.3±12	0.002

*PostT: Posttreatment, 8W: One month after the end of treatment *Friedman Test*

Tab. 7: PDI Intergroup Evaluations

	Laser Group	Control Group	p
PostT	16.6±15	18.7±11	0.416
8W	10.5±10	15.3±12	0.150

*PostT: Posttreatment, 8W: One month after the end of treatment *Mann Whitney U Test*

Intragroup Evaluations

There was no statistically significant decrease in the intergroup evaluation performed both at the posttreatment and in the first month follow up (p=0.416, p=0.150; p<0.05 respectively). (Table 7).

Discussion

Results of our study showed improvement resting and activity VAS values at posttreatment and 8th week in LG. In the CG improvements continued only in activity at the 8th week. In SF-36 evaluation, intragroup comparison of physical values; significant improvement was observed at posttreatment and at the 8th week in LG. In the intragroup comparison of PDI values, improvement was observed in both groups at the 8th week.

It is thought that PFPS is more common in women. In general, women have more joint laxity than men. This results in a reduction in joint proprioception, which creates susceptibility to injury in connective tissues and ligaments. In addition, structural differences such as pelvis width, femoral anteversion, quadriceps (Q) angle, quadriceps strength, sitting with the legs in adducted position, wearing high-heeled shoes, and slight knee flexion required during walking are also risk factors for PFPS. The effects of estrogen and other female sex hormones on connective tissue and changes in hormones may also contribute to the development of PFPS (1). Q angle defined by Hvid is an average of 14° in men and 17° in women. Hvid et al, evaluated Q angles of 29 patients with patellofemoral complaints in their study. As a result of the measurements, the Q angles were found to be higher in women than in men (12). In addition, Christou (13) and Willson (14) stated in their study that the development of PFPS is more common in women compared to men. In our study, there were 31 women (77.5 %) and 9 men. These results are consistent with the data indicating that PFPS is more common in women.

In the clinical evaluation of patients diagnosed with PFPS, it is seen that the majority of individuals are young and active women between the ages of

11 and 40 (4). In a randomized study conducted by Balcı et al., the mean age of the hip internal rotation group was 39.1±8.0 years and the mean age of the external rotation group was 36.1±8.7 years (15). In our study, the mean age was 40±9.8 years in CG and 44±6 years in LG, close to the results of this study. The average age of the patients in our study seems to be slightly higher when compared with the literature.

In addition to many factors, excessive weight is also responsible for the pathogenesis of PFPS (2). Since the increase in patellofemoral joint reactive power will increase patellofemoral joint stress, the symptoms become more pronounced. People with high body mass index (BMI) are more likely to have PFPS. It is stated that weight loss reduces stress on the patellofemoral joint (16). Higher BMI is present in PFPS in adults (17). In our study, the average BMI of the patients is 27.6±5 kg/m^2 and the groups show a homogeneous distribution in terms of BMI. BMI of the patients consisted of overweight patients in accordance with the literature.

The first step in the treatment of PFPS is to strengthen the VMO in order to provide the dynamic balance of the patella. Herrington et al., compared quadriceps strengthening exercises with and without weight transfer in their randomized controlled study. In the study conducted on 45 male patients between the ages of 18-35, knee extension exercises were given to the 1st group, leg press exercises in sitting position were given to the 2nd group and no treatment was applied to the CG. As a result, statistically significant reduction in pain, increase in muscle strength and functional performance were observed in both exercise groups compared to the CG. It has been observed that quadriceps exercises performed both by with and without weight transfer significantly increase clinical results in patients with PFPS (16). Considering these results, quadriceps strengthening exercises were applied as open and closed kinetic chain in our treatment program without discrimination. In our study, pretreatment manual muscle strength values increased by 6 % in both groups, without statistical difference.

Decreased knee extension strength may also contribute to the formation of PFPS (5). Bakhtiary et al., divided 32 female patients with patellar chondromalacia into straight leg raising and mini-squat exercise groups. In addition to the pretreatment evaluations, thigh circumference was also measured from 5 and 10 centimeters above the patella. In the results, the difference between the right and left thigh circumference shows VMO atrophy. In the comparisons made in both groups 3 weeks after the treatment, a significant increase was observed in the values at 5 and 10 centimeters in the mini squat group (18). In our study, the same exercise program was given to CG and LG and it was checked by verbal questioning whether the exercises were performed regularly. Pain control is an important follow-up criterion in PFPS, and it is known to be affected by exercise. In our study, exercise was not a factor that created differences between groups, as both groups performed their exercises regularly. In the comparison, when the measurements made on 5 and 10 centimeters above the patella were compared, it was observed that there was no statistically significant difference in both groups.

Recently, many researchers have suggested an association between hip weakness or impaired motor control and PFPS. Poor hip control leads to abnormal patella friction, increased patellofemoral joint stress, and stress on the joint cartilage. Robinson et al., investigated the effectiveness of the hip strengthening program among 20 female patients aged 12-35 with unilateral knee pain complaints and the CG. Hip abduction, extension, and external rotation muscle strengths were measured in both groups. As a result, the hip muscle strength of the patients with PFPS was significantly lower compared to the healthy controls (19). In a cross-comparative study by Bolgla et al., they investigated whether decreased hip muscle strength caused femoral internal rotation and increased hip adduction and knee valgus in women diagnosed with PFPS. 18 female patients diagnosed with PFPS and 18 healthy female controls were compared. Hip abduction and external rotation muscle strength was evaluated in the pretreatment. Hip and knee kinematics of the patients were evaluated with a standardized stair step test. As a result, significant weakness was found in the hip muscles of patients with PFPS. Based on this, optimizing the muscle functions of the hip abductors and external rotators, preventing femoral movements from applying greater lateral force on the patella or reducing the existing lateral forces may be a possible treatment method for treatment of PFPS. Adding hip abductors and external rotators to the quadriceps strengthening program provides additional benefits as well as reduction in pain felt during functional activities after the six-week treatment program (20). In our study, the increase in hip abduction muscle strength of the patients was 5 % in CG and 6 % in LG. There was an increase in both groups and the groups had no superiority to each other.

ITB plays both a dynamic and passive role in the patellofemoral joint. Although ITB adheres to the tensor fascia proximally, joins vastus lateralis distally. A large part of the lateral retinaculum (superficial oblique and deep transverse part) comes from the ITB. Therefore, ITB provides lateral stabilization through indirect ways. Tense ITB adheres to the patella via the lateral retinaculum and increases lateral patellar shift, patellar tilt, and compression. Hudson et al., compared 12 patients with PFPS with 12 healthy subjects in a case-control study. ITB flexibility was evaluated by the Ober test. When the two groups were compared with each other, it was observed that patients with PFPS had tense ITB (21). In a cohort study, Tyler et al., included 35 patients (29 females, 6 males) in a 6-week treatment program. They investigated whether improvements in hip strength and flexibility are associated with a decrease in patellofemoral pain. Hip flexion, abduction, adduction muscle strength, Thomas and Ober tests results, VAS, activities of daily living and exercise evaluations were made at the beginning and end of the treatment. Strength and flexibility exercises focused on hip given to the patients. Improvements in hip flexion strength combined with increased ITB and iliopsoas flexibility were associated with excellent results in patients with PFPS (22). In our study, no statistical difference was found between the groups in the evaluations of pretreatment and posttreatment in ITB flexibility measurements.

Studies have generally grouped ITB, quadriceps, and hamstring flexibility together rather than under individual headings. Shortness of the hamstring muscle is related to the clinical features of the disease because hamstring shortness causes increased knee flexion, which increases patellofemoral joint friction forces. White et al., compared the hamstring flexibility of patients with PFPS between the ages of 18-35 and those in the healthy CG in their cross-comparative study. In the study, patients with PFPS were divided into 11 (6 males, 5 females) people, and the CG as 25 (12 females, 13 males) people. Hamstring shortness was evaluated by measuring the popliteal angle using the passive knee extension method. As a result, hamstring lengths of patients with PFPS were shorter than the CG (23). Piva et al. examined the differences in lower extremity muscle strength and flexibility on 30 patients (17 females, 13 males) in their case-control study. When patients with PFPS were compared with healthy CG, it was observed that the hamstring and quadriceps flexibility of patients with PFPS was significantly limited (24). Witvrouw et al. examined 282 students in terms of intrinsic and extrinsic characteristics in their two-year prospective study. During this period, 24 out of 282 students developed PFPS, but there was no significant difference in hamstring length between individuals with and without PFPS (25). In our study, no statistically significant relationship was found between hamstring flexibility and PFPS.

DDLT is a physical therapy modality used because of its analgesic and anti-inflammatory effects (26). In our study, we aimed to investigate the effectiveness of 830 nm Ga-As-Al laser in patients diagnosed with PFPS. Rogvi-Hansen et al. recruited 40 patellar chondromalacia patients to DDLT in their randomized, double-blind study. Ga-As (real and placebo) laser application was performed 8 times by the physiotherapist for 5 weeks. Pain localization, quality, intensity, how the pain affects the patient's mood, walking, sleep, work, and sports activities were evaluated in pretreatment and posttreatment. As a result, no statistically significant reduction in chondromalacia symptoms was observed in both groups (27). In a study conducted by Crossley et al., 89 articles were searched, and the effectiveness of various physical therapy applications were evaluated in 16 appropriate studies. As a result, no evidence supporting the treatment efficacy of DDT was found in the treatment of PSAS (28).

It has been shown that even in a small number of patient groups with a diagnosis of PFPS, statistically significant changes can be detected in pain evaluations using VAS performed after treatment (29). Based on this, it is correct to evaluate the pain and response to treatment with VAS. Crossley et al., divided 71 people into physical therapy group and CG in their randomized double-blind study. A standardized treatment program consisting of 6 sessions in total was applied once a week. In the evaluation, the most severe and usual pains experienced by the participants in the previous week were taken into consideration. In the physical therapy group (n=33), a significant reduction was found in mean pain, worst pain and disability compared to the CG (30). In a randomized controlled study in which Bily et al. compared the effectiveness of two different treatment programs in 38 patients with PFPS, they applied a physiotherapy program for 12 weeks in one group, and muscle stimulation with electricity in the other group with a physiotherapy program. The pain assessment of the patients was made with VAS. 36 patients completed the 12-week follow-up period. After 12 weeks of treatment, a statistically significant reduction in pain was observed in both groups, and the reduction in pain and improvement in function continued during the 1-year follow-up (5). Bjordal et al. examined 11 articles in their review. In these articles, DDLT was applied to the knee, temporomandibular and facet joints at the recommended dosage range. Results showed a significant decrease in the level of pain as a result of DDLT (31). Similar to the literature, in our study, resting and activity VAS values decreased in both groups during posttreatment and 1-month follow-up. Only in CG, this decrease did not continue in the first month control at rest.

The chronic pain associated with PFP often interferes with work, daily activities, and exercise, leading to reductions in both quality of life and overall physical activity (32). Piva et al. evaluated function and pain in patients with PFPS in their study. 74 patients diagnosed with PFPS were included in the study and participated in the physical therapy program. After the evaluations were completed, the patients were taken to the standardized physical therapy program. In the evaluation made in the 2nd month follow-up after the treatment, a significant statistical change was observed in both pain and function

(33). In SF-36 intragroup physical evaluation, significant improvement was observed in LG in posttreatment and first month follow-up. In mental comparison, there was no statistically significant change in intra and inter group comparison in both groups. In PDI evaluation, in intragroup comparison, improvement was observed in both groups in the first month follow-up, but there was no difference in the intergroup comparison.

Conclusion

DDLT used in the treatment of patients with PFPS caused a decrease in resting, activity pain value and QoL physical assessment in posttreatment and one month after the end of treatment. When the disability levels were evaluated, improvement was observed in posttreatment and one month after the end of treatment in both groups, but the superiority of the groups to each other was not determined.

References

1. Kuran, B., & Doğu, B. (2009). Ön diz ağrılarında tanı ve tedavi yaklaşımları. *Turkish Journal of Physical Medicine and Rehabilitation, 55*(1), 20-25.

2. Çubukçu, D., & Sarsan, A. (2008). Patellofemoral ağrı sendromunun rehabilitasyonu. *Rheumatism, 23*(1), 18-23.

3. Yılmaz, B., Alaca, R., Göktepe, S. A., Möhür, H., Kalyon, T. A. (2001). Patellofemoral ağrı sendromunda izokinetik egzersiz programının fonksiyonel kapasite ve ağrı üzerindeki etkisi. *Turkish Journal of Physical Medicine and Rehabilitation, 47*(5), 5-11.

4. Aydın A. T. (1995). Patellofemoral eklem hastalıkları (semptomatoloji, klinik tanı ve ayırıcı tanı). *Acta Orthopaedica et Traumatologica Turcica, 29*(5), 372-375.

5. Bily, W., Trimmel, L., Mödlin, M., Kaider, A., & Kern, H. (2008). Patellofemoral ağrı sendromu için antrenman programı ve ilave elektrik kas uyarımı: Bir pilot çalışma. *Archives of Physical Medicine Rehabilitation, 3*(4), 264-271.

6. Crossley, K. M., Callaghan, M. J., & van Linschoten, R. (2016). Patellofemoral pain. *British Journal of Sports Medicine, 50*(4), 247-250. doi:10.1136/bjsports-2015-h3939rep

7. Clijsen, R., Brunner, A., Barbero, M., Clarys, P., & Taeymans, J. (2017). Effects of low-level laser therapy on pain in patients with musculoskeletal disorders: A systematic review and meta-analysis. *European Journal*

of Physical and Rehabilitation Medicine, 53(4), 603-610. doi:10.23736/
S1973-9087.17.04432-X

8. Tait, R. C., Chibnall, J. T., Krause, S. (1990). The pain disability
index: Psychometric properties. *Pain, 40*(2), 171-182. doi:10.1016/
0304-3959(90)90068-o

9. Uğurlu, M., Uğurlu, G. K., Erten, Ş., Kaymak, S. U., & Çayköylü, A. (2016).
Reliability and factorial validity of the Turkish version of the pain disability
index in rheumatic patients with chronic pain. *Archives of Rheumatology,
31*(3), 265-271. doi:10.5606/ArchRheumatol.2016.5750

10. Ware, J. E., & Sherbourne, C. D. (1992). "The MOS 36-item short form
health survey", I. conceptual framework and item selection. *Medical Care,
30*(6), 473-483.

11. Koçyiğit, H., Aydemir, O., Fisek, G., Olmez, N., Memis, A. (1999). Validity
and reliability of Turkish version of short form 36: A study of a patients
with romatoid disorder. *Drug and Therapy, 12*, 102-106.

12. Hvid, I., & Andersen, L. I. (1982). The quadriceps angle and its relation
to femoral torsion. *Acta Orthopaedica Scandinavica, 53*(4), 577-579.
doi:10.3109/17453678208992261

13. Christou, E. A. (2004). Patellar taping increases vastus medialis oblique
activity in the presence of patellofemoral pain. *Journal of Electromyography
and Kinesiology, 14*(4), 495-504. doi:10.1016/j.jelekin.2003.10.007

14. Willson, J. D., & Davis, I. S. (2008). Lower extremity mechanics of females
with and without patellofemoral pain across activities with progressively
greater task demands. *Clinical Biomechanics, 23*(2), 203-211. doi:10.1016/
j.clinbiomech.2007.08.025

15. Balcı, P., Tunay, V. B., Baltacı, G., & Atay, A. Ö. (2009). The effects of
two different closed kinetic chain exercises on muscle strength and
proprioception in patients with patellofemoral pain syndrome. *Acta
Orthopaedica Et Traumatologica Turcica, 43*(5), 419-425. doi:10.3944/
AOTT.2009.419

16. Skinner, H. B. (2007). *Current diagnosis & treatment in orthopedics.*
California: Mc Graw-Hill.

17. Hart, H. F., Barton, C. J., Khan, K. M., Riel, H., & Crossley, K. M. (2017). Is
body mass index associated with patellofemoral pain and patellofemoral
osteoarthritis?   A   systematic   review   and   meta-regression   and
analysis. *British Journal of Sports Medicine, 51*(10), 781-790. doi:10.1136/
bjsports-2016-096768

18. Bakhtiary, A. H., & Faterni, E. (2008). Open versus closed kinetic chain
exercises for patellar chondromalacia. *British Journal of Sports Medicine,
42*(2), 99-102. doi:10.1136/bjsm.2007.038109

19. Robinson, R. L., & Nee, R. J. (2007). Analysis of hip strength in females seeking physical therapy treatment for unilateral patellofemoral pain syndrome. *The Journal of Orthopaedic and Sports Physical Therapy*, 37(5), 232-238. doi:10.2519/jospt.2007.2439

20. Bolgla, A. L., Malone, T. R., Umberger, B. R., & Uhl, T. L. (2008). Hip strength and hip and knee kinematics during stair descent in females with and without patellofemoral pain syndrome. *The Journal of Orthopaedic and Sports Physical Therapy*, 38(1), 12-18. doi:10.2519/jospt.2008.2462

21. Hudson, Z., & Darthuy, E. (2009). Iliotibial band tightness and patellofemoral pain syndrome: A case control study. *Manual Therapy*, 14(2), 147-151. doi:10.1016/j.math.2007.12.009

22. Tyler, T. F., Nicholas, S. J., Mullaney, M. J., & McHugh, M. P. (2006). The role of hip muscle function in the treatment of patellofemoral pain syndrome. *The American Journal of Sports Medicine*, 34(4), 630-636. doi:10.1177/0363546505281808

23. White, L. C., Dolphin, P., & Dixon, J. (2009). Hamstring length in patellofemoral pain syndrome. *Physiotherapy*, 95(1), 24-28. doi:10.1016/j.physio.2008.05.009

24. Piva, S. R., Goodnite, E. A., & Childs, J. D. (2005). Strength around the hip and flexibility of soft tissues in individuals with and without patellofemoral pain syndrome. *The Journal of Orthopaedic And Sports Physical Therapy*, 35(12), 793-801. doi:10.2519/jospt.2005.35.12.793

25. Witvrouw, E., Lysens, R., Bellemans, J., Cambier, D., & Vanderstraeten, G. (2000). Intrinsic risk factors for the development of anterior knee pain in an athletic population a two-year prospective study. *The American Journal of Sports Medicine*, 28(4), 480-489. doi:10.1177/03635465000280040701

26. Huang, Z., Ma, J., Chen, J., Shen, B., Pei, F., & Kraus, V. B. (2015). The effectiveness of low-level laser therapy for nonspecific chronic low back pain: A systematic review and meta-analysis. *Arthritis Research & Therapy*, 17(1), 360. doi:10.1186/s13075-015-0882-0

27. Rogvi-Hansen, B., Ellitsgaard, N., Funch, M., Dall-Jensen, M., & Prieske J. (1991). Low level laser treatment of chondromalacia patellae. *International Orthopaedics*, 15(4), 359-361. doi:10.1007/BF00186879

28. Crossley, K., Bennell, K., Green, S., & McConnell, J. (2001). A systematic review of physical interventions for patellofemoral pain syndrome. *Clinical Journal of Sport Medicine*, 11(2), 103-110. doi:10.1097/00042752-200104000-00007

29. Bennell, K., Bartam, S., Crossley, K., & Green, S. (2000). Outcome measures in patellofemoral pain syndrome: Test retest reliability and

inter-relationships. *Physical Therapy in Sport, 1*(2), 32-41. doi:10.1054/ptsp.2000.0009

30. Crossley, K., Bennell, K., Green, S., Cowan, S., & McConnell, J. (2002). Physical therapy for patellofemoral pain: A randomized, double-blinded, placebo-controlled trial. *The American Journal of Sports Medicine, 30*(6), 857-865. doi:10.1177/03635465020300061701

31. Bjordal, J. M., Couppé, C., Chow, R. T., Tunér, J., & Ljunggren, E. A. (2003). A systematic review of low level laser therapy with location-specific doses for pain from chronic joint disorders. *The Australian Journal of Physiotherapy, 49*(2), 107-116. doi:10.1016/s0004-9514(14)60127-6

32. Crossley, K. M., Zhang, W. J., Schache, A. G., Bryant, A., & Cowan, S. M. (2011). Performance on the single-leg squat task indicates hip abductor muscle function. *The American Journal of Sports Medicine, 39*(4), 866–873. doi:10.1177/0363546510395456

33. Piva, S. R., Fitzgerald, G. K., Wisniewski, S., & Delitto, A. (2009). Predictors of pain and function outcome after rehabilitation in patients with patellofemoral pain syndrome. *Journal of Rehabilitation Medicine, 41*(8), 604-612. doi:10.2340/16501977-0372

Pelin Pişirici, Leyla Ataş Balcı, and Seda Akkoyun

The Effect of Instrument Assisted Soft Tissue Mobilization Technique on Proprioception and Balance in Individuals with Non-specific Neck Pain - Pilot Study

Abstract

Objective: To investigate the acute effect of instrument assisted soft tissue mobilization (IASTM) technique applied to cervical region muscles on balance and proprioception in individuals with non-specific neck pain (NSNP).

Materials and Methods: A total of 20 individuals with NSNP, 11 women and 9 men, between the ages of 20-40 years old (mean age 27.80±13.67), who had pain for at least 3 months were included in the study. The pain intensity levels during the resting, activity and night, disability levels, cervical range of motion (ROM), proprioception and static, dynamic balance measurements were evaluated before and after the application with a visual analog scale (VAS) of 10 centimeters, neck disability index (NDI), CROM (Cervical Range Of Motion) device and Biodex balance device, respectively. After the warm-up exercise program, IASTM technique was applied to right and left side cervical muscles for 8 minutes with Graston Technique® (GT®) instruments.

Results: After the application, a statistically significant increase was observed in the ROM measurements of cervical flexion, extension, right and left lateral flexion, right and left rotation and, in the static and dynamic overall, anteroposterior and mediolateral balance performances (p<0.05 for all). While a significant increase was observed on the right side (p=0.005), no statistically significant difference was found on the left side (p=0.162) in the proprioception measurements.

Conclusion: It has been found that myofascial release applied with IASTM technique to the individuals with NSNP causes an increase in cervical ROM and balance. In the proprioception evaluation, a statistically significant improvement was observed only on the dominant side.

Keywords: Graston Technique, Instrument Assisted Soft Tissue Mobilization, Non-specific Neck Pain, Postural Stability, Proprioception

Introduction

Sensorimotor control refers to the control of the central nervous system (CNS) on movement, balance, posture, and joint stability. Well-adapted motor movements require robust and well-integrated information from the somatosensory system, including proprioceptive, visual, and vestibular senses. The muscles of the cervical region, especially the suboccipital muscles, are the most important structures that provide proprioceptive information since they contain a large number of mechanoreceptors (1). Non-specific neck pain (NSNP) is defined as pain, without any signs of major structural pathology and is not caused by any specific problem such as trauma, fracture, tumor, infection or inflammation in the posterior and lateral region of the neck between the superior nuchal line of the neck and the spinous process of the first thoracic vertebra (2). Problems may occur in proprioception, balance, and range of motion in acute and chronic cervical pathologies (1,3,4). Therefore, patients with NSNP have problems in head and neck posture, function of neck muscles, proprioception, and balance (5,6). As a result of proprioception changes that caused by pain, inadequacies may be experienced in planning, control, and timing of body movements. Any change in cervical proprioception can affect the person's posture, standing and walking performance, and increase the risk of injury in sports activities (7,8).

Although there are various approaches for the treatment of NSNP, no gold standard treatment method has been determined yet (9). Patient education, recommendations for high activity level, ergonomic arrangements, medical therapy, manual therapy, local and epidural injections, massage, acupuncture, ozone therapy, orthotics, physical therapy agents, traction, laser, and various exercise routines are commonly used approaches in the treatment of NSNP (2). Despite all treatment approaches, there is a 50-85 % improvement in symptoms. However, the complete recovery cannot be achieved. In addition, symptoms appear to recur within 1-5 years (10).

In recent years, effects of soft tissue mobilization techniques on proprioception and balance in the individuals with musculoskeletal disorders have been investigated (11-14). The reason for the increased interest in soft tissue mobilization techniques is the large number of mechanoreceptors in the structure of the fascia. Because of that fascia is defined as an organ of stability and mechanoregulation (15). Instrument assisted soft tissue mobilization (IASTM) technique, one of the fascial mobilization techniques, is a treatment approach created by James Cyriax. Although there are many instruments and techniques used under different names for soft tissue mobilization, the most used one in the literature is Graston Technique® (GT®) (16,17). The heat generated by the frictional force, created by the instruments, reduces tissue viscosity. At the same time, because of stimulation of the mechanoreceptors that exposed to mechanical stress with this technique, the proprioceptive data which sent to CNS changes and the tension in the damaged tissue decreases. The increase of ROM and the healing process begin in the damaged soft tissue (18,19).

A multimodal approach has been proposed to evaluate changes in sensori-motor control, as no single approach can address all aspects of sensorimotor function (20). The sensorimotor control can be evaluated indirectly with the assessments of proprioception and balance. Proprioception is evaluated by the acuity of repositioning the head, which is defined as the ability to return the head to neutral position after active movements (21-23).

There has been no study examining the effect of soft tissue mobilization with GT® on the balance and proprioception of the cervical region. This study is a pilot study was conducted to investigate the acute effect of IASTM technique on proprioception and balance in the individuals with NSNP.

Materials and Methods

This study was approved by the "Ethics Committee Decision" dated 19.07.2019 and numbered 10840098-604.01.01-E.33227 by the Non-Invasive Clinical Research Ethics Committee of İstanbul Medipol University. It was carried out in Bahçeşehir University, Faculty of Health Sciences, Physiotherapy and Rehabilitation Laboratory. All participants were informed about the study and their written consents were obtained.

Participants

The universe of the study includes the students, academic and administrative staff of Bahçeşehir University. The study included 20 individuals aged between 20 and 40, who had pain for at least 3 months, had at least 10 % loss in cervical rotation ROM, had the neck disability index (NDI) score ≤15/50, and diagnosed NSNP. Pain related to a specific cause such as acute cervical pain, fracture, spondylolisthesis, disc herniation and cervical stenosis; neurological, endocrinological, orthopedic diseases, other systemic diseases that may affect balance; surgical procedure history due to past neck pain, congenital anomalies and pregnancy were the exclusion criteria.

Participants' age, body weight, height, body mass index, gender, disease history and neck pain durations were recorded. The hand which the participants signed the voluntary consent form was accepted as the dominant extremity, and verbal confirmation was also obtained.

Evaluations

The pain intensity levels of the individuals during the rest, activity and night were evaluated with the 10-centimeter Visual Analogue Scale (VAS) (24) and the disability levels due to neck pain determined by the NDI (25) before the GT° application.

Visual Analogue Scale: It is a scale between 0 and 10 points. 0 corresponds to no pain, 10 corresponds to unbearable pain. It is a scale that has been validated for use in the pathologies of cervical region, in which the patient self-evaluates the pain intensity at the moment of evaluation (26).

Neck Disability Index: Each question is scored between 0 and 5 in the scale consisting of ten sub-divisions that evaluate the effect of neck pain on the daily living activities of the individual, including pain severity, personal care, lifting, reading, headache, attention, work, driving, sleep and leisure activities. The total score ranges from 0 (no disability) to 100 (severe disability). NDI was developed by Vernon et al. In 1991 (25), and its Turkish validity and reliability study was conducted by Aslan et al. in 2008 (27).

Cervical Range of Motion Measurements: It was measured with CROM (Cervical Range of Motion) device (Spine Products, basic version, Performance Attainment Associates, Roseville, MN, USA). CROM is an inclinometer system that takes advantage of gravity and magnetic effect. It is an instrument consisting of two inclinometers related to gravity in the sagittal and frontal planes, an inclinometer with magnetic needle attached from the top in the horizontal plane, a magnetic collar, an arm with a ruler in centimeters and a vertebral fixing arm with a scale system. The CROM device has been proven to be a valid and reliable device for measuring cervical ROM (28-30). This study was conducted with reference to the protocol used by Audette et al. (30). Participants were asked to sit in a stable chair, with both feet fully supported on the ground, and their hands on their thighs. The shoulders and torso were fixed with straps to allow movement only in the neck. The participants were first asked to look straight ahead, then move their head in the direction the researcher wanted, without moving the shoulders and torso. Cervical ROM was evaluated by taking the average of three random ordered measurement of the flexion, extension, right and left lateral flexion and rotation of the neck. Before any measurement was recorded, a trial was done once in each direction to let the participants learn the procedure and the movements in which the interval was measured.

Proprioception Assessment: The assessment of proprioception with the CROM device has been proven to be a reliable clinical method (21,22). Head repositioning accuracy (HRA) to neutral that we used in our study is a method frequently used in the literature (21,22,31). HRA is the ability of reposition the neck to the neutral position with the eyes closed after the 30° of cervical rotation. This study was conducted with reference to the protocol used by

Wibault et al. (21). This protocol has previously been proven to be valid for detecting differences between healthy individuals and individuals with neck pathology (32). Participants were placed in a fixed chair without back support, with both feet fully supported on the ground, and a CROM device was placed on their head. The neutral head position is the point where the inclinometer of the CROM device reads as 0° in the primary plane of the movement. This point has been accepted as the starting and reference point. Individuals were asked to close their eyes, memorize the starting position, actively rotate their head to 30° and return their heads to the starting position without any speed restriction, but with maximum precision. After rotating to the right and left three times, respectively, the joint position sense error (JPSE) was recorded and averaged in degrees.

Balance Assessment: The Biodex Balance System (BBS) (Biodex 945-302, Biodex Medical Systems Inc., Shirley, New York, USA) was used for the objective evaluation of the static and dynamic balance. BBS is a valid and reliable device for the assessment of the static and dynamic balance (33). In the device, which can allow free movement in the anterior-posterior (AP) and medial-lateral (ML) planes, it can be difficult to stay in stable on the 20° inclined platform with eight different resistances. Overall stability index (OSI), anteroposterior stability index (APSI) and mediolateral stability index (MLSI) show overall, anterior-posterior, and right-left balance ability, respectively. Increasing scores in BBS indicates a decrease and a deterioration in balance (34). Balance assessments of the participants were made with bare feet with their eyes open and their hands on their hips. In the assessment of the static postural balance, the participants were asked to keep the moving black dot that they see on the screen in the center for 20 seconds after the trial period of one minute. In the assessment of dynamic balance, the difficulty level of the platform was chosen as 4. The average of the OSI, APSI and MLSI scores of the individuals were recorded by taking 3 measurements, each lasting 20 seconds and having 10 seconds rest time between them.

Intervention

Before soft tissue mobilization with GT° instruments, a mild warm-up program consisting of cervical ROM exercises was applied to the participants to make the tissue ready for application. Each exercise was done for 30 seconds and 3 times in total. While exercising, it was desired to avoid pain and to maintain of the correct posture. The application protocol was determined by a GT° certified physiotherapist, with reference to the GT° user manual (35).

Suboccipital muscles, cervical extensors, scalene muscles, upper trapezius, and sternocleidomastoid muscles were scanned with GT® instruments, problematic areas were detected, and application focused on damaged soft tissues. A total of 8 minutes was applied, 4 minutes on the right and left sides.

Statistical Analysis

The statistical analysis of the study was performed using the SPSS 22.0 (SPSS Inc., Chicago, II., USA) package program. The mean, standard deviation, median and percentage were calculated in the measurement data. After measuring the normality test, Wilcoxon Test, one of the non-parametric tests, was used for the analysis of the data. The sample size is based on the difference in the JPSE in neck rotation in the chronic neck pain (CNP) patients and asymptomatic. In the calculation made with G*Power, it was seen that 58 individuals with 2° (80 %) difference, 80 % power, 95 % confidence and 2.78 standard deviation were required to participate. By increasing the sample size to 64, a dropout rate of 10 % was allowed (36). This study is a pilot study with a sample size of 20 in order to evaluate preliminary results before conducting a randomized controlled study.

Results

Eleven of the participants were female (55 %) and 9 (45 %) were male, with an average age of 27.80 (13.67) years. Their mean height was 172.45 (11.19) centimeters, their mean weight was 68.40±16.77 kilograms, and their mean body mass index was 22.77 (4.06). Their mean pain duration was 24.69 (32.39) months. Their mean pain intensities, according to VAS, were 4.05 (1.95) at the rest, 4.65 (2.41) during the activity and 2.85 (2.36) centimeters at the night. Their mean NDI score was 9.90 (4.27). All participants were right-handed. Demographic characteristics of the participants were shown in Table 1.

Range of Motion

The statistically significant differences were observed in the comparison of the pre-treatment and post-treatment measurements of the cervical flexion, extension, right lateral flexion, left lateral flexion, right rotation, and left rotation (p<0.05) (Table 2).

Balance and Proprioception

A statistically significant difference was found in the comparison of OSI, APSI and MLSI scores of the participants before and after the treatment (p<0.05).

Tab. 1: Descriptive Characteristics of Participants

Variables		Mean (SD)
Age		27.80 (13.67)
BMI		22.77 (4.06)
VAS (rest)		4.05 (1.95)
VAS (activity)		4.65 (2.41)
VAS (night)		2.85 (2.36)
NDI		9.90 (4.06)
		n (%)
Gender	Female	11 (55 %)
	Male	9 (45 %)
Dominant side	Right	20 (100 %)
	Left	0 (0 %)

SD: Standard Deviation; BMI: Body Mass Index; VAS: Visual Analogue Scale; NDI: Neck Disability Index

While there was a significant difference in the proprioception measurements of the right rotation in comparison of the pre- and post-treatment ($p<0.05$), no statistically significant difference was found in the proprioception measurements of the left rotation ($p>0.05$) (Table 2).

Discussion

As a result of the literature review, this is the first study investigating the effect of GT° treatment applied to the cervical region on proprioception, balance, and ROM in individuals with NSNP. In our study, it was determined that the myofascial release protocol applied according to the GT° user manual (35) had statistically positive effects on the participant's dominant side proprioception, static and dynamic balance, and ROM.

Proprioception

Muscle spindles are found in high density in the cervical region, especially in the suboccipital region, which has 200 muscle spindles per 1 gram of muscle. The importance of the cervical region is better understood when this number is compared with the lumbrical muscle of the thumb, where there are 16 muscle spindles per 1 gram. Trauma, functional impairment of receptors, changes in muscle spindle sensitivity, and changes in the nervous system caused by high

Tab. 2: Comparison of Pre- and Post-intervention Measurements of the Range of Motion, Balance and Proprioception

Variables	Pre Mean (SD)	Post Mean (SD)	Change Mean (SD)	p^*
Flexion	58.80 (9.09)	67.55 (9.82)	-3.655	**0.000**
Extension	62.10 (10.82)	69.90 (11.22)	-3.253	**0.001**
Right Lateral Flexion	39.45 (6.76)	47.90 (9.07)	-3.517	**0.000**
Left Lateral Flexion	42.25 (5.81)	50.60 (10.12)	-3.572	**0.000**
Right Rotation	57.15 (15.83)	62.85 (14.39)	-2.202	**0.028**
Left Rotation	59.75 (20.93)	68.65 (17.64)	-2.708	**0.007**
Overall Dynamic	1.23 (0.86)	0.96 (0.55)	-2.421	**0.015**
Overall Static	0.44 (0.24)	0.30 (0.12)	-2.653	**0.008**
AP Dynamic	0.83 (0.64)	0.64 (0.37)	-2.063	**0.039**
AP Static	0.32 (0.18)	0.23 (0.09)	-2.507	**0.012**
ML Dynamic	0.74 (0.46)	0.55 (0.37)	-2.715	**0.007**
ML Static	0.20 (0.14)	0.11 (0.07)	-2.667	**0.008**
Proprioception of Right Rotation	3.95 (4.34)	0.25 (1.11)	-2.797	**0.005**
Proprioception of Right Rotation	2.9 (3.65)	1.35 (3.18)	-1.399	0.162

*SD: Standard Deviation; AP: Anteroposterior; ML: Mediolateral; *Wilcoxon Signed Ranks Test p<0.05*

amounts of pain cause deterioration in afferent information from cervical receptors. Dysfunction of cervical receptors can alter afferent input by altering the integration, timing, and setting of sensorimotor control in neck diseases. In patients with neck pain, evaluation of the sensorimotor control is as important as performing the lower extremity proprioceptive training following the ankle or knee injury (5).

There is no definitive evidence in the literature about proprioception in individuals with CNP. While some studies gave different JPSE (4,31,37), others did not find a difference between the people with CNP and asymptomatic controls (22,38). Reid et al. stated that individuals with JPSE have 3°-4° of deficit (4). As well as Kristjansson et al. found JPSE as 3.33° (1.42) in individuals with insidious neck pain (31). This means that greater JPSE is seen in cervical region pathologies (21). In our study, in accordance with this information, pre-treatment JPSE were determined as 3.95° (4.34) in right rotation and 2.9° (3.65) in left rotation.

GT° is an approach that creates a significant increase in flexibility by creating pressure and friction on myofascia. In addition, the intrafascial receptors are stimulated with the mechanical stress applied by the instruments. The tension in the motor units connected to the tissue changes with the proprioceptive input which sent to the CNS (18,39). In order to observe the changes in ROM and proprioception more clearly after GT° application, the condition of having 10 % ROM loss was added to the inclusion criteria. Faulkner et al. stated that self-myofascial release improves the physical awareness of the person, the joint sensitivity, the function of proprioceptors, balance, and muscle strength (40). Similarly, Cho et al. found that self-myofascial release was increased the muscle flexibility and joint proprioception (41). Like the literature, in our study, it is found that there is an increase in cervical ROM, right-sided proprioception and balance after GT° application. It is thought that the lack of significant change in left-sided proprioception after the application may be related to the fact that the dominant sides of the participants are right-sided.

Balance

IASTM is used for myofascial release and stimulation of motor nerves (39), as well as providing sensory input for joint position. These sensory inputs ensure the proper body alignment (42). Schaefer et al. demonstrated that the application of dynamic balance training and GT° for twice a week for 4 weeks gave the most effective results in ROM, pain, and disability in individuals with chronic ankle instability (14). Kim et al showed that, in their study on football players, exercise and GT° application 5 days a week for 12 weeks increased balance besides the positive effects on isokinetic strength measurement, muscle fatigue and physical fitness (42). In our study, in accordance with the results of these studies, a statistically significant increase was observed in the static and dynamic balance performances of the participants. Whether the GT° directly improves the dynamic postural stability is unknown, but an increase in ROM, reduction in pain, and increased function may contribute to improvement. Improvements in balance may be related to the newly acquired ROM and flexibility since it provides more flexibility and more mobility (14). Our study contributes to the literature as it is the first study examining the acute effect of the GT° on balance.

Range of Motion

Adequate ROM is required for optimal musculoskeletal function. As a result of the loss of ROM and decrease in flexibility, people become susceptible to various musculoskeletal diseases (19). The goal of increasing flexibility is generally to prevent injury, improve performance, and provide recovery after injury (43). Many studies have shown that GT° application causes an increase in ROM (14,44,45). While some of these studies include combined treatment applications between 3 and 12 weeks (14,46-48), some studies have found a significant increase in ROM after single session application (39,42,44). In our study, a statistically significant increase was obtained in all cervical ROM in accordance with these studies.

Conclusion

As far as we know, this is the first study about the application of GT° to the cervical region muscles in individuals with NSNP. This study is our first step to fill the gap in the literature. Our study is a pilot study in which acute results are evaluated. In future studies evaluating the effectiveness of GT° application, the relationship between the changes in proprioception and the dominant side should also be examined. Also, the effectiveness of only GT° and the combinations of the GT° application and exercise on the NSNP should be investigated.

References

1. Röijezon, U., Clark, N. C., & Treleaven, J. (2015). Proprioception in musculoskeletal rehabilitation. Part 1: Basic science and principles of assessment and clinical interventions. *Manual Therapy*, 20(3), 368-377. doi:10.1016/j.math.2015.01.008

2. Hidalgo, B., Hall, T., Bossert, J., Dugeny, A., Cagnie, B., & Pitance, L. (2017). The efficacy of manual therapy and exercise for treating non-specific neck pain: A systematic review. *Journal of Back and Musculoskeletal Rehabilitation*, *30*(6), 1149-1169. doi:10.3233/BMR-169615

3. Page, P., Frank, C., & Lardner, R. (2009). *Assessment and treatment of muscle imbalance: The janda approach*. Windsor, Ontario, Canada: Human Kinetics.

4. Reid, S. A., Callister, R., Katekar, M. G., & Rivett, D. A. (2014). Effects of cervical spine manual therapy on range of motion, head repositioning, and balance in participants with cervicogenic dizziness: A randomized controlled trial. *Archives of Physical Medicine and Rehabilitation*, *95*(9), 1603-1612. doi:10.1016/j.apmr.2014.04.009

5. Treleaven, J. (2008). Sensorimotor disturbances in neck disorders affecting postural stability, head and eye movement control. *Manual Therapy*, *13*(1), 2-11. doi:10.1016/j.math.2007.06.003

6. Saadat, M., Salehi, R., Negahban, H., Shaterzadeh, M. J., Mehravar, M., & Hessam, M. (2018). Postural stability in patients with non-specific chronic neck pain: A comparative study with healthy people. *Medical Journal of the Islamic Republic of Iran*, *32-33*. doi:10.14196/mjiri.32.33

7. Okhravi, S. M., Zavveyeh, M. K., Kalantari, K. K., Baghban, A. A., & Karimi, M. T. (2015). A study on the effects of general fatigue on head and neck proprioception in healthy young adults. *Ortopedia, Traumatologia, Rehabilitacja*, *17*(1), 1-6. doi:10.5604/15093492.1143513

8. Amiri Arimi, S., Ghamkhar, L., & Kahlaee, A. H. (2018). The relevance of proprioception to chronic neck pain: A correlational analysis of flexor muscle size and endurance, clinical neck pain characteristics, and proprioception. *Pain Medicine*, *19*(10), 2077-2088. doi:10.1093/pm/pnx331

9. Tsakitzidis, G., Remmen, R., Dankaerts, W., & Van Royen, P. (2013). Non-specific neck pain and evidence-based practice. *European Scientific Journal*, *9*(3), 1-19.

10. Haldeman, S., Carroll, L., Cassidy, J. D., Schubert, J., & Nygren, A. (2008). The bone and joint decade 2000-2010 task force on neck pain and its associated disorders. *European Spine Journal*, *17*(Suppl 1), 5-7. doi:10.1007/s00586-008-0619-8

11. David, E., Amasay, T., Ludwig, K., & Shapiro, S. (2019). The effect of foam rolling of the hamstrings on proprioception at the knee and hip joints. *International Journal of Exercise Science*, *12*(1), 343-354.

12. Junker, D., & Stöggl, T. (2019). The training effects of foam rolling on core strength endurance, balance, muscle performance and range of motion: A

randomized controlled trial. *Journal of Sports Science & Medicine, 18*(2), 229-238.

13. Lee, C. L., Chu, I. H., Lyu, B. J., Chang, W. D., & Chang, N. J. (2018). Comparison of vibration rolling, nonvibration rolling, and static stretching as a warm-up exercise on flexibility, joint proprioception, muscle strength, and balance in young adults. *Journal of Sports Sciences, 36*(22), 2575-2582. doi:10.1080/02640414.2018.1469848

14. Schaefer, J. L., & Sandrey, M. A. (2012). Effects of a 4-week dynamic-balance-training program supplemented with graston instrument-assisted soft-tissue mobilization for chronic ankle instability. *Journal of Sport Rehabilitation, 21*(4), 313-326. doi:10.1123/jsr.21.4.313

15. Myers, T. W. (2009). *Anatomy trains: Myofascial meridians for manual and movement therapists.* London: Elsevier Health Sciences.

16. Sevier, T. L., & Wilson, J. K. (1999). Treating lateral epicondylitis. *Sports Medicine, 28*(5), 375-380. doi:10.2165/00007256-199928050-00006

17. Fowler, S., Wilson, J. K., Sevier, T. L. (2000). Innovative approach for the treatment of cumulative trauma disorders. *Work, 15*(1), 9-14.

18. Schleip, R. (2003). Fascial plasticity-a new neurobiological explanation part 2. *Journal of Bodywork and Movement Therapies, 7*(2), 104-116. doi:10.1016/S1360-8592(02)00076-1

19. Kim, J., Sung, D. J., & Lee, J. (2017). Therapeutic effectiveness of instrument-assisted soft tissue mobilization for soft tissue injury: Mechanisms and practical application. *Journal of Exercise Rehabilitation, 13*(1), 12-22. doi:10.12965/jer.1732824.412

20. Izquierdo, T. G., Pecos-Martin, D., Girbés, E. L., Plaza-Manzano, G., Caldentey, R. R., Melús, R. M., ... Falla, D. (2016). Comparison of cranio-cervical flexion training versus cervical proprioception training in patients with chronic neck pain: A randomized controlled clinical trial. *Journal of Rehabilitation Medicine, 48*(1), 48-55. doi:10.2340/16501977-2034

21. Wibault, J., Vaillant, J., Vuillerme, N., Dedering, Å., & Peolsson, A. (2013). Using the cervical range of motion (CROM) device to assess head repositioning accuracy in individuals with cervical radiculopathy in comparison to neck-healthy individuals. *Manual Therapy, 18*(5), 403-409. doi:10.1016/j.math.2013.02.004

22. Treleaven, J., Peterson, G., Ludvigsson, M. L., Kammerlind, A. S., & Peolsson, A. (2016). Balance, dizziness and proprioception in patients with chronic whiplash associated disorders complaining of dizziness: A prospective randomized study comparing three exercise programs. *Manual Therapy, 22*, 122-130. doi:10.1016/j.math.2015.10.017

23. Duray, M., Şimşek, Ş., Altuğ, F., & Cavlak, U. (2018). Effect of proprioceptive training on balance in patients with chronic neck pain. *Ağrı-The Journal of The Turkish Society of Algology, 30*(3), 130-137. doi:10.5505/agri.2018.61214

24. Gross, A. R., Paquin, J. P., Dupont, G., Blanchette, S., Lalonde, P., Cristie, T., ... Bronfort, G. (2016). Exercises for mechanical neck disorders: A Cochrane review update. *Manuel Therapy, 24.* 25-45. doi:10.1016/j.math.2016.04.005

25. Vernon, H., & Mior, S. (1991). The neck disability index: A study of reliability and validity. *Journal of Manipulative and Physiological Therapeutics, 14*(7), 409-415.

26. MacDowall, A., Skeppholm, M., Robinson, Y., & Olerud, C. (2018). Validation of the visual analog scale in the cervical spine. *Journal of Neurosurgery. Spine, 28*(3), 227-235. doi:10.3171/2017.5.SPINE1732

27. Aslan, E., Karaduman, A., Yakut, Y., Aras, B., Simsek, I. E., & Yaglý, N. (2008). The cultural adaptation, reliability and validity of neck disability index in patients with neck pain: a Turkish version study. *Spine, 33*(11), E362-E365. doi:10.1097/BRS.0b013e31817144e1

28. Tousignant, M., de Bellefeuille, L., O'Donoughue, S., & Grahovac, S. (2000). Criterion validity of the cervical range of motion (CROM) goniometer for cervical flexion and extension. *Spine, 25*(3), 324-330. doi:10.1097/00007632-200002010-00011

29. Dhimitri, K., Brodeur, S., Croteau, M., Richard, S., & Seymour, C. J. (1998). Reliability of the cervical range of motion device in measuring upper cervical motion. *Journal of Manual & Manipulative Therapy, 6*(1), 31-36. doi:10.1179/jmt.1998.6.1.31

30. Audette, I., Dumas, J. P., Côté, J. N., & De Serres, S. J. (2010). Validity and between-day reliability of the cervical range of motion (CROM) device. *Journal of Orthopaedic & Sports Physical Therapy, 40*(5), 318-323. doi:10.2519/jospt.2010.3180

31. Kristjansson, E., Dall'Alba, P., & Jull, G. (2003). A study of five cervicocephalic relocation tests in three different subject groups. *Clinical Rehabilitation, 17*(7), 768-774. doi:10.1191/0269215503cr676oa

32. Treleaven, J., Jull, G., & Sterling, M. (2003). Dizziness and unsteadiness following whiplash injury: Characteristic features and relationship with cervical joint position error. *Journal of Rehabilitation Medicine, 35*(1), 36-43. doi:10.1080/16501970306109

33. Arnold, B. L., Schmitz, R. J. (1998). Examination of balance measures produced by the biodex stability system. *Journal of Athletic Training, 33*(4), 323-327.

34. İnanır, A., Okan, S., & Yıldırım, E. (2013). Postural stability and fall risk in rheumatoid arthritis. *Cukurova Medical Journal, 38*(1), 72-77.

35. Carey-Loghmani, M.T., Schrader, J. W., Hammer, W. I. (2014). *Clinical foundations for graston technique® adapted from: Graston technique® m1 instruction manual.*

36. Jull, G., Falla, D., Treleaven, J., Hodges, P., & Vicenzino, B. (2007). Retraining cervical joint position sense: The effect of two exercise regimes. *Journal of Orthopaedic Research, 25*(3), 404-412. doi:10.1002/jor.20220

37. Cheng, C. H., Wang, J. L., Lin, J. J., Wang, S. F., & Lin, K. H. (2010). Position accuracy and electromyographic responses during head reposition in young adults with chronic neck pain. *Journal of Electromyography and Kinesiology, 20*(5), 1014-1020. doi:10.1016/j.jelekin.2009.11.002

38. Rix, G. D., & Bagust, J. (2001). Cervicocephalic kinesthetic sensibility in patients with chronic, nontraumatic cervical spine pain. *Archives of Physical Medicine and Rehabilitation, 82*(7), 911-919. doi:10.1053/apmr.2001.23300

39. Markovic, G. (2015). Acute effects of instrument assisted soft tissue mobilization vs. foam rolling on knee and hip range of motion in soccer players. *Journal of Bodywork and Movement Therapies, 19*(4), 690-696. doi:10.1016/j.jbmt.2015.04.010

40. Faulkner, J. A., Larkin, L. M., Claflin, D. R., & Brooks, S. V. (2007). Age-related changes in the structure and function of skeletal muscles. *Clinical and Experimental Pharmacology and Physiology, 34*(11), 1091-1096. doi:10.1111/j.1440-1681.2007.04752.x

41. Cho, S. H., & Kim, S. H. (2016). Immediate effect of stretching and ultrasound on hamstring flexibility and proprioception. *Journal of Physical Therapy Science, 28*(6), 1806-1808. doi:10.1589/jpts.28.1806

42. Kim, D. H., & Lee, J. J. (2018). Effects of instrument-assisted soft tissue mobilization technique on strength, knee joint passive stiffness, and pain threshold in hamstring shortness. *Journal of Back and Musculoskeletal Rehabilitation, 31*(6), 1169-1176. doi:10.3233/BMR-170854

43. Baker, R. T., Nasypany, A., Seegmiller, J. G., & Baker, J. G. (2013). Instrument-assisted soft tissue mobilization treatment for tissue extensibility dysfunction. *International Journal of Athletic Therapy and Training, 18*(5), 16-21. doi:10.1123/ijatt.18.5.16

44. Laudner, K., Compton, B. D., McLoda, T. A., & Walters, C. M. (2014). Acute effects of instrument assisted soft tissue mobilization for improving posterior shoulder range of motion in collegiate baseball players. *International Journal of Sports Physical Therapy, 9*(1), 1-7.

45. Hammer, W. I., & Pfefer, M. T. (2005). Treatment of a case of subacute lumbar compartment syndrome using the graston technique. *Journal of Manipulative and Physiological Therapeutics, 28*(3), 199-204. doi:10.1016/j.jmpt.2005.02.010

46. Black, D. W. (2010). Treatment of knee arthrofibrosis and quadriceps insufficiency after patellar tendon repair: A case report including use of the graston technique. *International Journal of Therapeutic Massage & Bodywork, 3*(2), 14-21.

47. Solecki, T. J., & Herbst, E. M. (2011). Chiropractic management of a postoperative complete anterior cruciate ligament rupture using a multimodal approach: A case report. *Journal of Chiropractic Medicine, 10*(1), 47-53. doi:10.1016/j.jcm.2010.07.005

48. Solecki, T. J., & Hostnik, K. D. (2012). Chiropractic management of a patient with postoperative lateral retinacular release using a multimodal approach: A case report. *Journal of Chiropractic Medicine, 11*(1), 42-48. doi:10.1016/j.jcm.2011.10.003

Semih Özdemir, Hasan Kerem Alptekin, and Mirsad Alkan

Effects of Kinesio Taping on Balance and Performance in Healthy Adults with Dynamic Knee Valgus

Abstract

Objective: This research aims that, assess to immediate effects of kinesio taping on balance and performance in healthy adults with dynamic knee valgus.

Materials and Methods: Thirty healthy individuals with dynamic knee valgus (DKV) and without any medical history were included in this study. Individuals randomly separated in three groups which are kinesio tape group (KG) (n=10), placebo group (PG) (n=10) and control group (CG) (n=10). Muscle facilitation technique applied on gluteus medius muscle in KG, that repeated with plaster tape in PG. Handheld digital dynamometer MicroFet2® used for measure to gluteus medius muscle strength and OptoJump Next® used for vertical jump tests. Frontal Plan Projection Angle (FPPA) measured with cam for assess to DKV at the same time with vertical jump test. Balance assessed with Star Balance Excursion Test (SEBT). Pre-test and post-test method used for statistics. Changes between groups tested with once Kruskal Wallis Test then Mann-Whitney U Test and in group changes tested with Wilcoxon Test.

Results: Fifteen male and fifteen female who ages 25.07±2.54 included in this study. In group analysis significantly showed that; FPPA decreased, Gluteus Medius Strength and vertical jump height increased in KG; FPPA decreased and SEBT increased on anterior direction in PG; SEBT increased on anterior direction in CG (p<0.05). Between group analysis significantly showed that; FPPA lower and Gluteus Medius Strength higher in KG than PT and CG (p<0.05).

Conclusion: Muscle facilitation technique applied on gluteus medius muscle in healthy adults with dynamic knee valgus decreased FPPA and improved parameters related to balance and performance.

Keywords: Kinesio Tape, Dynamic Knee Valgus, Star Balance Excursion Test, Muscle Strength, Vertical Jump Tests

Introduction

Dynamic knee valgus is an abnormal movement pattern in the lower extremity during weight-bearing activities. This abnormal movement pattern is characterized by internal rotation and adduction in the hip joint and medial dodge in the knee (1). This medial dodge in the knee is affected by the decreasing

of muscle strength and causes many disorders such as anterior cruciate ligament (ACL) injuries, patellofemoral pain syndrome (PFPS) (2-4). The muscle
structure which surrounding the knee joint provides dynamic stabilization
for this joint (5). The gluteus medius muscle is an important factor for pelvic
stabilization and continuity of knee kinematics (6). Gluteus medius muscle
weakness when functional conditions, causes dynamic valgus in the ipsilateral lower extremity (7-10). The gluteus medius muscle is the most important
hip abductor for control the dynamic knee valgus (11). Gluteus medius muscle
is formed with anterior, middle, and posterior fibers. Weakness especially the
posterior fibers of the gluteus medius, will lead to increased femoral internal
rotation and knee valgus angle (12-15). Past studies declared that muscle
strength decreasing in hip girdle may affect knee mechanics (16,17).

Kinesio tape method was developed by Kenzo Kase in 1976 in Japan. Kinesio
tapes were made with different materials from other tapes. It stimulates the
somatic receptors and promotes the increase inputs of mechanoreceptors and
proprioceptive receptors. These increases cause many mechanical and physiological effects such as decreased pain, increased circulation, muscle inhibition
and facilitation (18-20).

This study aims that, providing lower DKV angle with the more active
gluteus medius and improved neuromuscular control on knee and hip girdles
with the way that facilitate to gluteus medius muscle using kinesio tape. It is
researched that these effects of kinesiology taping on the hip and knee area
results in DKV, performance and balance.

Moreover, this study will be show that whether or not kinesio tape effect
for fightback to ACL and other knee injuries. Addition that if it effects to precautions for preventive rehabilitation from this injury shows us how its work.
The results will present with Kinesio Tape effect on performance and balance.

Materials and Methods

In the study, which was designed with a randomized placebo-controlled prospective single-blind study model, placebo control was performed by taping
with plaster. Three group names which are KG, PG, CG were written on paper
by researcher and chosen with closed paper method by participants.

Sample selection was made from students and employees of Bahçeşehir
University who suffer with dynamic knee valgus as a result of posture analysis
without any known health problems. 15 women and 15 men totally 30 volunteers were included in the study. Inclusion and exclusion criteria of this study

Tab. 1: Inclusion and Exclusion Criteria

Inclusion Criteria	Exclusion Criteria
– Asymptomatic Dynamic Knee Valgus – Frontal Plan Projection Angle that greater than 13° in women and 8° in men – Being in the ages between 18-30 – Body Mass Index between 18.5-25 kg/m² – Being physically active	– History of neurological diseases – History of systemic diseases – Injury of lower extremity last in the 1 year or surgical incisions – Pregnancy or suspicion of pregnancy – Medical drugs or sedatives used in las 48 hours – History of any allergies

showed in Table 1 and in Figure 1 a flow chart shows detailed information about the study plan.

A demographic data for which included questions for ask to age, gender, weight, shoes size, dominant extremity, medical history, and medication were completed by participants before inclusion. Candidate participants according to demographic data form also completed to IPAQ and they were assessed for DKV with FPPA measurement. FPPA was measured with 2D analysis of single leg squat test. Measurements were performed on dominant side. Study data were gained date between 1 March 2020 and 1 June 2020.

IPAQ is a data collection tool which was developed for determine to physical activity level and used in scientific researches (21). IPQA is a method which recommended from world health organization. (22). IPAQ evaluates physical activities which longer than 10 minutes in the last seven days in terms of frequency, duration (minutes) and intensity with this, it based on the calculation of the metabolic equivalent (MET) value which spent with physical activities. 1 MET indicates the amount of oxygen consumption while sitting or resting (23). IPAQ consists of 7 questions. It has been translated into Turkish and its reliability and validity level has been tested (21). In the study, IPAQ was applied for evaluate to physical activities of individuals. Results categorized with a weekly METs consumption values which less than 600 is low, between 601 and 3,000 are minimally active, over 3,000 are active. The minimally active and active individuals were included in this study.

FPPA measured with single leg squat test (SLST) record with Logitech c920 Pro HD cam. Records transferred to computer interface and analyzed.

DKV measured with 2D analyzes. 2D FPPA was evaluated and recorded in degrees when knee flexion was 60° during a single leg squat. In order to

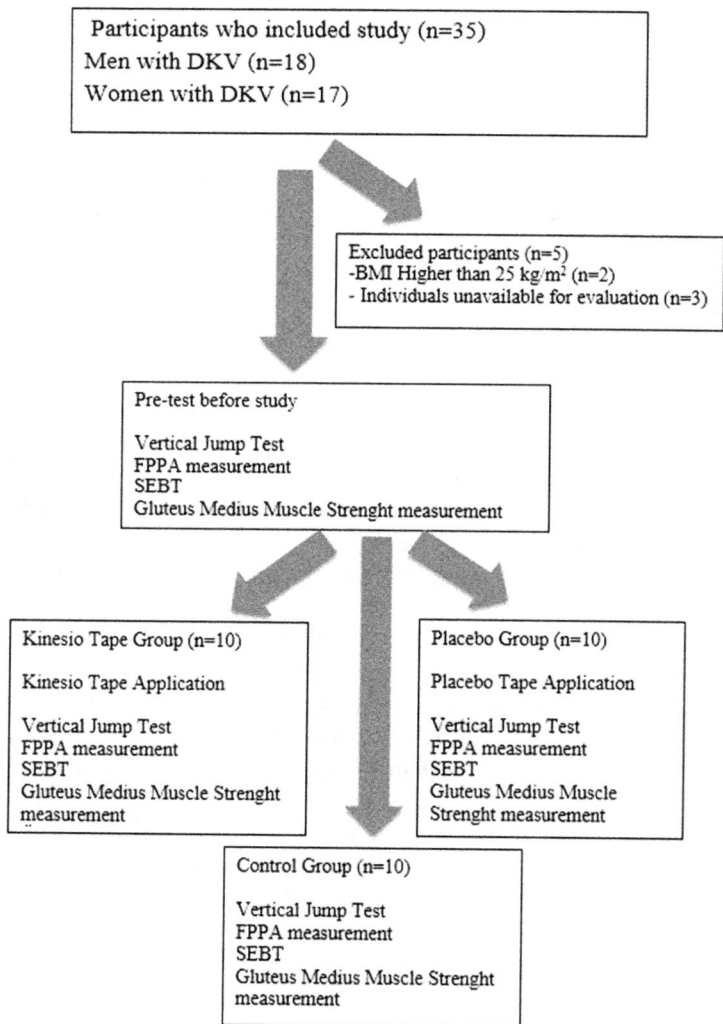

Fig. 1: Flow Chart

find 2D FPPA in the knee, reflective markers with a diameter of 9 mm were placed in two SIAS, midpoint of the knee and the midpoint of the ankle malleoli of the participants (8,24) and FPPA was determined by these marks. 2D FPPA can be measured with two cameras and its reliability and validity level has been tested (3,11). For the unilateral landing task, this angle should be in the range of 5-12° for women and 1-9° for men (8), participants whose knee valgus angles exceeding these ranges were included in the study. The camera was positioned 3 meters away in front of participants and 45 cm height form the floor (24). There were three trials conducted and the average of these was taken as a single data.

During the data collection phase, a track was created and used to measure these in order; vertical jump height with a photoelectric sensor based computerized system, muscle strength with digital handheld dynamometer, balance with SEBT. Each taping method was applied by a physiotherapist who completed the necessary trainings for the application. Taping applications were performed with recommended directions in the literature. Implementation and data collection took approximately 90 minutes in total for each individual and done in the same day. Flow diagram is given in attachment. Before the tests performed in the study, stretching exercises were applied to the quadriceps femoris muscle and hamstring muscle and Calf muscles for 20 seconds for 5 repetitions in order to reduce the risk of injury.

OptoJump Next device which developed by Micro Gate company was used for vertical jump measurement. In the past, its reliability and validity level has been tested (25). Vertical jump height measurement was performed with according to the Drift protocol which ready for use in the software interface. According to the test protocol, 5 consecutive vertical jumps were performed on single leg which dominant. It was requested to try to reach the maximum height for all jumps. The flight height of the participants was calculated in centimeters (cm) by the sensors of the device. Participants placed their hands on their contralateral shoulder for eliminate to arm swing affects to jumping parameters. The maximum, minimum and average height values of vertical jump series has been recorded for each participant.

For the assessment of DKV, FPPA measurements were made with the camera which working simultaneously with the "OptoJump Next" device. In the analyzes, the FPPA value before the highest jump height was recorded in degrees (°) with the computer software which specific to the "OptoJump Next" device (Figure 2).

The Star Excursion Balance Test (SEBT) has been tested for validity and reliability and can be used to evaluate dynamic balance quickly and easily.

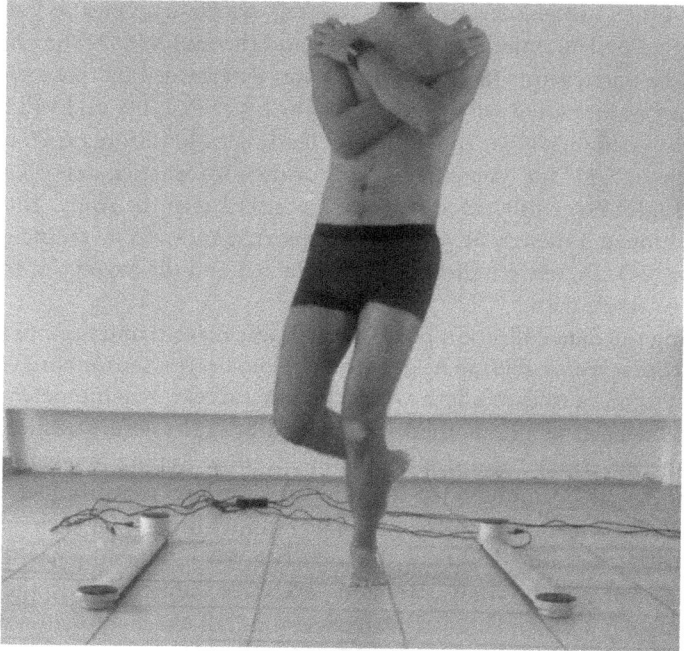

Fig. 2: FPPA Measurement and Vertical Jump Test

This test performed with 8 bars which originate from same point and draws on the floor. These bars are 100 cm, and they are lying 8 different directions from origin point with the 45° angles in between each of them. These different directions are as follows; anterior, anteromedial, anterolateral, medial, lateral, posterior, posteromedial, posterolateral (26). This test is performed as participant trying to reach maximum on each bar in an order with one lower extremity while single leg stance at origin point (27). Participants places their hands-on crista iliaca during testing. Dominant foot places on origin point and non-dominant foot moves on bars without floor contact. Maximum reached points were recorded in cm for each way. It was requested turn back on the bar to origin point again after maximum reaching point. Then they across to next bar with clockwise. The test was conducted for three times, with the one-minute breaks between each test (Figure 3).

Isometric muscle strength of gluteus medius was measured with microfet2 handheld dynamometer. The reliability and validity research of the device

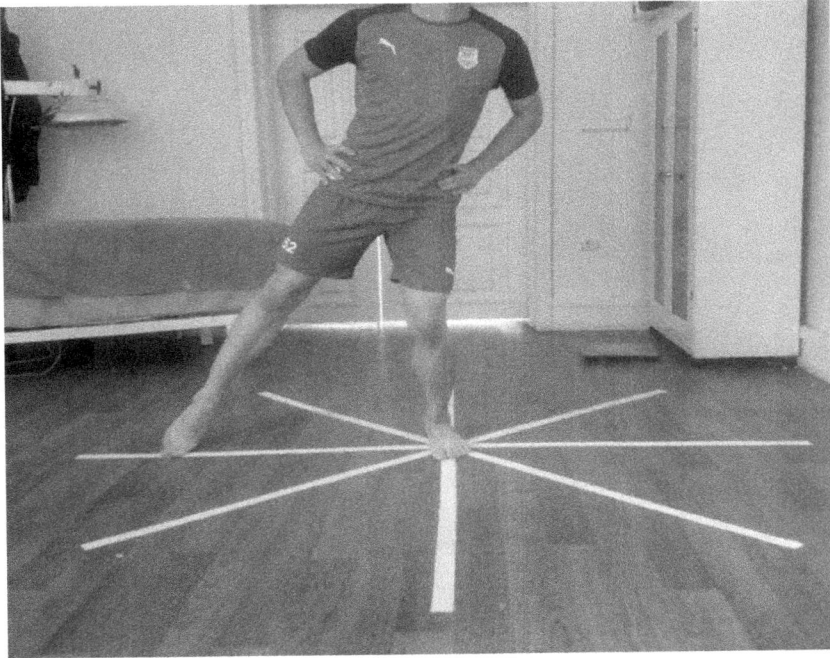

Fig. 3: Star Excursion Balance Test

has been done. In the past, its reliability and validity level has been tested. Measurement is performed while participant with lateral lying position and device fixed on 5 cm proximal to the knee line with an inelastic belt (28). Measurements were repeated for 3 times and the highest value was recorded in kgf. (Figure 4).

Placebo tape application was started from the tuberosity of tibia and goes parallel on the middle fibers of gluteus medius muscle. Plaster tape was used with zero tension for placebo application (Figure 5).

Kinesio tape application was made for the anterior and posterior fibers of the gluteus medius muscle. Facilitation technique was applied the form of I band for both fibers. Kinesio Tex Gold tape used for the application.

When taping on anterior fibers of the gluteus medius, the anchor part of the tape was attached to the crista iliaca in a neutral position from lateral of SIAS. Then, hip joint was positioned in adduction and extension and tape was applied with 15-35 % tension, the other end was applied slightly distal to the

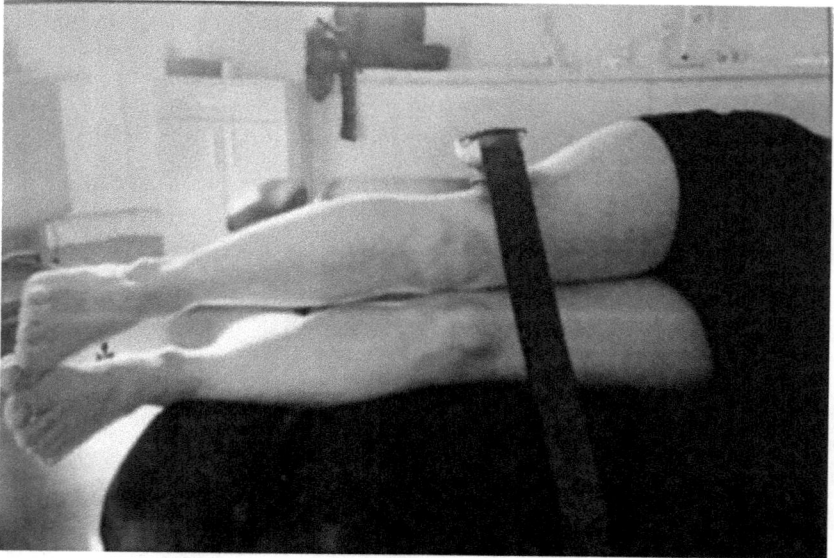

Fig. 4: Gluteus Medius Isometric Muscle Test (28)

trochanter major without stretching the tape. Tape was activated with the hip joint was stretched position (Figure 6).

When taping on posterior fibers of the gluteus medius, the anchor part of the tape was attached to the crista iliaca in a neutral position from lateral of SIPS. Then, hip joint was positioned in adduction and extension and tape was applied with 15-35 % tension, the other end was applied slightly distal to the trochanter major without stretching the tape. Tape was activated with the hip joint was stretched position.

Results

Arithmetic Average (Art. Avg.), Standard Deviation (SD), Ordered Average (Ord. Avg.) values were used for the statistical analysis of the data. The distribution of the data was evaluated with the Kolmogorov Smirnov Test with 95 % confidence interval. In the statistical analysis of non-parametric data pretest and posttest changes of the groups was evaluated with Kruskal Wallis Test and Mann Whitney U Test.

Comparison of post test results of KG and PG showed in Table 2. There were no significant changes detected (p>0.05).

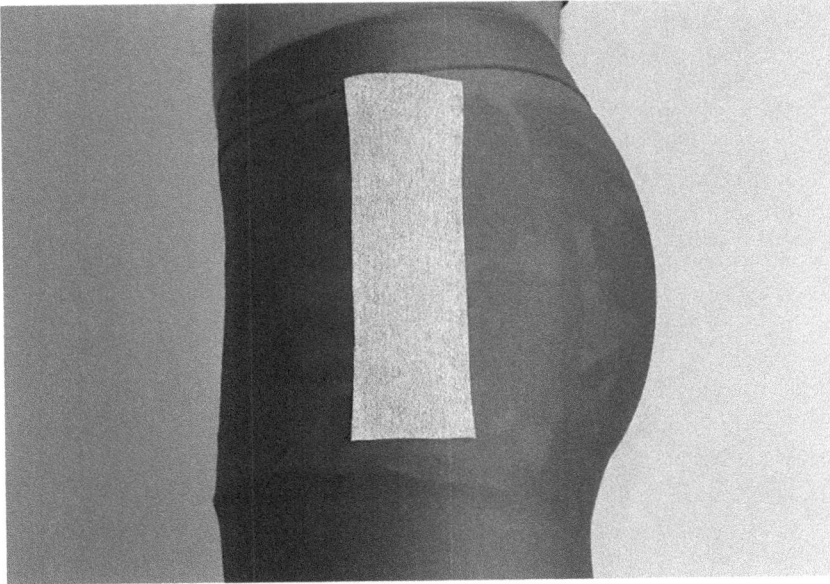

Fig. 5: Placebo Tape Application

Comparison of post test results of KG and CG showed in Table 3. There were no significant changes detected (p>0.05).

Comparison of post test results of PG and CG showed in Table 4. There were no significant changes detected (p>0.05).

Comparison of Pre-Test and Post-Test Results in Between Groups showed in Table 5. According to Kruskal Wallis Test results of average of difference value; there were significant changes on FPPA and gluteus medius muscle strength (p<0.05). There were no significant changes for other parameters (p>0.05).

Comparison of Pre-Test and Post-Test Differences in Between KG with PG showed in Table 6. There were no significant changes between groups according to average of difference values (p>0.05). On the other side, there were significant changes with decrease of FPPA and increase of gluteus medius muscle strength in favor of the KG according to ordered average values (p<0.05). There were no significant changes between groups according to ordered average values (p>0.05).

Comparison of Pre-Test and Post-Test Differences in Between KG with CG showed in Table 7. There were no significant changes between groups according

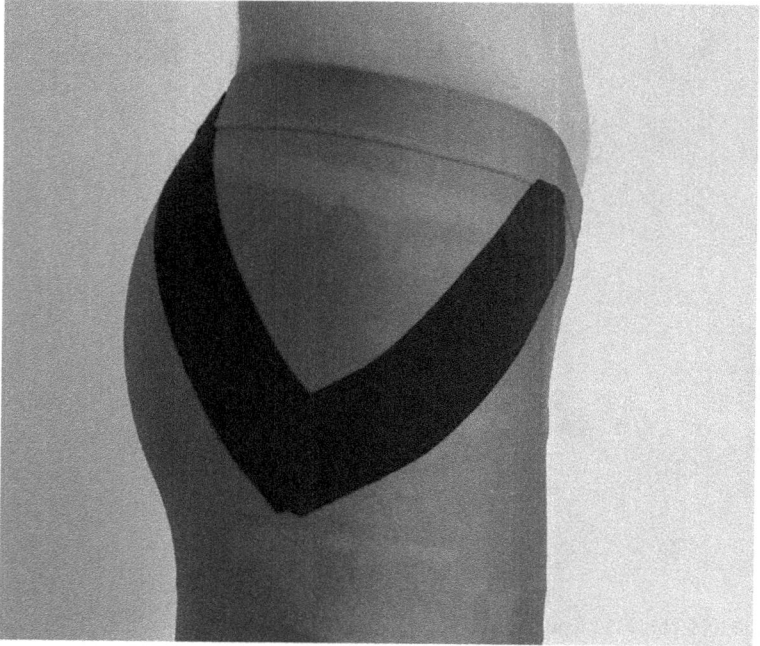

Fig. 6: Kinesio Tape Application

to average of difference values (p>0.05). On the other side, there were significant changes with increase of gluteus medius muscle strength, increase of SEBT on medial direction and decrease of FPPA in favor of the KG according to ordered average values (p<0.05). There was no significant change between groups according to ordered average values (p>0.05).

Comparison of Pre-Test and Post-Test Differences in Between PG with CG showed in Table 8. There was no significant chance between groups according to average of difference values (p>0.05). There was no significant change between groups according to ordered average values (p>0.05).

Discussion

Literature searched on indexed journals in PubMed with keywords that kinesio tape, dynamic knee valgus, frontal plan projection angle, balance, performance, vertical jump test, gluteus medius and star balance excursion test

Tab. 2: Comparison of Post Test Results of KG and PG

Data	Groups	Art. Avg.±SD	Ord.Avg.	U	Z	P
Vertical Jump	KG	3.94±2.33	10.2	47	-0.227	0.821
	PG	3.62±1.78	10.8			
FPPA	KG	12.9±3.00	8.95	34.5	-1.176	0.24
	PG	14.03±2.09	12.05			
Gluteus Medius	KG	47.19±9.18	12.35	31.5	-1.399	0.162
	PG	41.77±8.74	8.65			
Anterior	KG	68.37±11.02	10.35	48.5	-0.113	0.91
	PG	70.5±8.36	10.65			
Posterior	KG	68.3±8.15	10.2	47	-0.227	0.821
	PG	68.27±7.6	10.8			
Medial	KG	74.07±7.94	10.75	47.5	-0.189	0.85
	PG	74.5±8.67	10.25			
Lateral	KG	58.17±7.6	11.95	35.5	-1.097	0.272
	PG	56.03±5.54	9.05			
Anterolateral	KG	65.93±10.31	11.05	44.5	-0.416	0.677
	PG	65.03±6.43	9.95			
Anteromedial	KG	74.43±9.08	10.2	47	-0.227	0.82
	PG	74.9±9.68	10.8			
Posterolateral	KG	63.8±9.56	10.1	46	-0.303	0.762
	PG	62.57±7.07	10.9			
Posteromedial	KG	69.13±10.03	10.55	49.5	-0.038	0.97
	PG	69.17±7.53	10.45			

Art. Avg.: Measured Arithmetic Mean Value, Ord. Avg.: Ordered Average, S.D.: Standard Deviation U: Mann Whitney U value z: Z value P: Significance Level, FFPA: Frontal Plan Projection Angle

in dates between 1 and 2 Oct. 2019. It has been detected current literature insufficient for evidence on these dates. It has been decided current literature insufficient for gain to evidence on these dates.

That were statistically assessed BMI, ages, IPAQ parameters and FPPA values of all three groups and there was no significant change between groups for these parameters (p>0.05). So, it has been seen that participants separated with homogeneity in all groups.

Pre-test and post-test results showed that gluteus medius muscle strength was significantly higher in KG than both of PG and CG (p<0.05). So, it has been thought that there was no placebo effect with KT on muscle strength.

Tab. 3: Comparison of Post Test Results of KG and CG

Data	Groups	Art. Avg.±SD	Ord.Avg.	U	Z	P
Vertical Jump	KG	3.94±2.33	10.45	49.5	-0.038	0.97
	CG	3.65±1.40	10.55			
FPPA	KG	12.9±3	8	25	-1.892	0.058
	CG	14.87±2.62	13			
Gluteus Medius	KG	47.19±9.18	11.4	41	-0.68	0.496
	CG	42.73±6.72	9.6			
Anterior	KG	68.37±11.02	10.45	49.5	-0.038	0.97
	CG	71.43±3.93	10.55			
Posterior	KG	68.3±8.15	10.5	50	0.00	1.00
	CG	69.03±13.27	10.5			
Medial	KG	74.07±7.94	10.9	46	-0.303	0.762
	CG	74.63±7.48	10.1			
Lateral	KG	58.17±7.6	10.95	45.5	-0.34	0.734
	CG	57.23±7.34	10.05			
Anterolateral	KG	65.93±10.31	10.4	49	-0.076	0.94
	CG	67.67±3.42	10.6			
Anteromedial	KG	74.43±9.08	9.55	40.5	-0.718	0.473
	CG	75.83±7.99	11.45			
Posterolateral	KG	63.8±9.56	9.8	43	-0.529	0.597
	CG	64.9±10.52	11.2			
Posteromedial	KG	69.13±10.03	10.25	47.5	-0.189	0.85
	CG	70.77±8.9	10.75			

Art. Avg.: Measured Arithmetic Mean Value, Ord. Avg.: Ordered Average, S.D.: Standard Deviation U: Mann Whitney U value z: Z value P: Significance Level, FFPA: Frontal Plan Projection Angle

Rajasekar et al. declared that Kinesio tape application on gluteus medius muscle was increased muscle strength and decreased DKV with significance (p<0.05) (29). This study showed similar results with ours and this is only study which found by us about to effects of kinesio tape application on gluteus medius to DKV.

Andrade et al. and Pearce et al. researched kinesio taping effects on gluteus medius muscle strength. Both studies declared to significantly increased muscle strength similar with our results (p<0.05) (30,31).

Nunes et al. researched placebo effect of muscle facilitation technique of kinesio tape and they declared there were no placebo effects similar with our

Tab. 4: Comparison of Post Test Results of PG and CG

Data	Groups	Art. Avg.±SD	Ord.Avg.	U	Z	P
Vertical Jump	PG	3.62±1.78	9.95	44.5	-0.416	0.677
	CG	3.65±1.40	11.05			
FPPA	PG	14.03±2.09	9.6	41	-0.683	0.495
	CG	14.87±2.62	11.4			
Gluteus Medius	PG	41.77±8.74	9.8	43	-0.529	0.597
	CG	42.73±6.72	11.2			
Anterior	PG	70.5±8.36	10.65	48.5	-0.113	0.91
	CG	71.43±3.93	10.35			
Posterior	PG	68.27±7.6	10.75	47.5	-0.189	0.85
	CG	69.03±13.27	10.25			
Medial	PG	74.5±8.67	10.8	47	-0.227	0.82
	CG	74.63±7.48	10.2			
Lateral	PG	56.03±5.54	10.4	49	-0.076	0.94
	CG	57.23±7.34	10.6			
Anterolateral	PG	65.03±6.43	9.7	42	-0.605	0.545
	CG	67.67±3.42	11.3			
Anteromedial	PG	74.9±9.68	9.9	44	-0.454	0.65
	CG	75.83±7.99	11.1			
Posterolateral	PG	62.57±7.07	10.5	50	0	1
	CG	64.9±10.52	10.5			
Posteromedial	PG	69.17±7.53	10.3	48	-0.151	0.88
	CG	70.77±8.9	10.7			

Art. Avg.: Measured Arithmetic Mean Value, Ord. Avg.: Ordered Average, S.D.: Standard Deviation U: Mann Whitney U value z: Z value P: Significance Level, FFPA: Frontal Plan Projection Angle

results (32). Many past studies declared similar results with us for kinesio tape effect on muscle strength (33-35). Addition that Kanık et al. reported that kinesio tape application with fan technique, which uses for lymphedema, showed no significant change on muscle strength (36).

Csapo & Allegre et al. researched kinesio tape effects on muscle strength with 19 studies meta-analysis. These declared that 8 of 19 studies reported kinesio tape significantly effective on strength (p<0.05) and 11 of 19 studies reported no significant changes (p>0.05) (37).

Vertical jump test results were significantly higher in KG according to pre-test and posttest analysis (p<0.05) but there were no significant changes in each

Tab. 5: Comparison of Pre-Test and Post-Test Results in Between Groups

Data	Groups	Pre-Test Art. Avg.±SD	Pott-Test Art. Avg.±SD	Avg. of Difference	H	P
Vertical Jump	KG	3.41±2.01	3.94±2.33	0.53		
	PG	3.51±1.68	3.62±1.78	0.11	2.621	0.27
	CG	3.46±1.32	3.65±1.40	0.19		
FPPA	KG	14.6±3.52	12.9±3	-1.7		
	PG	14.4±2.12	14.03±2.09	-0.37	13.368	0.001
	CG	14.8±3.65	14.87±2.62	0.07		
Gluteus Medius	KG	42.11±8.23	47.19±9.18	5.08		
	PG	41.86±7.38	41.77±8.74	-0.08	12.41	0.002
	CG	41.83±6.75	42.73±6.72	0.9		
Anterior	KG	68.37±11.02	69.47±11.5	1.1		
	PG	69.03±8.31	70.5±8.36	1.47	0.899	0.638
	CG	69.87±4.34	71.43±3.93	1.57		
Posterior	KG	68.3±8.15	68.57±8.35	0.27		
	PG	68.37±7.34	68.27±7.6	-0.1	0.218	0.897
	CG	69.03±12.07	69.03±13.27	0		
Medial	KG	74.07±7.94	76.83±7.72	2.77		
	PG	74.23±8.57	74.5±8.67	0.27	5.067	0.079
	CG	74.17±7.29	74.63±7.48	0.47		
Lateral	KG	58.17±7.6	58.9±8.12	0.73		
	PG	59.97±5.63	56.03±5.54	-0.94	2.472	0.291
	CG	57.2±6.8	57.23±7.34	0.03		
Antero Lateral	KG	65.93±10.31	67.07±10.73	1.13		
	PG	65.1±6.42	65.03±6.43	-0.07	0.963	0.618
	CG	66.57±2.13	67.67±3.42	1.1		
Antero Medial	KG	74.43±9.08	73.87±9.84	-0.57		
	PG	75.07±11.42	74.9±9.68	-0.17	0.197	0.906
	CG	75.87±7.81	75.83±7.99	-0.03		
Postero Lateral	KG	63.8±9.56	62.77±13.4	-1.03		
	PG	63.93±5.76	62.57±7.07	-1.37	1.872	0.392
	CG	63.97±8.48	64.9±10.52	0.93		
Postero Medial	KG	69.13±10.03	69.77±10.62	0.63		
	PG	70±6.78	69.17±7.53	-0.83	1.243	0.537
	CG	70.7±9.11	70.77±8.9	0.07		

Art. Avg.: Measured Arithmetic Mean Value S.D.: Standard Deviation U: Mann Whitney U value z: Z value P: Significance Level, Avg. Of Difference: Arithmetic average of changes between pretest and posttest FFPA: Frontal Plan Projection Angle, H: Kruskal Wallis H value P: Significance Level, FFPA: Frontal Plan Projection Angle

Tab. 6: Comparison of Pre-Test and Post-Test Differences in Between KG with PG

Data	Groups	Avg. of Difference	Ord.Avg.	U	Z	P
Vertical Jump	KG	0.53	12.45	30.5	-1.475	0.14
	CG	0.11	8.55			
FPPA	KG	-1.7	6	5	-3.409	0.001
	CG	-0.37	15			
Gluteus Medius	KG	5.08	14.5	10	-3.024	0.002
	CG	-0.08	6.5			
Anterior	KG	1.1	10.15	46.5	-0.265	0.791
	CG	1.47	10.85			
Posterior	KG	0.27	11.25	42.5	-0.568	0.57
	CG	-0.1	9.75			
Medial	KG	2.77	12.85	26.5	-1.778	0.075
	CG	0.27	8.15			
Lateral	KG	0.73	12.15	33.5	-1.25	0.211
	CG	-0.94	8.85			
Anterolateral	KG	1.13	11.5	40	-0.757	0.449
	CG	-0.07	9.5			
Anteromedial	KG	-0.57	10.5	50	0.00	1.00
	CG	-0.17	10.5			
Posterolateral	KG	-1.03	10.85	46.5	-0.265	0.791
	CG	-1.37	10.15			
Posteromedial	KG	0.63	11.7	38	-0.908	0.364
	CG	-0.83	9.3			

Avg. of Difference: Arithmetic average of changes between pretest and posttest, Ord. Avg.: Ordered Average, U: Mann Whitney U value z: Z value P: Significance Level, FFPA: Frontal Plan Projection Angle

other groups and between all three groups (p>0.05). These results were insufficient to showed kinesio tape effects on vertical jump performance. Huang et al. researched placebo effect of kinesio tape on vertical jump and reported that no significant changes (p>0.05) (38). Magalhaes et.al researched performance effect of kinesio tape when 24 hour and 48 hours later then taping and reported that no significant changes (p>0.05) (39). Nakajima & Baldridge researched kinesio tape effects on vertical jump performance in healthy subjects and reported that no significant changes (p>0.05) (40). In our study vertical jump was performed on single leg so there was a difference seen in KG but if it examined with all three group there all results similar with others.

Tab. 7: Comparison of Pre-Test and Post-Test Differences in Between KG with CG

Data	Groups	Avg. of Difference	Ord.Avg.	U	Z	P
Vertical Jump	KG	0.53	12.1	34	-1.211	0.226
	CG	0.19	8.9			
FPPA	KG	-1.7	6.85	13.5	-2.763	0.006
	CG	0.07	14.15			
Gluteus Medius	KG	5.08	14.5	10	-3.024	0.002
	CG	0.9	6.5			
Anterior	KG	1.1	9.25	37.5	-0.945	0.345
	CG	1.57	11.75			
Posterior	KG	0.27	10.55	49.5	-0.038	0.97
	CG	0	10.45			
Medial	KG	2.77	13.2	23	-2.044	0.041
	CG	0.47	7.8			
Lateral	KG	0.73	12.35	31.5	-1.402	0.161
	CG	0.03	8.65			
Anterolateral	KG	1.13	9.9	44	-0.454	0.65
	CG	1.1	11.1			
Anteromedial	KG	-0.57	9.9	44	-0.454	0.65
	CG	-0.03	11.1			
Posterolateral	KG	-1.03	9.35	38.5	-0.87	0.384
	CG	0.93	11.65			
Posteromedial	KG	0.63	11.7	38	-0.908	0.364
	CG	0.07	9.3			

Avg. of Difference: Arithmetic average of changes between pretest and posttest, Ord. Avg.: Ordered Average, U: Mann Whitney U value z: Z value P: Significance Level, FFPA: Frontal Plan Projection Angle

Our results about FPPA cause to thought that kinesio tape may use for decreasing injury risk origins from DKV when playing in sports competition, working hardly or in other risky activities. It is necessary future studies with crowded populations for clear result and evidence.

SEBT is a reliable test for evaluate to dynamic balance (41). Our SEBT results showed that there were no significant changes in all SEBT directions for any group (p>0.05). Controversary that, many past studies declared that kinesio tape application were significantly improved to dynamic balance (42-44).

Tab. 8: Comparison of Pre-Test and Post-Test Differences in Between PG with CG

Data	Groups	Avg. Of Difference	Ord.Avg.	U	Z	P
Vertical Jump	PG	0.11	9.85	43.5	-0.492	0.622
	CG	0.19	11.15			
FPPA	PG	-0.37	8.7	32	-1.363	0.173
	CG	0.07	12.3			
Gluteus Medius	PG	-0.08	10.2	47	-0.227	0.821
	CG	0.9	10.8			
Anterior	PG	1.47	9.7	42	-0.605	0.545
	CG	1.57	11.3			
Posterior	PG	-0.1	10.25	47.5	-0.19	0.85
	CG	0	10.75			
Medial	PG	0.27	9.65	41.5	-0.645	0.519
	CG	0.47	11.35			
Lateral	PG	-0.94	9.8	43	-0.53	0.596
	CG	0.03	11.2			
Anterolateral	PG	-0.07	9.4	39	-0.832	0.406
	CG	1.1	11.6			
Anteromedial	PG	-0.17	10.1	46	-0.303	0.762
	CG	-0.03	10.9			
Posterolateral	PG	-1.37	8.65	31.5	-1.402	0.161
	CG	0.93	12.35			
Posteromedial	PG	-0.83	9.8	43	-0.531	0.596
	CG	0.07	11.2			

Avg. of Difference: Arithmetic average of changes between pretest and posttest, Ord. Avg.: Ordered Average, U: Mann Whitney U value z: Z value P: Significance Level, FFPA: Frontal Plan Projection Angle

Conclusion

There were limited results and insufficient number of studies which designed with similar method of our study in the literature. It shows the importance of our research. Current studies focused on other muscles than gluteus medius in subjects with DKV.

Results showed that kinesio tape application increased muscle strength of gluteus medius and decreased FPPA without placebo effects. In addition to that, there are no changes on balance and performance with kinesio taping. According to these results, researchers thought that kinesio tape can be used for prevention from ACL or PFPS injuries which related with DKV.

References

1. Powers, C. M. (2010). The influence of abnormal hip mechanics on knee injury: A biomechanical perspective. *Journal of Orthopaedic & Sports Physical Therapy, 40*(2), 42-51. doi:10.2519/jospt.2010.3337

2. Hickey, A., Hopper, D., Hall, T., & Wild, C. Y. (2016). The effect of the mulligan knee taping technique on patellofemoral pain and lower limb biomechanics. *The American Journal of Sports Medicine, 44*(5), 1179-1185. doi:10.1177/0363546516629418

3. Ugalde, V., Brockman, C., Bailowitz, Z., & Pollard, C. D. (2015). Single leg squat test and its relationship to dynamic knee valgus and injury risk screening. *PM & R, 7*(3), 229-235. doi:10.1016/j.pmrj.2014.08.361

4. McLean, S. G., Walker, K., Ford, K. R., Myer, G. D., Hewett, T. E., & van den Bogert, A. J. (2005). Evaluation of a two dimensional analysis method as a screening and evaluation tool for anterior cruciate ligament injury. *British Journal of Sports Medicine, 39*(6), 355-362. doi:10.1136/bjsm.2005.018598

5. Hall, S. J. (2012). *Basic biomechanics.* New York: The McGraw-Hill Companies.

6. Mascal, C. L., Landel, R., & Powers, C. (2003). Management of patellofemoral pain targeting hip, pelvis, and trunk muscle function: 2 case reports. *Journal of Orthopaedic & Sports Physical Therapy, 33*(11), 647-660. doi:10.2519/jospt.2003.33.11.647

7. Dischiavi, S. L., Wright, A. A., Hegedus, E. J., & Bleakley, C. M. (2019). Rethinking dynamic knee valgus and its relation to knee injury: Normal movement requiring control, not avoidance. *Journal of Orthopaedic & Sports Physical Therapy, 49*(4), 216-218. doi:10.2519/jospt.2019.0606

8. Herrington, L., & Munro, A. (2010). Drop jump landing knee valgus angle; normative data in a physically active population. *Physical Therapy in Sport, 11*(2), 56-59. doi:10.1016/j.ptsp.2009.11.004

9. Schmitz, R. J., Shultz, S. J., & Nguyen, A. D. (2009). Dynamic valgus alignment and functional strength in males and females during maturation. *Journal of Athletic Training, 44*(1), 26-32. doi:10.4085/1062-6050-44.1.26

10. Schmitz, R. J., Ficklin, T. K., Shimokochi, Y., Nguyen, A. D., Beynnon, B. D., Perrin, D. H., & Shultz, S. J. (2008). Varus/valgus and internal/external torsional knee joint stiffness differs between sexes. *The American Journal of Sports Medicine, 36*(7), 1380-1388. doi:10.1177/0363546508317411

11. Maia, M. S., Carandina, M. H. F., Santos, M. B., & Cohen, M. (2012). Association of the knee dynamic valgus in the stair descent test with the hip range of motion of medial rotation. *Revista Brasileira de Medicina do Esporte, 18*(3), 164-166. doi:10.1590/S1517-86922012000300005

12. Osborne, H. R., Quinlan, J. F., & Allison, G. T. (2012). Hip abduction weakness in elite junior footballers is common but easy to correct quickly: A prospective sports team cohort based study. *Sports Medicine, Arthroscopy, Rehabilitation, Therapy & Technology, 4*(1), 1-8. doi:10.1186/1758-2555-4-37

13. Donatelli, R. A. (2007). *Sports-specific rehabilitation.* St. Louis Missouri: Churchill Livingstone Elsevier.

14. Baker, R. L., & Fredericson, M. (2016). Iliotibial band syndrome in runners: Biomechanical implications and exercise interventions. *Physical Medicine and Rehabilitation Clinics, 27*(1), 53-77. doi:10.1016/j.pmr.2015.08.001

15. Sahrmann, S. (2011). *Movement system impairment syndromes of the extremities, cervical and thoracic spines.* St. Louis, Missouri: Elsevier Mosby.

16. Ferber, R., Kendall, K. D., & Farr, L. (2011). Changes in knee biomechanics after a hip-abductor strengthening protocol for runners with patellofemoral pain syndrome. *Journal of Athletic Training, 46*(2), 142-149. doi:10.4085/1062-6050-46.2.142

17. Nakagawa, T. H., Moriya, É. T., Maciel, C. D., & Serrão, F. V. (2012). Trunk, pelvis, hip, and knee kinematics, hip strength, and gluteal muscle activation during a single-leg squat in males and females with and without patellofemoral pain syndrome. *Journal of Orthopaedic & Sports Physical Therapy, 42*(6), 491-501. doi:10.2519/jospt.2012.3987

18. Bicici, S., Karatas, N., & Baltaci, G. (2012). Effect of athletic taping and kinesiotaping® on measurements of functional performance in basketball players with chronic inversion ankle sprains. *International Journal of Sports Physical Therapy, 7*(2), 154-166.

19. Kahanov, L. (2007). Kinesio taping®, part 1: An overview of its use in athletes. *International Journal of Athletic Therapy and Training, 12*(3), 17-18. doi:10.1123/att.12.3.17

20. Kase, K., Wallis, J., & Kase, T. (2003). *Clinical therapeutic applications of the kinesio taping method.* Tokyo: Ken Ilkai Co. Ltd.

21. Saglam, M., Arikan, H., Savci, S., Inal-Ince, D., Bosnak-Guclu, M., Karabulut, E., & Tokgozoglu, L. (2010). International physical activity questionnaire: Reliability and validity of the Turkish version. *Perceptual and Motor Skills, 111*(1), 278-284. doi:10.2466/06.08.PMS.111.4.278-284

22. Craig, C. L., Marshall, A. L., Sjöström, M., Bauman, A. E., Booth, M. L., Ainsworth, B. E., ... Oja, P. (2003). International physical activity questionnaire: 12-country reliability and validity. *Medicine & Science in Sports & Exercise, 35*(8), 1381-1395. doi:10.1249/01.MSS.0000078924.61453.FB

23. Keleş, I., & Boduroğlu, Y. (2007). Kalp hastalıklarında tanı ve tedavinin yönlendirilmesinde egzersiz testi. *Clinic Medicine, 3*(3), 12-22.

24. Scholtes, S. A., & Salsich, G. B. (2017). A dynamic valgus index that combines hip and knee angles: Assessment of utility in females with patellofemoral pain. *International Journal of Sports Physical Therapy, 12*(3), 333-340.

25. Glatthorn, J. F., Gouge, S., Nussbaumer, S., Stauffacher, S., Impellizzeri, F. M., & Maffiuletti, N. A. (2011). Validity and reliability of optojump photoelectric cells for estimating vertical jump height. *The Journal of Strength & Conditioning Research, 25*(2), 556-560. doi:10.1519/JSC.0b013e3181ccb18d

26. Gribble, P. A., Hertel, J., & Plisky, P. (2012). Using the star excursion balance test to assess dynamic postural-control deficits and outcomes in lower extremity injury: A literature and systematic review. *Journal of Athletic Training, 47*(3), 339-357. doi:10.4085/1062-6050-47.3.08

27. Yanagisawa, O., Futatsubashi, G., & Taniguchi, H. (2018). Side-to-side difference in dynamic unilateral balance ability and pitching performance in Japanese collegiate baseball pitchers. *Journal of Physical Therapy Science, 30*(1), 58-62. doi:10.1589/jpts.30.58

28. Karagözoğlu, D. (2015). *Patellofemoral ağrı sendromunda medial ve lateral hamstringlerin kas aktivasyonunun ve aktivasyon zamanının dinamik olarak değerlendirilmesi ve fizyoterapinin etkisi.* (Doctoral dissertation). Hacettepe University, Ankara, Turkey.

29. Rajasekar, S., Kumar, A., Patel, J., Ramprasad, M., & Samuel, A. J. (2018). Does kinesio taping correct exaggerated dynamic knee valgus? A randomized double blinded sham-controlled trial. *Journal of Bodywork and Movement Therapies, 22*(3), 727-732. doi:10.1016/j.jbmt.2017.09.003

30. Andrade, G. M., Ismania, C., Cyrillo, F. N., & Fukuda, T. Y. (2014). Effects of kinesio taping on gluteus medius muscle strength and electrical activity. *Physical Therapy in Sport, 15*(2), e3. doi:10.1016/j.ptsp.2013.12.012

31. Pearce, B., Olivier, B., Mtshali, S., & Becker, P. J. (2015). Gluteus medius kinesio-taping: The effect on torso-pelvic separation, ball flight distance and accuracy during the golf swing. *South African Journal of Sports Medicine, 27*(4), 97-101. doi:10.17159/2413-3108/2015/v27i4a1262

32. Nunes, G. S., de Noronha, M., Cunha, H. S., Ruschel, C., & Borges Jr, N. G. (2013). Effect of kinesio taping on jumping and balance in athletes: A crossover randomized controlled trial. *The Journal of Strength & Conditioning Research, 27*(11), 3183-3189. doi:10.1519/JSC.0b013e31828a2c17

33. Mostaghim, N., Jahromi, M. K., Shirazzi, Z. R., & Salesi, M. (2016). The effect of quadriceps femoris muscle Kinesio Taping on physical fitness indices in non-injured athletes. *The Journal of Sports Medicine and Physical Fitness, 56*(12), 1526-1533.

34. Zhang, S., Fu, W., Pan, J., Wang, L., Xia, R., & Liu, Y. (2016). Acute effects of Kinesio taping on muscle strength and fatigue in the forearm of tennis players. *Journal of Science and Medicine in Sport, 19*(6), 459-464. doi:10.1016/j.jsams.2015.07.012

35. Vercelli, S., Sartorio, F., Foti, C., Colletto, L., Virton, D., Ronconi, G., & Ferriero, G. (2012). Immediate effects of kinesiotaping on quadriceps muscle strength: A single-blind, placebo-controlled crossover trial. *Clinical Journal of Sport Medicine, 22*(4), 319-326. doi:10.1097/JSM.0b013e31824c835d

36. Kanik, Z. H., Citaker, S., Demirtas, C. Y., Bukan, N. C., Celik, B., & Gunaydin, G. (2019). Effects of kinesio taping on the relief of delayed onset muscle soreness: A randomized, placebo-controlled trial. *Journal of Sport Rehabilitation, 28*(8), 781-786. doi:10.1123/jsr.2018-0040

37. Csapo, R., & Alegre, L. M. (2015). Effects of kinesio® taping on skeletal muscle strength-a meta-analysis of current evidence. *Journal of Science and Medicine in Sport, 18*(4), 450-456. doi:10.1016/j.jsams.2014.06.014

38. Huang, C. Y., Hsieh, T. H., Lu, S. C., & Su, F. C. (2011). Effect of the kinesio tape to muscle activity and vertical jump performance in healthy inactive people. *Biomedical Engineering Online, 10*, 70. doi:10.1186/1475-925X-10-70

39. Magalhães, I., Bottaro, M., Freitas, J. R., Carmo, J., Matheus, J. P., & Carregaro, R. L. (2016). Prolonged use of kinesiotaping does not enhance functional performance and joint proprioception in healthy young males: Randomized controlled trial. *Brazilian Journal of Physical Therapy, 20*(3), 213-222. doi:10.1590/bjpt-rbf.2014.0151

40. Nakajima, M. A., & Baldridge, C. (2013). The effect of kinesio® tape on vertical jump and dynamic postural control. *International Journal of Sports Physical Therapy, 8*(4), 393-406.

41. Gribble, P. A., Hertel, J., & Denegar, C. R. (2007). Chronic ankle instability and fatigue create proximal joint alterations during performance of the Star Excursion Balance Test. *International Journal of Sports Medicine, 28*(3), 236-242. doi:10.1055/s-2006-924289

42. Celenay, S. T., & Kaya, D. O. (2019). Immediate effects of kinesio taping on pain and postural stability in patients with chronic low back pain. *Journal of Bodywork and Movement Therapies, 23*(1), 206-210. doi:10.1016/j.jbmt.2017.12.010

43. Mostert-Wentzel, K., Swart, J. J., Masenyetse, L. J., Sihlali, B. H., Cilliers, R., Clarke, L., ... Steenkamp, L. (2012). Effect of kinesio taping on explosive muscle power of gluteus maximus of male athletes. *South African Journal of Sports Medicine, 24*(3), 75-80. doi:10.7196/sajsm.261

44. Tekin, D., Agopyan, A., & Baltaci, G. (2018). Balance training in modern dancers: Proprioceptive-neuromuscular training vs kinesio taping. *Medical Problems of Performing Artists, 33*(3), 156-165. doi:10.21091/mppa.2018.3022

Ahu Kürklü, Pınar Doğan, and Merve Tarhan

Comparison of the Public's Social Distance toward Syrian Refugees and Perceptions of Access to Healthcare Services: İstanbul Sample

Abstract

Objective: This study was planned with the aim of comparing social distance of society towards Syrian refugees with perceptions about access to health care services.

Materials and Methods: The descriptively planned research was completed with 2426 individuals attending hospital at least once themselves or with first degree relatives who received nursing care living in counties in İstanbul from 1 January - 15 March 2017 and who agreed to participate in the research. Data collection tools used the information form containing information about patient and relative ages, sex, and educational level, Bogardus Social Distance Scale (SDS) and healthcare services access perception survey. Data obtained in the research were analyzed using the SPSS program. Appropriate tests were used based on the distribution of data.

Results: Mean age of participants was 36.1±11.4 years, with the majority of individuals in Generation Y, 55.9 % were female, 44.7 % were high school graduates, 37.9 % resided in İstanbul 2nd region and 69.7 % had moderate income levels. Among participants, 25.3 % stated they or a first degree relative had chronic disease, while 74.8 % were satisfied with service in the health facility they attended. Additionally, 68.8 % of participants waited mean 42.09±38.46 minutes before examinations or tests. Total mean points obtained from the SDS were identified as 65.28±26.11. When the status of living in the same street as Syrian refugees, risk in terms of security of this situation, and effect of presence of refugees on level of health service received and time allocated to them by health personnel are compared with mean SDS of participants, statistically significant differences were identified (p<0.05).

Conclusion: Most participants had moderate social distance to refugees and thought that the presence of refugees delayed their access to health services and lowered the level of health services.

Keywords: Refugee, Social Distance, Health Services

Introduction

Item 14 of the Universal Declaration of Human Rights states that everyone has the right to seek and to enjoy asylum from persecution in other countries. If the asylum-seeker's request for asylum is accepted by the country of refuge, this person is called a refugee (1). Civil war has been continuing in Syria from 2011 to the present. According to Human Rights Watch report, 470,000 people have died in this civil war, while 4.8 million people were forced to abandon their homes and are living as refugees in a variety of countries (2). According to Ministry of Interior General Directorate of Migration Management, 3,695,944 Syrians refugees are living in Turkey under temporary protection (3).

Considering a significant portion of refugees, with a variety of needs like housing, education, health and employment, comprise women and children who are accepted as a vulnerable group, the importance of health services among these needs further increases (4). Attendance at health services by this population is due to physical situations like infections, gastrointestinal and pulmonary disorders, early age, and risky pregnancies, along with psychological reasons like post-traumatic stress disorder (5).

Turkey has important responsibilities in offering the health services required by refugees. Syrian refugees registered in Turkey can benefit from health services and medication stated within the scope of the Health Practice Statement (SUT) led by preventive health services, especially, without any charge (6). However, this situation has caused a significant increase in intensity in accessing health services in Turkey, led by cities which house dense refugee groups (7). According to ORSAM records, state hospitals especially in border provinces provide 30-40 % of their total services to Syrian individuals.

This situation has caused a variety of problems like capacity problems in terms of physical conditions, professional burnout of health personnel and language problems. Additionally, the free treatment and medications determined for refugees, and the lack of contributory share paid by citizens of the Republic of Turkey but not by refugees have led to additional costs in Social Security Institution (SGK) expenditure and negatively affected social peace (8). Studies in provinces with dense population of asylum-seekers like Ankara and Kilis determined perceptions about the difficulty of accessing public health services, especially among Turkish citizens (9-11).

One of the provinces where refugees live densely, though not registered, is İstanbul. According to data from the Directorate of Migration Management, there are 555,179 refugees living in İstanbul (3). Due to similar reasons, this situation has the potential to create an intensity which may affect access to health services of Turkish citizens from different generations in İstanbul.

In this study, the aim was to determine the perception of access to health care among individuals living in İstanbul caused by Syrian refugees and social distance. The research questions are listed as follows.

- What is the level of social distance between participants and Syrian refugees?
- What are the individual traits affecting the social distance of participants?
- How do participants think Syrian refugees have affected health services?

Materials and Methods

This study with descriptive qualities was completed in İstanbul from 1 January - 15 March 2017. The population for the research comprised individuals living in İstanbul aged over 18 years, while the sample comprised volunteer individuals who attended hospital at least once themselves or with first degree relatives and received care. The size of the sample group noted the age group, number of each sex within the group and the sample's representative features considering the age and sex population distribution for İstanbul province in Turkish Statistical Institute data from 2017. Sample size was determined as 2426 volunteer individuals by taking α=0.10 and effect size=0.05.

Collection of data used a survey form comprising three sections of Personal Information Form, the Social Distance Scale, and a survey to determine perceptions of access to health services prepared in accordance with the literature by the researchers.

Personal Information Form: The first section comprised 10 open-ended questions about the participant's age, sex, educational level, region of residence, mean income level, whether they or their first degree relative had chronic disease, most recent service received from any health organization and information related to waiting period when receiving this service.

Social Distance Scale: Developed by Bogardus (1925), validity and reliability were investigated by Arkar (1991) and the Social Distance Scale comprises two cases and questions related to these cares. The scale has 7-point Likert type responses from absolutely not disturbed: 1, does not disturb: 2, does not disturb at all: 3, does not matter: 4, slightly disturbed: 5, disturbed: 6, absolutely disturbs: 7 and comprises 14 questions. Arkar determined the scale had reliability coefficient of 0.88 when tested with the Cronbach alpha method. In this study the Cronbach alpha coefficient was determined as 0.95. The scale is assessed based on total points, with higher points indicating more social distance.

Perception of Access to Healthcare Services: The survey questions were created by the researchers according to literature information and comprised questions about the individual's contact with Syrian refugees during attendance in health organizations, refugees use of health services and any problems the individual encountered in access to health services (1,9,12-14).

Before beginning the study, ethical permission was granted by İstanbul Medipol University Ethics Committee. Individuals participating in the study were given information about the topic and provided verbal consent. Responding to the survey form took 10-15 minutes and data was collected by the researchers with the face-to-face interview method.

Data obtained in the study were evaluated using SPSS Inc. SPSS for Windows, Version 21.0 Chicago, IL, ABD (Statistical Package for the Social Sciences) program. Categoric variables are given as number and percentage; continuous variables are given as mean and standard deviation. The Mann-Whitney U test was used to compare ranked means from two independent groups, while Kruskal Wallis analysis was used to compare scale means in more than two independent groups. If significance was determined at the end of Kruskal Wallis analysis, the Mann-Whitney U test was used in order to find the group or groups causing the difference. Reliability analysis found the Cronbach alpha value. Significance was accepted as 0.05.

Results

The individual characteristics of participants are shown in Table 1. Participants were determined to have mean points of 65.28±26.11 (min: 14, max: 98) on the social distance scale.

Comparison of individual characteristics of participants with rank means received on the social distance scale found those in the baby boomer (BB) generation 10 % (KW=12.287; p=0.002), men 44.1 % (z=-4.470; p=0.000), primary school graduates 26.4 % (KW=1.054; p=0.000), living in İstanbul 2nd region 37.9 % (KW=6.132; 0.047), with low monthly income 12.2 % (KW=6.117; p=0.047), with chronic disease 25.3 % (z=-3.062; p=0.002), receiving services from private hospitals 25.4 % (KW=27.188; p=0.000) and receiving services without waiting 25.5 % (KW=47.688; p=0.000) were determined to have high social distance at statistically significant level (Table 1).

When participants were investigated for perception of access to health services due to Syrian refugees, 69.1 % lived on the same street/avenue as a Syrian, 58.5 % thought living in the same region represented a security threat, 60.6 % thought public services were affected due to refugees, 56 % thought health services were affected due to refugees, 69.5 % saw a refugee receiving health services, 51.7 % thought the presence of refugees in health services affected the quality of health services, 59.4 % thought refugees lengthened waiting durations, 49.8 % thought they shortened the duration of health service and 48.4 % thought the quality of health care services reduced due to refugees (Figure 1).

Tab. 1: Comparison of the Average Distance from the Social Distance Scale with Individual Characteristics of the Participants

Individual Characteristics		Number	Percentage	Range Average	Test and p degree
Generations	Baby boomer generation	243	10.0	1350.57	KW=12.287
	X generation	991	40.8	1175.51	p=0.002
	Y generation	1192	49.1	1217.14	
Age Groups Age average (36.1±11.4) (Min;19, Max; 72)	25 age and below	645	26.6	1130.74	KW=49.417
	26-35 age	449	18.5	1332.95	p=0.000
	36-45 age	920	37.9	1146.31	
	46 age and over	412	17.0	1362.92	
Gender	Female	1355	55.9	1157.07	Z=-4.470
	Male	1071	44.1	1284.90	p=0.000
Education Levels	Primary education	640	26.4	1287.96	KW=11.054
	Secondary education	1085	44.7	1201.40	p=0.004
	University education	701	28.9	1164.25	
Region of Residence	İstanbul First District	661	27.2	1159.76	KW=6.132
	İstanbul Second District	919	37.9	1247.64	p=0.047
	İstanbul Third District	846	34.9	1218.41	
Monthly Income	Low	295	12.2	1267.61	KW=6.117
	Middle	1691	69.7	1221.67	p=0.047
	High	440	18.1	1145.81	
Situation that Chronic Diseases	Yes	614	25.3	1288.19	Z=-3.062
	No	1812	74.7	1188.19	p=0.002

(continued on next page)

Tab. 1: Continued

Individual Characteristics		Number	Percentage	Range Average	Test and p degree
Health Care Institutions that Provide Services	State Hospital	1328	54.7	1218.53	KW=27.188
	Private Hospital	617	25.4	1297.39	p=0.000
	University Hospital	259	10.7	1148.99	
	Family Medicine	222	9.2	1025.49	
Satisfaction from the Health Institution	Yes	1815	74.8	1198.02	Z=-1.878
	No	611	25.2	1259.47	p=0.060
Waiting Time in the Health Institution	Never Expect	618	25.5	1356.84	
	15 minutes and below	440	18.1	1148.58	KW=47.688
	15-30 minutes	840	34.6	1132.55	p=0.000
	30-60 minutes	185	7.6	1333.83	
	60 minutes and over	343	14.1	1171.85	
	Total	2426	100.0		

Comparison of the Public's Social Distance toward Syrian Refugees

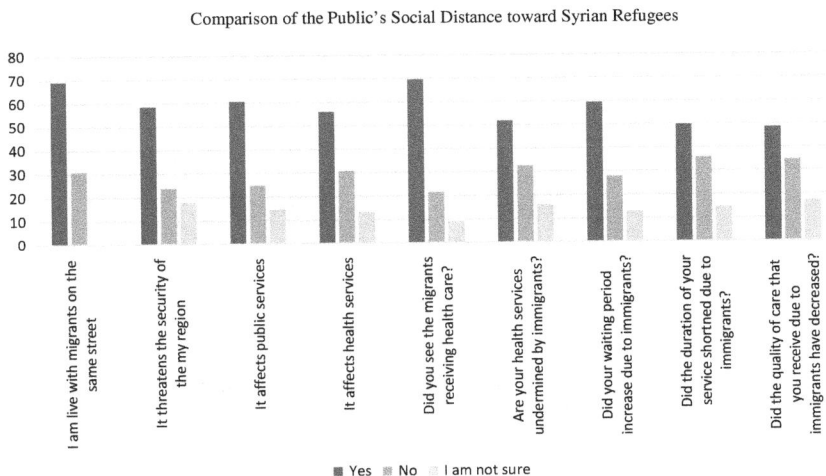

Fig. 1: Comparison of the Average Distance from the Social Distance Scale with Perceptions of Reaching to Health Services Due to Syrian Migrants of the Participants

When the distribution of perceptions about access to health services due to Syrian refugees and rank means obtained from the SDS of participants are compared, all parameters were found to differ by statistically significant levels (p<0.05) (Figure 1). Accordingly, those that lived in the same street, thought that Syrian refugees represented a threat to the region of residence, thought public and health services they received were affected due to migrants, and thought the quality of services received in the health service was affected by migrants were determined to have high social distance.

When the generation of participants is compared with rank means for statements on the social distance scale, apart from the statements "I would rent my home to a Syrian family", "I would be neighbors with a Syrian family" and "I would be served by a hairdresser or barber who was a Syrian individual", individuals in the BB generation were found to have statistically significantly high levels of social distance for all items (p<0.05) (Table 2).

Discussion

Turkey hosts refugees forced to leave their country due to safety until secure living conditions can be provided in their own countries. However, 4.51 % of the total population are refugees in the country, which has caused a variety of difficulties to be encountered with provision of public services, especially

Tab. 2: Comparison of Sequence Averages of Social Distance Scale Items with Generations of Participants (n=2426)

Social Distance Scale Items	BB Gen.	X Gen.	Y Gen.	Test	p Degree
Sitting side by side on the bus	1340.79	1170.42	1223.37	KW=12.581	**p=0.002**
To be together in a 7-hour journey	1360.96	1190.81	1202.30	KW=12.806	**p=0.002**
Shopping at a grocery store	1325.94	1185.90	1213.53	KW=8.231	**p=0.016**
Run as a doorman in your apartment	1340.32	1178.82	1216.48	KW=10.932	**p=0.004**
Renting your house	1293.66	1193.24	1214.00	KW=4.456	p=0.108
Join the family meeting	1348.76	1179.75	1213.98	KW=12.069	**p=0.002**
Playing a game like playing cards, okey, bingo	1389.83	1166.73	1216.43	KW=21.408	**p=0.000**
Talking about matters in the country	1336.59	1193.20	1205.29	KW=9.353	**p=0.009**
Talking about the thing that bother people.	1356.15	1179.20	1212.93	KW=13.941	**p=0.001**
Being a neighbor next door	1289.84	1187.20	1219.80	KW=4.674	p=0.097
Service as a hairdresser / barber	1255.58	1195.24	1220.11	KW=1.811	p=0.404
Share the same room at work	1315.29	1189.45	1212.75	KW=6.841	**p=0.033**
Living in the same house	1331.10	1170.94	1224.91	KW=11.493	**p=0.003**
Being close relatives	1323.87	1186.78	1213.21	KW=10.515	**p=0.005**

in cities where refugees live intensely. Leading these difficulties is the potential perception that Syrian refugees using the health services negatively affect access and quality of health services for Turkish citizens. In our study, supporting these potential perceptions, most participants had moderate-high level of social distance toward Syrian refugees. Additionally, due to the presence of Syrian refugees in nearly all regions in İstanbul, it was thought that Syrian individuals living in the same street/neighborhood caused a security problem and that they negatively affected public and health services. When identifications by Ertem (15) are noted, considering the health services most required by refugees are diagnosis and treatment of endemic diseases, immunization services, safe and sufficient nutrition, surveillance of children's growth and development, women's health, check-ups for chronic disease and mental health services, it appears these individuals require health services at all levels. In this situation, intense use is experienced at all levels of the health services and it is predicted to cause disruption in the provision of health services. Additionally, the increased incidence of infectious diseases like polio and measles, with much reduced incidence in Turkey, especially in border provinces may cause anxiety for society. The poor living conditions of refugees increase their risks in terms of infectious diseases and this situation may form a threat to the health of the local public (16,17).

The majority of participants in our study stated that waiting durations in health services were long due to Syrian refugees and that the quality of health services they received had lowered (Figure 1). A study by Erdoğan (18) stated that one out of every three disruptions mentioned by the regional public was inability to access health services. In Turkey, hospitals, and public health centers (PHC) were designated in camps created in cities close to Syria to meet the health requirements of Syrian refugees. Additionally, apart from these camps, health services are provided in İstanbul, Mersin, İzmir, Gaziantep, Adana, Bursa, Amasya, Ankara, Kayseri, Kahramanmaraş, Kilis and Osmaniye provinces and in 42 migrant health units (15). Since April 2011, nearly 5 million people have applied to receive services in public health centers in camps run by Disaster and Emergency Management (AFAD) and clinics in hospitals and nearly 1 million of these people were referred to hospitals. Hospitals provide clinical service to nearly 6 million people, with nearly 480,000 referred to other hospitals, nearly 325,000 patients operated and nearly 150,000 births (19). This intensity has caused a significant increase in offering services and costs. According to AFAD data (20), Turkey has used nearly 8 billion dollars of resources for Syrian asylum-seekers. This resource used in Turkey makes it the country with highest humanitarian aid in proportion to national income with

0.21 % of the Gross National Product assigned to humanitarian aid according to the Global Humanitarian Assistance Report prepared by the Development Initiative in the Geneva office of the United Nations in 2013. Supporting this, it was revealed that Syrian refugees caused 10 % additional costs to the health sector in Jordan and these services given free of charge increased the workload in the health centers and lowered service quality (21).

Before the Syrian crisis, the success of improvements in health service coverage and system performance in Turkey with the Health Transformation Program were at impressive levels (6,22,23). Turkey has taken a different approach toward Syrian refugees, using a moral-focused approach instead of a security-centered approach (24). To ensure local people access health services without effect on the health services received, the priority of preserving and developing the health of refugees should be accepted. Considering the cultural differences in relation to where these individuals came from, it is necessary to assess social and economic variables very well. Additionally, interventions like employing personnel who speak Arabic/Kurdish to solve the language problem, ensuring the refugees are registered in their region, providing education to women to solve problems related to fertility, monitoring chronic and infectious diseases and making their living areas healthier within the scope of supportive environment, will assist in reducing the load created by these individuals on the health system (25). Additionally, an important step will be to increase the number and quality of health facilities in order to meet the requirements of migrants (15).

Conclusion

According to the study results, individuals in the BB generation and with high socioeconomic level living in the second region of İstanbul have higher social distance. Individuals participating in the study thought that Syrian refugees negatively affected their access to health services and the quality of health services received.

With these conclusions, it is considered necessary that the effect of the presence of the refugees on society reaching health services and nursing care should be revealed through extensive research to be conducted in Turkey.

Sharing these results with related institutions and organizations is suggested to reduce the problems experienced.

References

1. Gültaç, A. S., & Balçık, P. Y. (2018). Suriyeli sığınmacılara yönelik sağlık politikaları. *Sakarya Tıp Dergisi, 8*(2), 193-204.

2. Human Rights Watch. (2017). Suriye 2016 olayları. Retrieved from https://www.hrw.org/tr/world-report/2017/country-chapters/298673

3. Göç İdaresi Genel Müdürlüğü. (n.d.). Geçici koruma. Retrieved from https://www.goc.gov.tr/gecici-koruma5638

4. Saleh, A., Aydın, S., & Koçak, O. (2018). A comparative study of Syrian refugees in Turkey, Lebanon, and Jordan: Healthcare access and delivery. *International Journal of Society Researches, 8*(14), 448-464. doi:10.26466/opus.376351

5. Vatansever, K. (2016). *Sığınmacıların kamplardaki sorunları*. Türk Tabipleri Birliği Yayınları, Ankara.

6. T.C. Sağlık Bakanlığı. (2012). *Türkiye sağlıkta dönüşüm programı değerlendirme raporu (2003-2011)*.

7. Ortadoğu Stratejik Araştırmalar Merkezi (ORSAM). (2015). *Suriyeli sığınmacıların Türkiye'ye etkileri*. Ankara: ORSAM Yayınları.

8. Özcan, T. (2016). Suriyeli mültecilerin sağlık sorunları ve çözüm önerileri. Retrieved from http://www.sdplatform.com/Dergi/975/Suriyeli-multecilerin-saglik-sorunlari-ve-bir-cozum-modeli.aspx

9. Taştan, C., Haklı, S. Z., & Osmanoğlu, E. (2017). *Suriyeli sığınmacılara dair tehdit algısı: önyargılar ve gerçekler*. Polis Akademisi Yayınları.

10. Paksoy, H. M., Koçarslam, H., Kılınç, E., & Tunç, A. (2015). Suriyelilerin ekonomik etkisi: Kilis ili örneği. *Birey ve Toplum Sosyal Bilimler Dergisi, 5*(1), 143-174.

11. Türk Tabipleri Birliği (TTB). (2014). *Suriyeli sığınmacılar ve sağlık hizmetleri raporu*, Türk Tabipleri Birliği Yayınları, Ankara.

12. Soysal, A., & Yağar, F. (2016). Suriyeli sığınmacılar konusunda Türkiye'nin sağlık hizmetlerindeki etkinliğinin değerlendirilmesi. II. Middle EAST Conferences. doi:10.2015/2015-8

13. Erdoğan, E., & Semerci, P. U. (2017). *Attitudes towards Syrians in Turkey-2017*. İstanbul Bilgi University-Center for Migration Research.

14. Korkmaz, A. Ç. (2014). Sığınmacıların sağlık ve hemşirelik hizmetlerinde yarattığı sorunlar. *Sağlık ve Hemşirelik Yönetimi Dergisi, 1*(1), 37-42.

15. Columbia Global Centers. (2015). Workshop on refugee health: Responding to changing health needs in complex emergencies. Retrieved from https://globalcenters.columbia.edu/events/workshop-refugee-health-responding-changing-health-needs-complex-emergencies

16. Berti, B. (2015). The Syrian refugee crisis: Regional and human security implications. *Strategic Assessment, 17*(4), 41-53.

17. Eskiocak, M., Marangoz, B., & Etiler, N. (2016). *Suriye, Türkiye ve Irak'ta savaşın bölgedeki bulaşıcı hastalıklara etkisi.* Türk Tabipleri Birliği Yayınları, Ankara.

18. Erdoğan, M. (2014). *Türkiye'deki Suriyeliler: toplumsal kabul ve uyum araştırması.* Ankara: Hacettepe Üniversitesi Göç ve Siyaset Araştırmaları Merkezi.

19. Afet ve Acil Durum Yönetimi Başkanlığı (AFAD). (n.d.). Barınma merkezlerinde son durum. Retrieved from https://www.afad.gov.tr/barinma-merkezlerinde-son-durum

20. Afet ve Acil Durum Yönetimi Başkanlığı (AFAD). (n.d.). Suriye raporları. Retrieved from https://www.afad.gov.tr/suriye-raporlari

21. Ortadoğu Stratejik Araştırmalar Merkezi (ORSAM). (2014). *Suriye'ye komşu ülkelerde Suriyeli mültecilerin durumu: bulgular, sonuçlar ve öneriler,* Ankara: ORSAM Yayınları.

22. Akıncı, F., Mollahaliloğlu, S., Gürsöö*Health Policy, 107*(1), 21-30. doi:10.1016/j.healthpol.2012.05.002

23. Atun, R., Aydın, S., Chakraborty, S., Sümer, S., Aran, M., Gürol, I., ... Ayar, B. (2013). Universal health coverage in Turkey: Enhancement of equity. *Lancet, 382*(9886), 65-99. doi:10.1016/S0140-6736(13)61051-X

24. Aras, N. E. G., & Mencutek, Z. S. (2015). The international migration and foreign policy nexus: The case of Syrian refugee crisis and Turkey. *Migration Letters, 12*(3), 193-208. doi:10.33182/ml.v12i3.274

25. İrgil, E. (2016). *Suriyeli sığınmacılarda bulaşıcı olmayan hastalıkların sorunu.* Ankara: Türk Tabipleri Birliği Yayınları.

Dilay Hacıdursunoğlu Erbaş, Fadime Çınar, and Fatma Eti Aslan

Researches Related Violence Against Healthcare Workers in Turkey: A Meta-analysis Study

Abstract

Objective: This meta-analysis was conducted to systematically review national studies that examine the risk factors, causes, and types of violence in healthcare workers and to evaluate the data obtained through the meta-analysis method.

Materials and Methods: Relevant research articles published on the subject between January 2014 and September 2019 were included in the evaluation. Google Scholar, ULAKBİM, Türk Medline, CINAHL, and ClinicalKey database were searched within English, and Turkish "healthcare workers", "healthcare staff", "violence", "hospital" and "Turkey" keywords by making various combinations and 4281 publications were reached in the first stage of the search. Eight studies that met the inclusion criteria were included in the study.

Results: The studies included in the study were three descriptive, three cross-sectional, one cross-sectional descriptive, and one retrospective observational cross-sectional. As a result of the examination aimed at determining the violence against healthcare workers, it was determined that The Violent Incident Form (VIF), white code notification form, and questionnaire form developed by the researchers were used. It was determined that verbal violence occurred in most of the studies, and female employees were at higher risk of being exposed to violence.

Conclusion: When the variables that are considered common in all studies are evaluated, it was found that there was no significant difference between the gender and the unit of study and violence, physical violence and being a physician negatively affected the violence. It is thought that this meta-analysis, which was made to determine the risk factors affecting violence in healthcare workers, which is a universal public health problem in the world and in our country, will be a guide for future studies. In this context, the necessity of experimental studies on the subject, as well as determination of risk factors, methods that can be used to prevent violence, and the level of evidence regarding the attitudes of healthcare professionals and patient relatives against violence were put forward.

Keywords: Healthcare Workers, Violence, Hospital, Turkey

Introduction

The violence that occurs with the existence of humanity is one of the leading social problems all over the world (1). In our daily life, all individuals from all over the world, regardless of age, gender, race, religion, language, education level, experience violence in all areas (2). Turkish Language Association defines violence as "using brute force to those with opposing views / the degree of an action, a power, intensity, hardness" (3). According to the World Health Organization (WHO), violence is defined as "threats or acts which, as a result of the deliberate use of force or physical force, will cause or have a high probability of causing injury, death, psychological harm, developmental disorder or deprivation against the person himself, another person, or a group or community"(4).

By the European Commission, workplace violence is defined as "the deterioration of safety, well-being or health of individuals due to being abused, threatened or attacked in situations related to their jobs, including commuting" (5,6). World Health Organization, International Labor Organization (ILO), and International Council of Nurses (ICN) evaluates workplace violence is an issue that should be dealt with primarily at the international level, and intervention policies should be developed; a great risk for the world with drugs, alcohol, smoking and HIV / AIDS worldwide; evaluated it as an important factor that threatens the provision of effective patient care (7). Sectors providing community service, exposure to violence in the workplace are risky sectors. These are health, transportation, education, prisons, retail, and accommodation/catering sectors (8). The Bureau of Work Statistics (BLS) shows that accidents, including staying away from work, occurs in the health and social services environment; also, it is stated that healthcare workers and social service workers constitute the riskiest group to be exposed to violence. Health and social service workers are exposed to the patient, patient relatives, and other health violence in the workplace (9,10).

Health services is a very special field of study that is carried out in close communication with the society. Healthcare professionals serve the whole society of all age groups and genders, and people in need of care who lose their ability to care for themselves due to illness, aging, or other conditions. Therefore, the health sector is at great risk due to the basic features of the services provided and the current working environment (5). Approximately 25 % of the violence reported in workplaces is seen in the health sector. More than half of healthcare workers are exposed to some forms of violence, such as verbal violence (11).

With the technological advances and the digitalization process, the effective dialog has remained in the background. As a result of increased access to information by health care providers, expectations in health service providers have also increased. Verbal threats, physical attacks, etc. against healthcare workers are a big risk for employees, and such attacks affect the life of the employees and their families (12).

In the report published by the Health and Social Workers Union; the rate of those who stated that they were exposed to verbal, psychological, or physical violence at least once during their professional life is 87 %, and the rate of those who stated that they have never been exposed to violence is 13 %. The rate of the participants who stated that they were subjected to verbal, psychological, or physical violence at least once in the last year is 82 % (13). According to the joint report entitled "workplace violence in the health sector", published by WHO, ILO, and ICN in 2002, more than 50 % of healthcare workers report that they are exposed to violence whenever they practice their profession (14). It has been reported that; violence in the health field is related to; poor communication between hospital staff and patients (93.0 %), insufficient quality of medical service (56.7 %), insufficient treatment (60.0 %), the notion that healthcare workers have a heavy workload (43.3 %) and disappointment due to high medical expenses (40.0 %) in Cai et al. (15) study. Considering the rates of violence against healthcare workers in different countries in the joint report of the World Health Organization, ILO, and ICN in 2002, when we look at the rates of violence against healthcare workers, in general, 3-17 % of employees have physical, 27-67 % verbal, 10-23 % psychological, 0.7-8 % have sexual content, 0.8-2.7 % have ethnic reported being subjected to violence (16).

In this study, it was aimed to systematically review national studies that examine the risk factors and causes of violence in healthcare workers and to evaluate the data obtained from the studies with meta-analysis method. It is thought that analyzing the risk factors, causes, and types of violence in healthcare workers and making meta-analysis will contribute to the literature by presenting collective information about the subject and will guide the studies to be done.

Research Questions

- Is gender a risk factor for violence in healthcare workers?
- Is profession a risk factor for violence in healthcare workers?
- Is working unit a risk factor for violence in healthcare workers?
- Is type of violence a risk factor for violence in healthcare workers?

Materials and Methods

Type, Place, and Duration of the Study

This research was conducted using the meta-analysis method, which is one of the quantitative research methods between January 2014 and September 2019.

Ethical Requirements

Since the research is a meta-analysis study, the literature review model was used. Since the literature search does not directly affect animals or humans, ethics committee approval was not obtained for the research.

Application Steps of the Study

The application steps of the study were classified on the basis of PRISMA (Preferred Reporting Items for Systematic Reviews and Meta-Analyzes statement) and MOOSE (Meta-analysis of Observational Studies in Epidemiology) criteria in the articles to be included in the meta-analysis. Articles that meet these criteria were determined and presented in Figure 1 and Table 1 (17-24).

Detailed Literature Review

In the study, keywords were determined in Turkey Science Terms' and Medical Subject Headings (MeSH Browser). The determined keywords were scanned in Prospero (International prospective register of systematic reviews), and it was checked whether the determined research topic had been researched before then registered to Prospero. The keywords "healthcare workers", "healthcare staff", "violence", "hospital", and "Turkey" determined for article searches were searched in the designated databases in English and Turkish. Articles published between January 2014 and September 2019 in Google Scholar, ULAKBİM, Türk Medline, CINAHL, and ClinicalKey databases were included in the evaluation.

In the first step, 4281 publications were reached in the search performed in five databases with the determined search strategy. After removing the repetitive, that does not fit the title and summary, the remaining articles were evaluated, and the articles to be included in the full-text reading were determined. Articles found unrelated to the subject were classified and excluded from the study. Eight studies that met the inclusion criteria were included in the study. The article search and screening diagram for the inclusion flow of the articles is presented in Figure 1 (25).

Searching Articles and Inclusion Criteria in Meta-analysis

- Studies with original articles,
- Articles are written only in English and Turkish in order to prevent language bias in the relevant subject,

Database research

Ulakbim (n=420), Cinahl (n=387), Türk Medline (n=1216), Google Scholar (n=1683), Clinicalkey (n=575)
4281 articles in total

Duplications (n=857)

Scanning

Sources scanned at the summary stage (n=3424)

Excluded in the summary phase (n=3387):
- Do not fit the sample group (n=227)
- Duplication (n=145)
- Not done in healthcare workers (n=45)
- Unrelated to the topic (n=2970)

Compliance review

Full text review (n=37)

Inclusion

Included (n=8)

Dismissed for indifference (n=29)

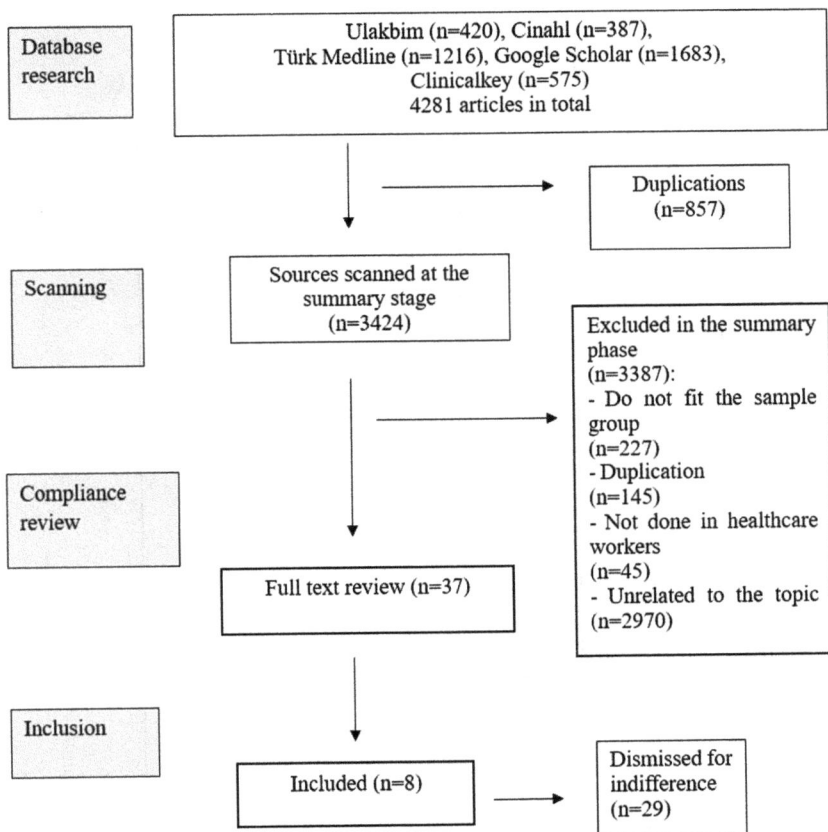

Fig. 1: Study Selection - PRISMA (Preferred Reporting Items for Systematic Reviews and Meta-analyses Statement)

- Full-text national articles published in a peer-reviewed journal on the subject,
- Articles published between January 2014 and September 2019 on violence in healthcare workers,
- Thesis studies on the subject and oral or poster presentations presented at congresses were not included in the study.

Tab. 1: Moose (Meta-analysis of Observational Studies in Epidemiology)

Name of the study	Authors and year of the study	Type of study	Sample Size	Gender	Profession	Working Unit	Type Of Violence	Quality evaluation score (A:9-12) (B:5-8) (C:1-4)
Violence to health care providers: purpose, attitude, and behavior	Yaşar et al. 2016	Descriptive	179	✓	✓	✓	✓	B
Workplace violence against health workers	Milet & Yanık 2017	Cross-sectional and descriptive	345	✓	✓	✓	✓	A
Violence towards health professionals: the case of Kilis city	Demiroğlu et al. 2015	Cross-sectional	252	✓	✓	✓	✓	B
Violence applied to health employees: an example of a private medical center.	Akça et al. 2014	Descriptive	92	✓	✓	✓	✓	A
Frequency of healthcare workers' exposure to violence in the city center of Sivas	Türkmenoğlu & Sümer 2017	Cross-sectional	496	✓	✓	✓	✗	B

Violence against healthcare professionals in Turkey: research in Ankara.	Yıldız 2019	Cross-sectional	429	✗	✗	✓	✗	B
Violence against healthcare workers in workplace: a case of university hospital	Bilişli & Hizay 2016	Descriptive	105	✓	✓	✓	✓	A
Violence against healthcare workers in light of white code data.	Egici & Öztürk 2018	Retrospective, observational section	209	✓	✓	✓	✓	B

Methodological Quality Assessment According to the Review, Coding, and Inclusion Criteria of Articles

Independent and detailed abstract and full-text readings of the articles were completed by two researchers/experts in order to prevent publication bias. The articles evaluated were coded according to their descriptive features. These defining features.

- Name of the study, authors, and year
- Type of study
- The sample size of the study
- Variables of gender, occupation, unit of work, and type of violence
- Quality evaluation score

Twelve of the research quality evaluation criteria proposed by Polit and Beck were used for the remaining eight publications after the review of the studies (26). These criteria allow a general evaluation based on the aims, sample characteristics, findings, and results of the studies. Each study was separately evaluated by the researchers over all of the criteria, and they were given "one point" if they fully met each article, and "zero points" when they failed to meet them. The scores that the study can get according to the criteria range from zero to 12. In the study, articles belonging to all subgroups were examined independently by two researchers, and articles scoring seven or more in the quality evaluation were evaluated as quality. Since studies evaluated with strong and medium quality will be included in the meta-analysis, a total of eight studies met this criterion and were included in the meta-analysis.

Evaluation of Main Outputs

The articles included in the study were analyzed according to the risk factors of violence seen in healthcare workers. Descriptive statistics were included in the analysis since the studies were not randomized controlled studies.

Data Analysis

In the analysis of the data, the licensed software "Comprehensive Meta-Analysis Academic (CMA)/Non-profit Pricing (Version 3)" was used. The data of all articles meeting the inclusion criteria and decided to be included in the study were entered into the CMA software, and the heterogeneity of the articles was evaluated. In the heterogeneity test, the random-effects model in the group analyzed with $p \leq 0.05$, and the fixed-effect model in the group analyzes with $p > 0.05$, effect sizes, study weights, 95 % confidence intervals, and the overall effect size was calculated all the studies. The statistical significance limit was accepted as p≤0.05 in the evaluation of the overall effect. Funnel Plot analysis was performed to test the publication bias, and the results of Classic Fail-Safe N and Tau coefficient calculations were used.

Results

Descriptive Findings

The studies included in the meta-analysis are three descriptive, three cross-sectional, one cross-sectional descriptive, and one retrospective observational cross-sectional, and it was determined that the publications were one for 2014, 2015, 2018, and 2019, and two for 2016 and 2017.

Characteristics of the Sampling Group in the Studies Considered

The sample size in the studies included in the meta-analysis was determined to be between 92 and 496.

Question Form Used in the Studies Evaluated

In the studies we included in this meta-analysis, it was determined that to assess violence in healthcare workers, two studies (23,24) white code notification form, one study (20) The Violent Incident Form (VIF), five studies (17-19,21,22) used a questionnaire developed by the researchers.

Risk Factors Causing Violence in Healthcare Professionals in the Studies Evaluated

In review studies, it was determined that the demographic characteristics, the status of seeing/witnessing violence, who was the perpetrator of the violence, the type, reasons, gender of the perpetrator, where the violence was perpetrated, and violent profession variables were examined. It was determined that the risk, which was considered to be common in all of the studies, was gender, profession, unit of work, and the type of violence and examination analysis of these factors was made.

Evaluation of Methodological Quality

In this meta-analysis, it was found that the agreement between coders was 82 % according to the quality assessment score. In the reliability analysis, Cohen's kappa is 0.84, 95 % confidence interval [Confidence Interval (CI) (CI: 0.767-0.873)]. Kappa value <0 worse fit than chance fit; 0.01-0.20 insignificant compliance; 0.21-0.40 poor compliance; 0.41-0.60 moderate compliance; 0.61-0.80 good fit and 0.81- 1.00 very good fit, or 0.75 and above excellent, 0.40-0.75 medium-good and below 0.40 is considered to be a poor fit. The kappa value (0.82) in this study shows that there is a very good level of agreement between encoders.

Analytical Findings

Among the risk factors that cause violence in healthcare workers it was determined to be positive with, the general effect size of gender on the development of violence is 1.318 (CI; 0.45-3.78; $p > 0.05$), the general effect size for the profession is 0.321 (CI; 0.21-0.48; $p < 0.05$), the general effect size for the unit studied is 1.318 (CI; 0.45-3.78; $p > 0.05$), and the general effect size for the type of violence is 0.158 (CI; 0.03-0.67; $p < 0.05$).

Gender

Within the heterogeneity test performed for the gender variable, which is a risk factor for violence in healthcare workers, the p-value was found to be less than 0.05, and the Q (68.042) value was found to be greater than the df value, and as a result of the individual studies included in the analysis, it was determined that the studies examined according to the gender variable, which is considered as a risk factor for violence in healthcare workers, have a heterogeneous structure. The I^2 statistic value was calculated as 92.65. As a result of the calculations, the effect size distribution was evaluated according to the random effects model (Table 2). With the analysis made according to the random-effects model, it was found that the general effect size of gender on the development of violence in healthcare workers was high and positive with a value of 1.318 (CI; 0.45-3.78; $p > 0.05$), in studies, it was determined that the effect of gender on the development of violence in healthcare workers was significant alone, but not statistically significant when considered together (Figure 2).

Profession

The heterogeneity test performed for the occupational variable, which is a risk factor for violence in healthcare workers, found the p-value less than 0.05 and the Q (15.150) value greater than the value corresponding to the df value and

Tab. 2: Heterogeneity Test Results for Gender Variable

Model	Number Studies	Point estimate	Effect size and 95% interval		Test of null (2-Tail)		Heterogeneity				Tau-squared			
			Lower limit	Upper limit	Z-value	P-value	Q-value	df (Q)	P-value	I-squared	Tau Squared	Standard Error	Variance	Tau
Fixed	6	0.913	0.710	1.174	0.710	0.478	68.04	5	0.000	92.652	1.494	1.292	9.381	1.19
Random	6	1.318	0.458	3.789	0.512	0.608								

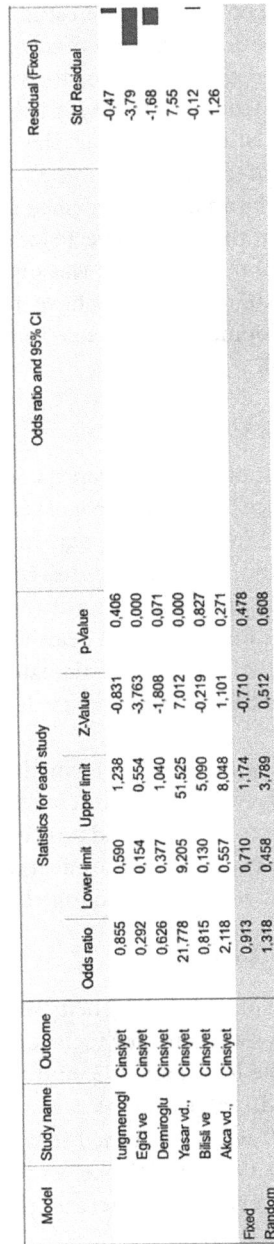

Model	Study name	Outcome	Statistics for each study					Odds ratio and 95% CI	Residual (Fixed)
			Odds ratio	Lower limit	Upper limit	Z-Value	p-Value		Std Residual
	turgmenogl	Cinsiyet	0.855	0.590	1.238	-0.831	0.406		-0.47
	Egici ve	Cinsiyet	0.292	0.154	0.554	-3.763	0.000		-3.79
	Demiroglu	Cinsiyet	0.626	0.377	1.040	-1.808	0.071		-1.68
	Yasar vd.,	Cinsiyet	21.778	9.205	51.525	7.012	0.000		7.55
	Bilisi ve	Cinsiyet	0.815	0.130	5.090	-0.219	0.827		-0.12
	Akca vd.,	Cinsiyet	2.118	0.557	8.048	1.101	0.271		1.26
Fixed			0.913	0.710	1.174	-0.710	0.478		
Random			1.318	0.458	3.789	0.512	0.608		

Fig. 2: Meta-analysis Diagram Showing the Impact Direction of the Research for the Gender Variable

as a result of the individual studies included in the analysis, it was determined that the studies examined according to the occupational variable, which is considered as a risk factor for violence in healthcare workers, have a heterogeneous structure. The I^2 statistic value was calculated as 66.99. As a result of the calculations, the effect size distribution was evaluated according to the random effects model (Table 3).

With the analysis performed according to the random-effects model, it was found that the overall effect size on the development of violence in healthcare workers of the profession was high and positive with a value of 0.321 (CI; 0.21-0.48; p<0.05), and studies have determined that the effect of the profession on the development of violence in healthcare workers is statistically significant (Figure 3).

Working Unit

As a result of the heterogeneity test for the unit variable, which is a risk factor for violence in healthcare workers, the p-value was found to be less than 0.05, and the Q (68.042) value was found to be greater than the df value, and as a result of the individual studies included in the analysis, it was determined that the studies examined according to the unit variable, which is considered as a risk factor for violence in healthcare workers, have a heterogeneous structure. The I^2 statistic value was calculated as 92.65. As a result of the calculations, the effect size distribution was evaluated according to the random effects model (Table 4).

With the analysis performed according to the random-effects model, the overall effect size of the unit studied on the development of violence in healthcare workers was high and positive with a value of 1.318 (CI; 0.45-3.78; p>0.05). It was determined that the effect was significant on its own, but not statistically significant when analyzed together (Figure 4).

Type of Violence

As a result of the heterogeneity test performed for the type of violence variable, which is a risk factor for violence in healthcare professionals, the p-value was found to be less than 0.05, and the Q (209.67) value was found to be greater than the df value, and as a result of the individual studies included in the analysis, It was determined that the studies examined according to the variable of the type of violence, which is considered as a risk factor for violence, had a heterogeneous structure. The I^2 statistic value was calculated as 97.61. As

Tab. 3: Heterogeneity Test Results for Profession Variable

Model	Number Studies	Effect size and 95 % interval			Test of null (2-Tail)		Heterogeneity				Tau-squared			
		Point estimate	Lower limit	Upper limit	Z-value	P-value	Q-value	df (Q)	P-value	I-squared	Tau Squared	Standard Error	Variance	Tau
Fixed	6	0.349	0.278	0.440	8.968	0.000	15.15	5	0.010	66.996	0.173	0.168	12.25	2.36
Random	6	0.321	0.213	0.486	5.380	0.000								

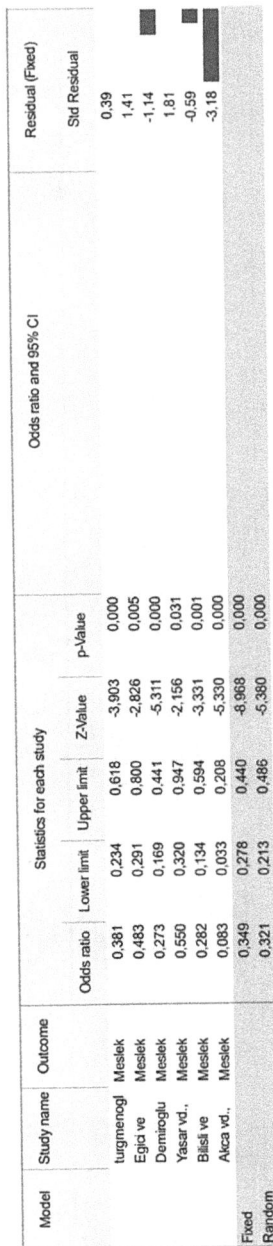

Model	Study name	Outcome	Statistics for each study					Odds ratio and 95% CI	Residual (Fixed)
			Odds ratio	Lower limit	Upper limit	Z-Value	p-Value		Std Residual
	turgmenogl	Meslek	0,381	0,234	0,618	-3,903	0,000		0,39
	Egici ve	Meslek	0,483	0,291	0,800	-2,826	0,005		1,41
	Demiroglu	Meslek	0,273	0,169	0,441	-5,311	0,000		-1,14
	Yasar vd..	Meslek	0,550	0,320	0,947	-2,156	0,031		1,81
	Bilsi ve	Meslek	0,282	0,134	0,594	-3,331	0,001		-0,59
	Akca vd..	Meslek	0,083	0,033	0,208	-5,330	0,000		-3,18
Fixed			0,349	0,278	0,440	-8,968	0,000		
Random			0,321	0,213	0,486	-5,380	0,000		

Fig. 3: Meta-analysis Diagram Showing the Impact Direction of the Research for the Profession Variable

Tab. 4: Heterogeneity Test Results for Working Unit Variable

Model	Number Studies	Effect size and 95 % interval			Test of null (2-Tail)		Heterogeneity				Tau-squared			
		Point estimate	Lower limit	Upper limit	Z-value	P-value	Q-value	df (Q)	P-value	I-squared	Tau Squared	Standard Error	Variance	Tau
Fixed	6	0.913	0.710	1.174	0.710	0.478	68.04	5	0.000	92.652	1.494	1.292	13.56	2.98
Random	6	1.318	0.458	3.789	0.512	0.608								

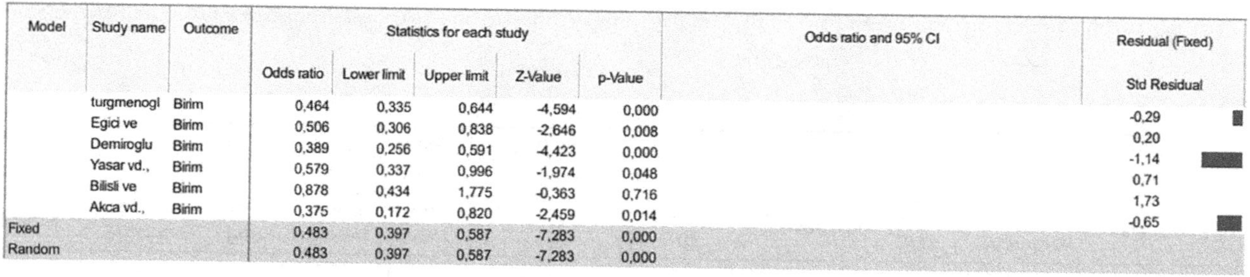

Model	Study name	Outcome	Statistics for each study					Odds ratio and 95% CI	Residual (Fixed)
			Odds ratio	Lower limit	Upper limit	Z-Value	p-Value		Std Residual
	turgmenogl	Birim	0.464	0.335	0.644	-4.594	0.000		-0.29
	Egici ve	Birim	0.506	0.306	0.838	-2.646	0.008		0.20
	Demiroglu	Birim	0.389	0.256	0.591	-4.423	0.000		-1.14
	Yasar vd.,	Birim	0.579	0.337	0.996	-1.974	0.048		0.71
	Bilsi ve	Birim	0.878	0.434	1.775	-0.363	0.716		1.73
	Akca vd.,	Birim	0.375	0.172	0.820	-2.459	0.014		-0.65
Fixed			0.483	0.397	0.587	-7.283	0.000		
Random			0.483	0.397	0.587	-7.283	0.000		

Fig. 4: Meta-analysis Diagram Showing the Impact Direction of the Research for the Unit of Study Variable

a result of the calculations, the effect size distribution was evaluated according to the random effects model (Table 5).

With the analysis performed according to the random-effects model, the general effect size of the type of violence on the development of violence in healthcare workers was high and positive with a value of 0.158 (CI; 0.03-0.67; $p<0.05$). It was determined that the effect was statistically significant (Figure 5).

Broadcast Bias

In the funnel scatter plot, which is also considered as a visual summary of the meta-analysis data set and shows the probability of publication bias, most of the eight studies included in the study are located very close to the combined effect size and at the bottom. Another way to determine publication bias in meta-analysis studies is to calculate Kendall's tau b coefficient. In the absence of publication bias, this coefficient is expected to be close to 1, and the two-tailed p-value does not make a significant difference, that is, the p-value is greater than 0.05 (27). Publication bias was not determined in studies that were meta-analyzed according to the values calculated in this statistic (Kendall's tau b=1.49; p=0.608).

Discussion

Violence against healthcare professionals is a global public health problem that is prominent around the world. Sectors that provide community services such as health, transportation, and education are risky sectors in terms of exposure to workplace violence (8). In health services, people in need of care, who lose the power to take care of themselves due to illness, aging, or other conditions, are provided to the whole society in all age groups and genders. Therefore, the health sector is at great risk due to the basic features of the services provided and the current working environment (5).

Although exposure to violence varies depending on the location of healthcare or social service and the type of organization, some risk factors include: working directly with people with a history of drug or alcohol use, patients or their relatives, working alone in a facility or patients' home, lack of environmental design that could prevent employees from escaping violence, poorly lit corridors, rooms, parking lots and other areas, lack of emergency communication tools, working in neighborhoods with high crime rates, working with inadequate staff and security personnel, long waiting times and

Tab. 5: Heterogeneity Test Results for Type of Violence Variable

Model	Number Studies	Effect size and 95% interval			Test of null (2-Tail)		Heterogeneity				Tau-squared			
		Point estimate	Lower limit	Upper limit	Z-value	P-value	Q-value	df (Q)	P-value	I-squared	Tau Squared	Standard Error	Variance	Tau
Fixed	6	0.218	0.175	0.271	13.67	0.000	209.6	5	0.000	97.615	3.181	2.236	4.998	3.26
Random	6	0.158	0.037	0.672	2.498	0.013								

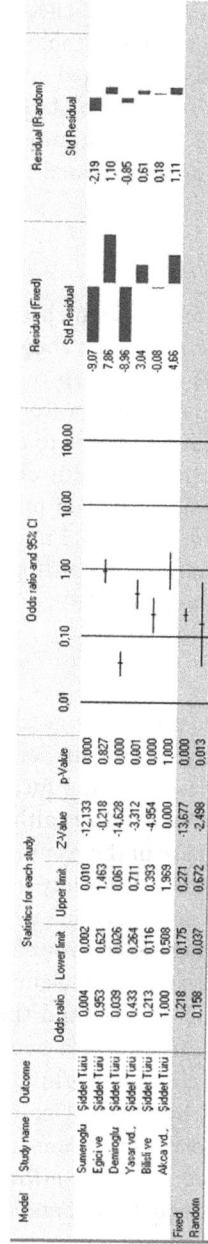

Fig. 5: Meta-analysis Diagram Showing the Impact Direction of the Research for the Type of Violence Variable

overcrowding, disturbing waiting rooms, the perception that violence is tolerated and that victims will not be able to report the incident to the police and/
or press criminal complaints (5,10).

Pain, destructive events, unusual environment, drugs that change the mind
and mood, and the progression of the disease can also cause agitation and
violent behavior (10). In terms of physical violence; Egici et al., 2-year (2016-
2017) data were evaluated, and 57 physical violence incidents were identified
(24). In the study conducted by Sossai et al. in a hospital in Italy, three-year
(2012-2015) data were evaluated, and only 36 injuries were found (28). These
data can be evaluated as important in terms of revealing the high level of violence against healthcare workers.

There are studies showing that gender is a risk factor for violence in healthcare workers and does not exist. Studies show that women in all kinds of violence; indicate a greater risk of becoming a victim; however, physical violence
is more common in men (29). In the study of Egici et al. (24), it was determined that men were more exposed to physical violence. In addition, when
the frequency of encountering violence is evaluated regardless of the types of
violence, it has been determined that women are exposed to violence more
frequently. In the study of Akça et al. (20), when looking at the descriptive
characteristics of the victims of violence; it has been stated that 85.7 % of them
are women and 14.2 % are men. In the study of Bilişci et al. (23); 45 % of the
personnel exposed to violence are male, and 55 % are female personnel, as a
result of the chi-square test conducted to investigate whether the genders of
healthcare workers who were subjected to physical or verbal violence show differences, it was determined that female nurses were exposed to more physical
or verbal violence than physicians and other healthcare personnel (X^2=11.442,
p<0.05). However, when the literature is examined, it is seen that male healthcare workers (59.2 %) are exposed to violence more than female employees
(40.8 %) among healthcare workers (30). Egici et al. (24) in his study; 55 %
(n=115) of those subjected to violence were women, in the study conducted by
Yaşar et al. (17), when "witnessing violence" and "exposure to violence" were
evaluated according to gender, it was found that male healthcare workers witnessed violence more than women (68.2 % and 43.5 %, respectively - p<0.05);
it was determined that there was no difference between the genders in terms
of exposure to violence (p>0.05). In the study of Demiroğlu et al. (19); no statistically significant difference was found between the healthcare professionals
participating in the study, such as gender, marital status, age, occupation,
duration of employment in the institution, and the state of being subjected to
violence in the last year (p>0.05). The high rate of exposure to physical violence

in women may be due to the fact that women become an easy target due to their physical weakness and that the majority of the sample in some studies consists of nurses (31). In our study, it was determined that the effect of gender on the development of violence in healthcare workers was significant by itself, but not statistically significant when analyzed together ($p>0.05$).

Healthcare workers are faced with all kinds of violence. In the joint report of WHO, ILO, and ICN for 2002, when we look at the rates of violence against healthcare workers in different countries, it has been reported that in general, 3-17 % of the workers are physical, 27-67 % verbal, 10-23 % psychological, 0.7-8 % sexual and 0.8-2.7 % were subjected to ethnic violence (4). Akça et al. (20), Türkmenoğlu et al. (21), and Egici et al. (24) in their studies; they explained that healthcare workers who were subjected to violence were exposed to verbal violence in the form of verbal threats or aggression. However, Egici et al. (24) reported that 30.90 % of the victims were simultaneously exposed to psychological violence and 29.80 % to physical violence. In the study of Yaşar et al. (17); of 175 participants who answered the question "Have you witnessed/exposed to violence in the last year?", 87 (47.7 %) stated that they witnessed violence, and 35 (20.1 %) had been exposed to violence. When the types of violence witnessed and exposed to were evaluated, it was determined that the type of violence witnessed and exposed most was "verbal violence" (89.8 % and 88.0 %, respectively). In the study conducted by Milet et al. (18) it was found that, 82.5 % of employees (n=193) who encountered violence were verbal, (n=25) 10.7 % was physical, (n=5) 6.4 % were psychological and 0.4 % of (n=1) were exposed to economic violence. Demiroğlu et al. (19) found that among the healthcare professionals exposed to violence, verbal abuse (38.9 %) and verbal threats (40.9 %) were the most common types of violence. In our study, it was determined that the effect of the type of violence on the development of violence in healthcare workers was statistically significant ($p<0.05$).

The situations where healthcare professionals are exposed to violence differ according to their profession. Egici et al. (24) in his study; it was stated that 117 (56 %) victims of violence were physicians, and hospital security personnel (n=21; 36.80 %) ranked first among the victims when evaluated in terms of occupational groups of those who were exposed to physical violence. In the study of Bilişci et al. (23), 59 % of those who reported verbal or physical violence incidents were physicians, 17 % were nurses, and 24 % were other healthcare workers. In the study of Türkmenoğlu et al. (21), it was determined that the frequency of exposure to violence in security guards (93.75 %) compared to other occupational groups (43.24 % 54.13) was found to be significantly higher (p=0.009). In our study, it was determined that the effect of the profession on the development of violence in healthcare workers was statistically significant (p<0.05). At this point, it can be thought that different professions' exposure to violence in the literature varies according to the type of violence and the sex of the healthcare worker exposed to violence.

Studies show that exposure to violence differs according to the unit of work. Egici et al. (24), although there is a statistical relationship between exposure to physical violence and the healthcare provider's gender, occupation, and the clinic where the employee is exposed to violence, it has been stated that the healthcare professionals who are exposed to violence most are those who work in the adult emergency service and that the most frequent violence is the adult emergency unit. In the study of Demiroğlu et al. (19); it was determined that the places where the violence occurred most were the examination room (23.1 %), the emergency service (20.8 %), the clinical service (19.2 %), the hospital corridor (15.1 %), and the patient waiting room (11.5 %) In the study of Yıldız et al. (22); While the areas most exposed to violence are emergency, surgical and internal services, and blood collection and injection departments, the departments with the lowest rates of violence are determined as intensive care and operating room, radiology and laboratories, respectively. Studies show that exposure to violence is generally higher in emergency services. The reason for this may be the high density of emergency clinics and the high-stress level of patients and their relatives in emergency services in general. In our study, it was determined that the effect of the working unit on the development of violence in healthcare workers was significant on its own, but not statistically significant when considered together (p>0.05).

Conclusion

To prevent violence except for factors that cannot be changed such as gender; it may be suggested to make violent punishments deterrent to healthcare workers, the importance of white code for healthcare workers, especially emergency service workers, to organize in-service training on dealing with stress, and to increase public service ads. We believe that making arrangements to make healthcare workers feel safe in terms of management, conducting studies on the success level after the arrangements for preventing violence, conducting studies with a high level of evidence including the reactions given at the end of violence and the recommendations of healthcare professionals will contribute to the literature.

References

1. Kuehn, B. M. (2010). Violence in health care settings on rise. *JAMA*, *304*(5), 511-512. doi:10.1001/jama.2010.1010

2. Al, B., Zengin, S., Deryal, Y., Gökçen, C., Yılmaz, D. A., & Yıldırım, C. (2012). Sağlık çalışanlarına yönelik artan şiddet. *The Journal of Academic Emergency Medicine*, *11*, 115-124. doi:10.5152/jaem.2012.033

3. Türk Dil Kurumu. (n.d.). Güncel Türkçe sözlük. Retrieved from https://sozluk.gov.tr/

4. World Health Organization (WHO). (2002). *World report on violence and health*. Geneva: WHO.

5. Cooper, C. L., & Swanson, N. (2002). *Workplace violence in the health sector. State of the art*. Geneva: International Labor Organization.

6. Milczarek, M. (2010). *Workplace violence and harassment: A European picture*. Luxembourg: Publications Office of the European Union.

7. International Labour Organization (ILO), International Council of Nurses, World Health Organization, & Public Services International. (2005). *Framework guidelines for addressing workplace violence in the health sector: The training manual*. Switzerland: ILO publications.

8. Kelloway, E. K., Catano, V. M., & Day, A. L. (2011). *People and work in Canada: Industrial and organizational psychology*. U.S.A.: Nelson Education.

9. Arnetz, J. E., Aranyos, D., Ager, J., & Upfal, M. J. (2011). Worker-on-worker violence among hospital employees. *International Journal of Occupational and Environmental Health*, *17*(4), 328-335. doi:10.1179/107735211799041797

10. Occupational Safety and Health Administration. (2016). *Guidelines for preventing workplace violence for healthcare and social service workers*. Washington: U.S. Department of Labor.

11. Di Martino, V. (2002). *Workplace violence in the health sector, country case studies. Brazil, Bulgaria, Lebanon, Portugal, South Africa, Thailand and an additional Australian study*. Geneva: WHO.

12. Greenlund, L. (2011). ED violence: Occupational hazard?. *Nursing Management*, *42*(7), 28-32. doi:10.1097/01.NUMA.0000398673.76876.a5

13. Sağlık-Sen. (2013). *Sağlık çalışanları şiddet araştırması*. Ankara: Sağlık-Sen Yayınları.

14. Nau, J., Halfens, R., Needham, I., & Dassen, T. (2009). The de-escalating aggressive behaviour scale: Development and psychometric

testing. *Journal of Advanced Nursing, 65*(9), 1956-1964. doi:10.1111/j.1365-2648.2009.05087.x

15. Cai, W., Deng, L., Liu, M., & Yu, M. (2011). Antecedents of medical workplace violence in South China. *Journal of Interpersonal Violence, 26*(2), 312-327. doi:10.1177/0886260510362885

16. Chen, W. C., Hwu, H. G., Kung, S. M., Chiu, H. J., & Wang, J. D. (2008). Prevalence and determinants of workplace violence of health care workers in a psychiatric hospital in Taiwan. *Journal of Occupational Health, 50*(3), 288-293. doi:10.1539/joh.L7132

17. Yaşar, Z. F., Durukan, E., Halibeyoğlu, B., Erdemir, I., Yöney, E. B., Kanat, A. C., & Aslan, Ö. (2016). Sağlık çalışanlarında şiddet, nedenler, tutumlar, davranışlar. *Adli Tıp Dergisi, 30*(2), 143-152. doi:10.5505/adlitip.2016.85619

18. Milet, M., & Yanık, A. (2017). Sağlık çalışanlarına karşı işyeri şiddeti. *Uluslararasi Sağlık Yönetimi ve Stratejileri Araştırma Dergisi, 3*(2), 25-36.

19. Demiroglu, T., Kilinc, E., & Atay, E. (2015). Sağlık çalışanlarına uygulanan şiddet: Kilis ili örneği. *Sağlık Bilimleri Dergisi, 24*, 49-55.

20. Akca, A., Yılmaz, A., & Isık, O. (2014). Sağlık çalışanlarına uygulanan şiddet: özel bir tıp merkezi örneği. *Ankara Sağlık Hizmetleri Dergisi, 13*(1), 1-12.

21. Türkmenoğlu, B., & Sümer, H. E. (2017). Sivas il merkezi sağlık çalışanlarında şiddete maruziyet sıklığı. *Ankara Medical Journal, 17*(4), 216-225. doi:10.17098/amj.364161

22. Yıldız, M. (2019). Türkiye'de sağlık çalışanlarına yönelik şiddet: Ankara ilinde araştırma. *Hacettepe Sağlık İdaresi Dergisi, 22*(1), 135-156.

23. Bilişli, Y., & Hizay, D. (2016). Sağlık çalışanlarına yönelik işyerinde şiddet: üniversite hastanesi örneği. *The Journal of Academic Social Science Studies, 52*, 473-486. doi:10.9761/JASSS3723

24. Eğici, M. T., & Öztürk, G. Z. (2018). Beyaz kod verileri ışığında sağlık çalışanlarına yönelik şiddet. *Ankara Medical Journal, 18*(2), 224-231. doi:10.17098/amj. 436537

25. Moher, D., Liberati, A., Tetzlaff, J., Altman, D. G., & Prisma Group. (2009). Preferred reporting items for systematic reviews and meta-analyses: The PRISMA statement. *British Medical Journal, 339*, b2535. doi:10.1136/bmj. b2535

26. Polit, D. F., & Beck, C. T. (2009). Literature reviews: Finding and reviewing research evidence. In *Essentials of nursing research appraising evidence for nursing practice* (pp. 169-193). China: Wolters Kluwer Health - Lippincott Williams & Wilkins.

27. Borenstein, M. (2006). Software for publication bias. In H. R. Rothstein, A. J. Sutton, & M. Borenstein (Eds.), *Publication bias in meta-analysis: Prevention, assessment and adjustments* (pp. 193-220). Great Britain: John Wiley & Sons Ltd. doi:10.1002/0470870168.ch11

28. Sossai, D., Molina, F. S., Amore, M., Ferrandes, G., Sarcletti, E., Biffa, G., ... Copello, F. (2017). Analysis of incidents of violence in a large Italian hospital. *La Medicina del Lavoro, 108*(5), 6005. doi:10.23749/mdl. v108i5.6005

29. Özcan, N., & Bilgin, H. (2011). Türkiye'de sağlık çalışanlarına yönelik şiddet: sistematik derleme. *Turkiye Klinikleri Journal of Medical Sciences, 31*(6), 1442-1456. doi:10.5336/medsci.2010-20795

30. Eker, H. H., Topcu, İ., Sahinoz, S., Ozder, A., & Aydin, H. (2011). Bir eğitim ve araştırma hastanesinde şiddet sıklığı. *Bidder Tıp Bilimleri Dergisi, 3*(3), 16-22.

31. Fallahi-Khoshknab, M., Oskouie, F., Najafi, F., Ghazanfari, N., Tamizi, Z., & Afshani, S. (2016). Physical violence against health care workers: A nationwide study from Iran. *Iranian Journal of Nursing and Midwifery Research, 21*(3), 232-238. doi:10.4103/1735-9066.180387

Emine Özdemir Aslan and Fatma Eti Aslan

Examination of Satisfaction of Patients Postoperative Nausea and Vomiting Management

Abstract

Objective: This study has been conducted to examine patients' satisfaction with post-operative nausea and vomiting management.

Materials and Methods: Phenomenological design, which is one of the qualitative research methods, has been utilized. After obtaining ethical suitability permission from Bahçeşehir University Clinical Researches Ethics Committee and institutional permission from the hospital where the study shall be conducted, an in-depth interview method has been used on ten patients who had a gastrointestinal system surgery. The data collected through leading questions have been recorded on a voice recorder. Themes were created via the analysis of the recorded data, and they have been evaluated.

Results: According to the findings obtained from the research, it has been detected that a great majority of the patients were not satisfied with the postoperative nausea and vomiting management. It has been determined that patients' personal traits, medical diagnoses, applied surgical treatment methods, and areas of surgery have affected the patients' satisfaction. It has been observed that risk factors influenced postoperative nausea and vomiting. It has been determined that experiencing nausea and vomiting before surgery affected patients' satisfaction with the postoperative nausea and vomiting management.

Conclusion: In this study, it has been determined that patients were not satisfied with the postoperative nausea and vomiting management. Depending on these results, it is suggested to establish personal management of nausea and vomiting postoperative treatment plan, plan all the implementations following the suggestions of Enhanced Recovery After Surgery Protocols, and for this study to be re-conducted with a larger sampling.

Keywords: Postoperative Care, Nausea, Vomiting, Satisfaction

Introduction

Nausea and vomiting are an important symptom of gastrointestinal disorders. Vomiting is the act of disgorging the contents of one's stomach and jejuna through the mouth via the contraction of abdominals and diaphragm. Generally, nausea occurs before vomiting and continues during vomiting (1). The integrated emergence of nausea and vomiting is called emesis. American

Society of Peri Anesthesia Nurses (ASPAN) defines it as nausea and vomiting which takes place in the first 24 hours after the surgery (2).

Postoperative nausea and vomiting that emerge shortly after the anesthesia has been recognized as a surgical problem since 1848. Postoperative nausea and vomiting still have a high incidence, albeit the many studies conducted on this area and the current antiemetic drugs (3). Postoperative nausea and vomiting are some of the most common and unwanted problems of anesthesia and surgery. After surgery, even the patients without any known risk factors carry 10 % of nausea and vomiting risk. This risk increases up to a rate between 61 % to 79 %, when accompanied by female gender, non-smoking, history of motion sickness, and postoperative narcotic analgesic usage (4).

Nausea and vomiting is an important problem that is encountered with a rate of 30 % (3) after surgery, which causes morbidity through wound dehiscence, bleeding, increased intracranial pressure, pulmonary aspiration, fluid-electrolyte disturbances, disruption of patient's nutrition and comfort, delayed discharge of the patient, unexpected hospitalizations, and decrease in the satisfaction of patients, thus delaying the recuperation (2). Even though the efforts to prevent nausea-vomiting and getting rid of these unwanted effects have been continuing for over centuries, it is pretty difficult to assert that an effective solution method has been developed.

It is known that recovery after surgery can be accelerated, mortality due to surgery and surgery-related complications can be reduced, and early discharge of patients due to fast recovery can be planned via an up-to-date approach to treatment and care in surgery and evidence-based practices (5). In this context, Enhanced Recovery After Surgery (ERAS) Protocols have been developed with evidence-based practices. ERAS protocol is defined as standardizing the psychological problems and organ dysfunctions caused by surgical trauma in individuals during the surgical process and maintaining physiology after surgery (6).

In the ERAS protocol, which has emerged towards the end of the 1990s through the publication of the conducted studies and has been developed later, there lie three main categories which being before surgery, during surgery, and after surgery. The protocol includes enhanced recovery pathways specialized in many different surgical specialties such as gynecologic surgery, gastrointestinal system surgery, gastrectomy surgery, bariatric surgery, and liver surgery. When considered generally, one of the most important topics in the ERAS protocol, which consists of 24 enhanced recovery pathways, is the multimodal postoperative nausea and vomiting management (7).

The rate of postoperative nausea and vomiting is between 25 and 35 %. It is known that this rate increases up to 70 % for the patients who had major abdominal surgery due to colorectal diseases (8). In addition to the frequent incidence of nausea and vomiting, this excepted or predicted problem must be prevented, and if cannot be prevented, it must be treated since it causes a lot of complications/problems such as disturbing the patient's comfort, delaying the recovery process, rehospitalization, pulmonary aspiration due to vomiting, surgical wound dehiscence, and dehydration in long-lasting vomiting. With all being said, our observations are in the direction that nausea and vomiting are not sufficiently deemed important. In addition to these observations, an answer to the question "What are the patients' thoughts who have experienced this process regarding the management of nausea-vomiting?" has been sought.

Materials and Methods

This study has been conducted to evaluate the patients' satisfaction with the postoperative nausea and vomiting management. To commence the research, ethical suitability permission from Bahçeşehir University Clinical Researches Ethics Committee and institutional permission from the hospital where the study was conducted have been obtained.

The type of research is the descriptive phenomenological design, which is one of the qualitative research methods. It has been conducted in the general surgery clinic of a training and research hospital in İstanbul that is affiliated to the Ministry of Health, between February 2019 and April 2019. In the studies with phenomenological design, which is one of the qualitative research methods, there is not a limitation for the sampling number (9). Data saturation is taken as a basis in this case. And the data saturation is determined by receiving similar answers to leading questions. The data saturation in the research has been provided with ten patients. The population of the study was composed of ten patients. In the literature, it is stated that nausea and vomiting are encountered more often after surgeries such as abdominal, eye, head, neck, gynecology (10). For this reason, patients who had a gastrointestinal system surgery operation (operated open or by laparoscopic method), which is a major surgery of the abdomen, have been included in the research. The patients who had an operation other than gastrointestinal system surgery, who were not in the orientation to be able to answer the questions, and who have not experienced nausea and vomiting were not included within the scoop of the research.

The data was collected through the face-to-face interview technique. The demographic, medical, and operative features of the patients were recorded to the patient identification form via an interview with the patient. Also, patients' anesthesia and surgery information were collected through their hospital records. Detailed notes were recorded by the researcher while the data was being collected with the form of the leading questions. The statements of the participants were recorded simultaneously with a voice recorder. The interviews conducted with the patients lasted between 25 and 30 minutes. Data were collected within one week after the surgery. In the research, themes were created through the analysis of the data that was collected via the form of the leading questions. The themes that were deduced following the findings were interpreted.

Results

The results obtained from this research are presented in two sections as the personal and medical features and the findings obtained via the leading questions.

Personal and Medical Features of the Patients

All of the surgeries have been performed with general anesthesia through anesthetics that are applied through the intravenous path. The average duration of surgery varied between 4 and 6 hours. Anesthesia has been applied simultaneously with the duration of surgery.

The age range of the patients that were included within the scope of the research has been determined as 34-69. Four of the participants were females. Their medical diagnosis was colon malign neoplasm and ileus (Table 1).

It has been determined that all of the patients had nausea, while four patients had vomiting accompanied by nausea. Two of the patients that experienced vomiting were diagnosed with ileus and they were females. The other two patients, on the other hand, were male patients that were diagnosed with colon cancer (Table 1).

After the evaluation of the satisfaction of the management of nausea and vomiting, it has been determined that six patients out of 10 patients (6/10, 60 %) were not satisfied with the management of nausea and vomiting.

In the research, four risk factors that could be the cause of nausea and vomiting have been examined, which are the state not smoking, nausea-vomiting history in the previous surgeries, motion sickness, and postoperative opioid usage. One patient had all of the risk factors (Table 2).

Tab. 1: Personal Features of Patients

Patient Codes	Age	Gender	Surgeries	Nausea	Vomiting
Patient A	42	Female	Bridectomy - Laparoscopic	+	+
Patient B	58	Female	Bridectomy - Laparoscopic	+	-
Patient C	58	Male	Transverse colon colostomy opening - Open	+	-
Patient D	58	Male	Rectum resection and colostomy opening - Open	+	+
Patient E	69	Male	Sigmoid colon resection - Laparoscopic	+	-
Patient F	65	Male	Hemicolectomy - Laparoscopic	+	-
Patient G	64	Male	Rectosigmoid colon resection - Laparoscopic	+	+
Patient H	34	Female	Bridectomy - Laparoscopic	+	+
Patient I	55	Male	Rectosigmoid colon resection - Laparoscopic	+	-
Patient J	55	Female	Hemicolectomy - Laparoscopic	+	-

Tab. 2: Risk Factors and Satisfaction Status of Postoperative Nausea and Vomiting

Patients	Nausea and vomiting in the previous surgeries	State of Motion Sickness	State of Smoking	Satisfaction status of the management of postoperative nausea and vomiting*
Patient A	+	+	1.5 pack/day	Satisfied
Patient B	+	-	Have never used	Unsatisfied
Patient C	-	-	1 pack/day	Unsatisfied
Patient D	+	-	1 pack/day	Very Satisfied
Patient E	+	-	Gave up 10 years ago	Unsatisfied
Patient F	+	-	Gave up 7 years ago	Unsatisfied
Patient G	-	-	15-16 cigarettes/day	Very Satisfied
Patient H	-	-	8-10 cigarettes/day	Very Satisfied
Patient I	+	-	1 pack/day	Unsatisfied
Patient J	-	+	Have never used	Unsatisfied

*In the hospital where the study took place, all patients are applied with postoperative antiemetic treatment.

Results Obtained via the Leading Questions

In this section, four themes have been established following the findings obtained via the leading questions.

Theme 1

State of Fear and Stress Before Surgery

It has been determined that a great majority of the patients experienced fear before surgery, but the reasons for their fear were different. Accordingly, the personal reasons for fear have been determined as follows (Patients with the codes C and F have stated that they did not experience fear.)

Patient A: *"Yes. Not because I did not know. I feared because I knew. I have experienced this illness in my guts before. Surgery once again. I vomit constantly already. I fear experiencing the same things because I know. People fear both what they know and what they don't..."*

Patient G: *"Human fears unintentionally with increasing age. As if death lurks near. More than myself, I think what my wife would do if anything happens to me. After all, this illness is cancer, isn't it..."*

Theme 2

State of Nausea and Vomiting

After examining the applications made in the research regarding the patients' state of experiencing nausea and vomiting, it has been detected that four patients experienced both nausea and vomiting, while the others experienced only nausea.

Patient D: *"I heaved and vomited just a little bit only when I drank water for the first time, my stomach was empty anyway, what is there to disgorge. But most of the time I felt sick at my stomach. I mean a lot."*

Patient G: *"I came round after leaving the surgery. I felt like that. First, I vomited, my wife called the nurse. They cleaned it up together. My stomach was already empty for the surgery, not a lot came out, but I mean I vomited anyways... I thought I wish I get up and go to the bathroom. I caused difficulty for the nurse..."*

Patient F: *"No I didn't vomit at all. I experienced nausea and dizziness for a bit, but I did not vomit. I got dizzy too when I felt sick at my stomach."*

To obtain information about the management of nausea and vomiting in the research, patients' treatment plans and patient answers were examined. It has been observed that in their treatment plans, antiemetic treatment was applied to all the patients who experienced nausea and vomiting. When the patient statements were examined, it has been detected that the patients were informed as "I am giving this treatment for you to vomit" while the treatments were getting executed.

Patient A: *"I couldn't eat without nausea and vomiting. I have been so tired of vomiting. My back muscles have ached due to vomiting. They attached an alimentary canal through my nose to feed me when I vomited too much. Only then I had low nausea."*
Has anything been done after the surgery?
"The nurse gave me medication. She immediately gave me medication when I vomited twice a bit. This vomiting medication will stop nausea, she said. In the evening of the surgery, she tried to make me stand up a little."

Patient D: *"The nurse gave me a medication for nausea. I felt a bit more relieved after having that medication. My eyes got a bit more open, so to say. I get uneasy when I feel sick at my stomach."*

Patient G: *"The nurse came into the room. They cleaned because I vomited. Many thanks to her..." She put me on a drip. This will take nausea away and lower the vomiting, she said.*

Patient H: *"I have been vomiting ever since I arrived at the hospital. They constantly gave me medications. Some helped, some were not enough. Then I was* *attached an alimentary canal through my nose. So that there would not be vomiting. That felt a bit better."*

It has been detected that most of the nurses particularly administrated medication to patients who suffered vomiting in addition to nausea, and the patients were informed about the administrated medications when vomiting and nausea occurred together. It has been determined that, while administrating medication, informing these 4 patients who suffered from vomiting affected their satisfaction levels.

Theme 3

State of Assessing the Healthcare Professionals' Approach Towards Nausea and Vomiting

After the assessment of nurses' standpoints regarding the patients' complaints of postoperative nausea and vomiting, it has been determined that generally, all the nurses take care of patients' nausea and vomiting.

Patient A: *"She seemed a bit bored. But what could she do, I have vomited so much that she grew tired of my complaints? I had been staying there for a week, always saying that I have nausea and vomiting. Yet she helped a lot. I did not see her grimacing even once. She gave me medication."*

Patient C: *"I did not tell the nurse. As I said, it is just a natural process, I said."*

Patient D: *"She's taken care of me a lot. She gave me medicament right away. She put me on a drip. She has taken care of my drip bag. She has taken care of me, God bless her."*

Patient F: *"I said I have some nausea when the nurse asked if I had any complaints. But not that much, I said. If it increases or if you vomit, tell me, she said. She did not do anything."*

Patient I: *"She said she was going to detach the canal from my nose. It would make you feel sick in the stomach as well, she said. She took it off. You are going to drink water in little amounts, she said."*

When the nurses' state of taking feedback and evaluating after nausea and vomiting treatment is examined, it has been determined most of them were in contact with the patients and kept an eye on them after the treatment.

Patient A: *"The nurse always came and asked. Even if she got bored, she always asked. Are you relieved, is it gone, she asked? She has taken care of me a lot."*

Patient B: *"She didn't do anything that she could evaluate my situation. They attached a canal to my nose for water, but it was the doctor who did that. She said let me know if you vomit, but she did not ask again since I did not vomit."*

Patient D: *"She gave me the medication first, then I slept a bit. She always asked my daughter, I have learned. She asked whether I am a bit better."*

Patient E: *"I guess since I did not vomit, the nurse did not ask. Nausea seems simpler."*

One of the patients stated that he/she only experienced nausea, and the nurse did not evaluate after the treatment because nausea on its own is considered simpler.

Theme 4

Effectiveness of the Applications Administered Regarding the Postoperative Nausea and Vomiting Management and the Satisfaction Status of these Applications

Four of the patients (Patients A, D, G, H) have stated that these applications were effective for postoperative nausea and vomiting.

Patient A: *"It, of course, affected me if I think about everything that has been done. My guts recovered. A bit of flatulence occurred. I did a number two, if you would excuse me saying so. My nausea has decreased as well. I was relieved after the flatulence"*

Patient D: *"I was very satisfied. This is a new hospital. The nurses are very good. The doctors are very good If God lets it, it will be so beautiful when I recover."*

Patient E: *"Not really. I have suffered nausea for two days. But I don't think they could do anything about it."*

Patient G: *"I have not vomited at all ever since I went back home after the surgery. The treatment was good, thanks to our doctors. Now there will be a cancer treatment, let us see. God gives the cure."*

Patient J: *"It affected me a bit. It neither passed nor got too bad."*

The satisfaction measurement has been utilized to evaluate the patients' satisfaction with the postoperative nausea and vomiting management. Patients have expressed their state of satisfaction expressed as follows.

Patient H: *"Nurse has taken care of me a lot. She asked. She administered my medications. I am very satisfied."*

After the assessment of the patients' answers, it has been determined that three of them were very satisfied, one was satisfied, and six were not satisfied. It has been determined that medication for nausea and vomiting was administrated to patients who were satisfied with the management of nausea and vomiting, and the medication application has increased their level of satisfaction. It has been detected that in-hospital pharmacological treatment has an important place for the patients' satisfaction with the management of nausea and vomiting.

Discussion

The rate of incidence of postoperative nausea and vomiting is between 25 and 35 %. For patients who had gastrointestinal system surgery, this rate can increase up to 70 % following the risk groups (8). It can cause aspiration of the puke, wound dehiscence, dehydration in cases of long-lasting vomiting, and fluid-electrolyte disturbances and/or insufficiency in patients. Also, nausea and vomiting form an unpleasant emotion in the patient. This unpleasant emotion disturbs the patient's comfort (11). In this study, out of the patients who have experienced nausea, six have stated that they were not satisfied with the postoperative nausea and vomiting management, albeit the antiemetic treatment. Without stumbling upon a similar study on this topic, ERAS Protocols suggest establishing nausea and vomiting treatment plan according to patients' risk groups. The fact that nausea and vomiting, which can cause many complications in the patient, is still unmanageable despite today's technology is quite thought-provoking.

All of the patients were administrated with antiemetic treatment and medication whose active ingredients are metoclopramide and ondansetron. According to the consensus guide, in the postoperative nausea and vomiting management, the usage of antiemetic agents such as ondansetron, dexamethasone, metoclopramide, tropisetron, dolasetron is effective in terms of preventing postoperative nausea and vomiting. Also, they are suggested to be given towards the end of the surgery or at the end of the surgery. In addition, the guide suggests the single or multiple usages of antiemetics primarily in accordance with risk groups (12). Also, Aşçı and Ömer suggest the usage of antiemetic agents such as ondansetron, dolasetron, granisetron, tropisetron at the end of the surgery for postoperative nausea and vomiting (13). Even though the antiemetics used in the hospital were among the antiemetic agents that the guides suggest, the fact that all the patients have experienced nausea and vomiting might indicate that all of the patients were administrated antiemetic prophylaxis without determining their risk groups, thus the treatment might have remained insufficient. The treatment and prevention of postoperative nausea and vomiting remaining insufficient have also reflected the patients' satisfaction results.

When the satisfaction levels were examined regarding the risk groups, in terms of management of nausea and vomiting, it has been observed that all of the patients with the highest satisfaction level had at least one risk factor, while two of them had more than one risk factors. In the literature, the expected risk factors of postoperative nausea and vomiting are the female gender, experiencing nausea-vomiting in the previous surgeries, motion sickness history, and opioid usage (14).

According to the results of the study, the patients' satisfaction with the postoperative nausea and vomiting management does not vary with regard to their ages. It is seen that the age of the patients with high satisfaction varies between 34 and 64. In the literature, it is stated that patients under the age of 50 are a risk group for nausea and vomiting, yet pediatric patients are apart from this group (15).

After the examination of the patients' answers, it has been determined that patients experience fear and stress due to reasons such as relapse of the disease, metastasis to another organ, not waking up after anesthesia, and leaving his/her family alone. Fear of death in surgery occurs due to reasons such as the body getting damaged due to surgery, anesthesia, disabilities after surgery, fear of the unknown (16). Also, in the literature, it has been observed that the female gender experience more anxiety, and patients aged over 60 experience more fear compared to other age groups. Dayılar et al. have asserted that concerns regarding the colon surgery lead up to more fear due to reasons such as postoperative cancer treatment, stoma opening, postoperative nausea and vomiting, and the expectation of ache (17). It has been detected that the reasons for fear in the study and the studies in the literature regarding this topic are similar. It has been observed that although all of the patients have experienced fear, it did not affect the satisfaction levels of the patients.

It has been detected that patients who were informed before the surgery experienced fear, yet that information did not affect their satisfaction level. Informing the patient before surgery reduces pain killer usage and postoperative anxiety, as well as increasing the satisfaction level. Informing and training the patient before surgery is the most important part of nursing since it contributes positively to the post-operation recovery process (18). It has been demonstrated in many studies that informing the patient before the surgery reduces the patient's post-operation stress and fear (19-22). It is supported by the literature that informing the patient about what the operation is and why it is done reduces the patient's fear and stress (23). The obtained findings did not demonstrate any similarity to the literature. The reason why this was the result concluded is thought to be due to the number of participated patients being low due to the nature of qualitative studies.

Conclusion

In this research, it has been determined that patients who were taken within the scoop of the research were not satisfied with the postoperative nausea and vomiting management; and personal features, medical diagnosis, and surgical treatment method and area affected the satisfaction of the management of nausea and vomiting.

Based on the data obtained, the following are suggested.

- Determining the risk of nausea and vomiting before the surgery,
- Informing the patients before surgery about the postoperative nausea and vomiting management,
- Establishing personal management of nausea and vomiting treatment plan for the postoperative nausea and vomiting management as indicated in the ERAS protocol,
- Using nonpharmacological methods in addition to pharmacological methods in the postoperative nausea and vomiting management,
- Reconducting the study with a larger sampling.

References

1. Aktaş, Y. Y., Gürçayır, D., & Atalay, C. (2018). Ameliyat sonrası bulantı kusma yönetiminde kanıta dayalı uygulamalar. *Dicle Tıp Dergisi, 45*(3), 341-351. doi:10.5798/dicletip.457268

2. Aygin, D. (2016). Bulantı ve kusma. In F. Eti Aslan & N. Olgun (Eds.), *Yoğun bakım seçilmiş semptom ve bulguların yönetimi* (pp. 217-241). İstanbul, Turkey: Akademisyen Tıp Kitabevi.

3. Khaled, H. S. A. (2015). *Postoperative nausea and vomiting an overview.* (Unpublished master's thesis), Ain Shams University, Egypt.

4. Jayaprasad, N., Chalil, V. S., & Akhtar, N. (2018). Post-operative nausea vomiting in laparoscopic cholecystectomy: A prospective, randomized, double blind comparative study of ramosetron and ondansetron. *International Journal of Scientific Research, 7*(2), 389-391.

5. Aksoy, A., & Vefikuluçay Yılmaz, D. (2018). Jinekolojik cerrahide kanıta dayalı uygulamalarda yeni bir yaklaşım: ERAS protokolü ve hemşirelik. *Türkiye Klinikleri Journal of Nursing Sciences Journal Identity, 10*(1), 49-58. doi:10.5336/nurses.2017-56268

6. Çilingir, D., & Candaş, B. (2017). Cerrahi sonrası hızlandırılmış iyileşme protokolü ve hemşirenin rolü. *Anadolu Hemşirelik ve Sağlık Bilimleri Dergisi, 20*(2), 137-143.

7. Gündoğdu, H. (2016). Cerrahi iyileşmenin hızlandırılması için modern teknikler. In F. Eti Aslan (Ed.), *Cerrahi bakım vaka analizleri ile birlikte* (pp. 455-470). İstanbul, Turkey: Akademisyen Tıp Kitabevi.

8. Dağıstanlı, S., Kalaycı, M. U., & Kara, Y. (2018). Genel cerrahide ERAS protokolünün değerlendirilmesi. *İstanbul Kanuni Sultan Süleyman Tıp Dergisi, 10*(Ek Sayı), 9-20. doi:10.5222/iksst.2018.43043

9. Erdoğan, S. (2017). Nitel araştırmalar. In S. Erdoğan, N. Nahcivan & N. Esin (Eds.), *Hemşirelikte araştırma süreç, uygulama ve kritik* (pp. 131-165). İstanbul, Turkey: Nobel Tıp Kitabevi.

10. Gülmez, S. (2017). Akupunkturun postoperatif bulantı kusmaya etkisi. (Unpublished master's thesis). Trakya University, Edirne, Turkey.

11. Apfel, C. C., Korttila, K., Abdalla, M., Kerger, H., Turan, A., Vedder, I., . . . Roewer, N. (2004). A factorial trial of six interventions for the prevention of postoperative nausea and vomiting. *The New England Journal of Medicine, 350*(24), 2441-2451. doi:10.1056/NEJMoa032196

12. Gan, T. J., Diemunsch, P., Habib, A. S., Kovac, A., Kranke, P., Meyer, T. A., . . . Tramer, M. R. (2014). Consensus guidelines for the management of postoperative nausea and vomiting. *Anesthesia & Analgesia, 118*(1), 85-113. doi:10.1213/ANE.0000000000000002

13. Aşçı, H., & Özer, M. K. (2011). Bulantı ve kusma için tedavi önerileri. *Süleyman Demirel Üniversitesi Sağlık Bilimleri Enstitüsü Dergisi, 2*(3), 160-165.

14. Pierre, S., & Whelan, R. (2013). Nausea and vomiting after surgery. *Continuing Education in Anaesthesia Critical Care & Pain, 13*(1), 28-32. doi:10.1093/bjaceaccp/mks046

15. Shaikh, S. I., Nagarekha, D., Hegade, G., & Marutheesh, M. (2019). Postoperative nausea and vomiting: A simple yet complex problem. *Anesthesia: Essays and Researches, 10*(3), 388-396. doi:10.4103/0259-1162.179310

16. Cimilli, C. (2001). Cerrahide anksiyete. *Klinik Psikiyatri Dergisi, 4*, 182-186.

17. Dayılar, H., Oyur, G., Kamer, E., Sarıçiçek, A., Cengiz, F., & Hacıyanlı, M. (2017). Evaluation of anxiety levels of patients before colon surgery. *Turkish Journal of Colorectal Disease, 27*, 6-10. doi:10.4274/tjcd.26122

18. Doğu, Ö. (2013). Cerrahi girişim planlanan hastaların eğitim gereksinimlerinin karşılanması ve eğitimin hasta bireyin psikolojik hazırlığına etkisi-Sakarya örneği. *Düzce Üniversitesi Sağlık Bilimleri Enstitüsü Dergisi, 3*(3), 10-13.

19. Gürlek, Ö., & Yavuz, M. (2013). Cerrahi kliniklerde çalışan hemşirelerin ameliyat öncesi hasta eğitimi uygulama durumları. *Anadolu Hemşirelik ve Sağlık Bilimleri Dergisi, 16*, 8-15.

20. Selimen, D., & Andsoy, I. I. (2011). The importance of a holistic approach during the perioperative period. *Association of Perioperative Registered Nurses-AORN Journal, 93*(4), 482-487. doi:10.1016/j.aorn.2010.09.029

21. Avşar, G., & Kaşıkcı, M. (2009). Ülkemizde hasta eğitiminin durumu. *Atatürk Üniversitesi Hemşirelik Yüksekokulu Dergisi, 12*(3), 67-73.

22. Uzun, Ö. (2000). Ameliyat öncesi hasta eğitimi. *Atatürk Üniversitesi Hemşirelik Yüksekokulu Dergisi, 3*(2), 36-45.

23. Taşdemir, A., Erakgün, A., Deniz, M. N., & Çertuğ, A. (2013). Preoperatif bilgilendirme yapılan hastalarda ameliyat öncesi ve sonrası anksiyete düzeylerinin state-trait anxiety inventory test ile karşılaştırılması. *Turkish Journal of Anaesthesiology and Reanimation, 41*(2), 44-49. doi:10.5152/TJAR.2013.11

Fatma Eti Aslan, Şebnem Çalkavur, Semra Bülbüloğlu, and
Neslihan Bektaş

Intervention Effectiveness: A Meta-analysis of the Central Line Bundles to Prevent Catheter-Related Bloodstream Infections

Abstract

Objective: The aim of this study is to review the effectiveness and contributions of preventive care bundles in the treatment of CRBSI in the ICU, and to systematize the evidence-based interventions via a meta-analysis.

Materials and Methods: Data sources; literature search was performed with "care bundle, nursing, care, central catheter, infection, catheter, central venous catheter-related bloodstream infection". Study selection: after establishing the criteria for inclusion into the meta-analysis, studies were selected. A meta-analysis was performed according to the Preferred Reporting Items for Systematic Review and Meta-Analysis (PRISMA) Protocol. Subsequently, all analyses made for meta-analysis calculations were recorded during the data coding phase: direct coding was implemented that analyzed sample numbers, arithmetic means, standard deviations, and research results. The positive effect size value indicates that the care bundle is more effective than traditional applications to prevent CRBSI. Data synthesis: MetaWin Statistical and The Comprehensive Meta-Analysis Software were employed to calculate effect size, variance, and group comparisons. In this meta-analysis an evaluation of effect size was realized according to the Cohen classification system (low between 0.20 and 0.50, medium between 0.50 and 0.80, higher than 0.80). The standardized effect size was used because of unusual characteristics and differences between measurement tools.

Results: According to this meta-analysis, central line bundles reduced CRBSI by 68 % in the ICU and 52 % in clinics. The studies in the meta-analysis show an average effect size at a high level, in homogenous distribution, and coherent with fixed effects. Central line bundles described in the literature with low achievement rates due to mixer variables were not included in the meta-analysis.

Conclusion: A Reformulation in the approach to CRBSI is required. The use and effectiveness of care bundles indicate the benefit of developing a guideline that decreases the rate of CRBSI, reduces complications, and increases the quality of health care.

Keywords: Care Bundle, Central Venous Catheter Related Bloodstream Infection, Central Catheter, Infection

Introduction

Health care-related infections in the Intensive Care Unit (ICU) have weakened the reliability of health care by increasing complications, adverse events, mortality, morbidity, hospital stay length, cost of care, the need for urgent care and antimicrobial therapy, as well as the use of immune-suppressive drugs and invasive techniques (1-7). Care bundles have been developed to protect catheter-related blood stream infections (CRBSI) (4-9). The care bundles prevent bloodstream infections related to the central venous catheter (CVC) and include the use of skin preparations with concentration greater than 0.5 % chlorhexidine, use of the subclavian or internal jugular vein rather than the femoral line, evaluation of the daily CVC requirement, using semi-permeable dressing cover or sterile gauze, following up on clinical guidelines, completing a CVC checklist, and hand hygiene.

Using care bundles improves the quality of health care (5-7). There are many research articles, meta analyses and systematic reviews which show the benefit of using care bundles among the literature (1-5). Specifically, some studies and meta analyses show various dressing covers such as silver impregnated and antimicrobial coating to have been used. In these studies, and meta analyses, the use of various CVCs is described that reduce bacteria colonization such as a CVC with miconazole rifampicin modified as well as pure polymer catheters or various uses of skin preparations (10-16). However, not knowing the statistical effect of care bundles on CRBSI causes two problems:

- It makes it difficult to envision new research.
- Variables which reduce the success of care bundles cannot be established.

In order to manage these problems, thorough experimental and randomized controlled trials (RCT) that provide empirical proof are needed in order to obtain quantifiable results of the effects of care bundles.

This study aims to measure the effects of care bundles via a meta-analysis which documents and compares the outcomes of experimental and randomized controlled studies conducted independently of one another.

Materials and Methods

Literature Search and Study Selection

We performed a meta-analysis according to the Preferred Reporting Items for Systematic Review and Meta-Analysis (PRISMA) Protocol (17) (Figure 1). The

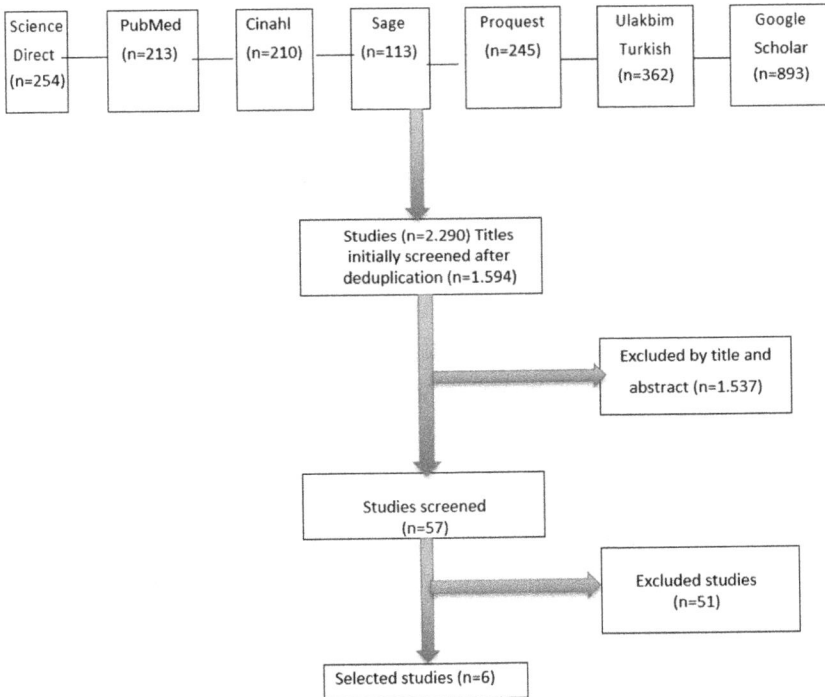

Fig. 1: Study Selection. *Preferred Reporting Items for Systematic Reviews and Meta-Analyses (PRISMA)*

US Centers for Disease Control and Prevention and Hospital Infection Control Practices Advisory Committee (HICPAC) developed evidence-based guidelines for the avoidance of catheter-related bloodstream infections. These were last revised in 2011 (18). Recommended interventions in catheter location and care for avoiding CRBSI comprise the use of correct vein and skin preparation techniques, hand hygiene, and daily evaluation of catheter requirements.

This meta-analysis began in 2011. We initiated the literature review using Medical Subject Headings (MeSH) in the CINAHL as well as PubMed, SAGE, ULAKBİM Turkish, Google Scholar, ProQuest and Science Direct databases for double-blind studies. The literature search was finalized in July 2017. Beyond these, we examined the references section of the current systematic reviews and meta-analyses in completing the literature search. The literature search was conducted by an experienced librarian. The criterion for including

Aslan et al.

research in the meta-analysis was experiments including a patient who had received CRBSI practices. Quasi-experimental studies or those without a control group were excluded.

Data Extraction

A Data Extraction Form was developed by the authors and the evaluations were made according to this form which recorded the year of the studies, the authors, the methodology, and the information about the experimental and control groups. Then, direct coding was done that analyzed sample numbers, arithmetic means, standard deviations, and research results. All analyses made for meta-analysis calculations were recorded during the data coding phase. All the authors checked the encodings to ensure data security. The positive effect size value indicates that the care bundle is more effective than traditional applications to prevent CRBSI and that is negative. Dependent Variables: The studies in the meta-analysis and the effect sizes calculated on the basis of the rates of CRBSI. Independent Variables: The units and clinics where the studies were carried out. The maintenance packages used in the studies are similar (Table 1). In experimental studies, dependent variables influence both independent and other variables.

Table 1 shows that the high-level distance of the mean effect on heterogeneity test $p<0.05$ and partition homogeneous that it was determined to comply with fixed effects model. Table 2 shows the homogeneous distribution value, average effect size and confidence interval.

Statistical Analysis

This meta-analysis employed the method of Intervention Effectiveness Meta-Analysis that to calculate the differences between the experimental and control groups. As Microsoft Office Excel 2016 supports the implementation of this technique, we used that software program for coding.

MetaWin Statistical and The Comprehensive Meta-Analysis Software were employed to calculate effect size, variance, and group comparisons. In this meta-analysis, evaluation of the effect size was carried out according to the Cohen classification system (low between 0.20 and 0.50, medium between 0.50 and 0.80, higher than 0.80) (19) (Table 2). The standardized effect size was used because of unusual characteristics and differences between measurement tools (20). Hedge g was used in calculating the effect size and the significance level was determined as 95 %, therefore used to fixed and random effect models. In

Tab. 1: The Studies Evaluation of Effectiveness in Subgroup Care Bundles to Prevent CRBSI

	Subgroups	N	Effect Percent (%)	Average Effect Size	Effect Size (95 % Confidence Interval)	
					Lower Limit	Top Limit
Work Field	Intensive care units	4	68	0.18	0.21	0.44
	Clinics	2	52	0.21	0.33	0.48

Tab. 2: Heterogeneity Distribution Value, Average Effect Size and Confidence Interval

Model type	N	Z	Heterogeneity Test P Value	Average Effect Size	Effect Size (95 % Confidence Interval)	
					Lower Limit	Top Limit
Fixed effects model	6	7.25	0.068	0.69	0.79	0.66
Random effects model	6	3.27	0.034	0.58	0.67	0.52

Study	Weight	IRR	Risk Ratio
		M-H, Random, 95% CI	M-H, Random, 95% CI
Marsteller et al. USA, 2012	17%	0.34 [0.23, 0.58]	
Sacks et al. USA, 2014	24%	0.35 [0.22, 0.56]	
Hebbar et al. USA, 2014	9%	0.24 [0.19, 0.31]	
Kaya et al. Turkey, 2016	11%	0.07[0.01,0.1]	
O'Nell et al. USA, 2016	21%	0.58 [0.32, 0.84]	
Gerceker et al. Turkey, 2017	18%	0.18[0.1,0.23]	
Total(95% CI)	%100	0.28[0.21-0.48]	

Heterogeneity: Tau^2=0.18;
Chi^2:514,71; df= 51 (p<0.05) I^2: 90%
Test of overall efect: Z=7.25(p<0.05)

0.01   0.1   1   10   100
Favours experimental   Favours contol

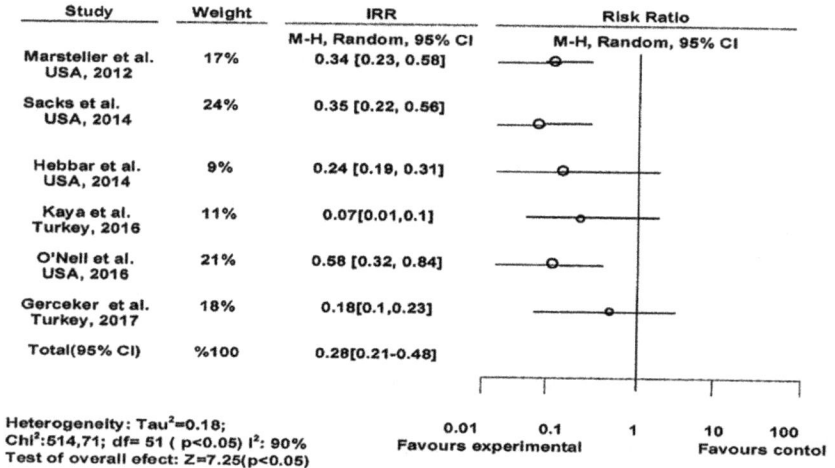

Fig. 2: Risk of Bias

heterogeneity test Q and I^2 tests, trying for risk of bias used to Orwin's Fail-safe N and TAU coefficient (21).

Results

Initially, we reviewed 2290 records. After the subsequent removal of 696 dupli-cates, the literature search contained 1594 studies, 1537 of which were excluded because of what we determined to be improper abstracts and titles. Ultimately, 51 articles were retrieved. The study selection was finalized with 6 studies (22-27), 3 of which were conducted in an ICU (22,23,25), 1 in a PICU (24), 2 in clinics (26,27). The studies were realized in the USA (22-24,26) and Turkey (25,27). CRBSI is a nosocomial disease that can be seen in all age groups, and care bun-dles were seen to be lifesavers also in all age groups (8). However, the dynamics of ICUs and clinics differ in that ICU patients are sedated and only healthcare professionals may touch the CVC. In the clinics, however, the CVC touch risk by patients and attendants is high.

Figure 2 shows intervention effectiveness of the central line bundle to pre-vent catheter- related bloodstream infections; all of the studies include risk of bias evaluation.

Intervention Effectiveness

Four RCT which are included in the meta-analysis have been documented and calculated in two experimental studies. In the literature, a total of 3367 patients formed the control group and 3666 patients formed the experiment group. While most studies detailed the numbers of the control and experiment groups, some neglected to provide such information. Some researchers did not provide descriptions of the specific practices included in the care bundles, but even in such instances it was indicated that care bundles had been practiced on each patient regularly. O'Neil et al. (26) report the use of needle free connectors, Kaya et al. (25) the use of a CVC checklist, and Gerceker et al. (27) the use of a sterilized Tegaderm in both groups. It has been determined that care bundles reduced CRBSI by 68 % in the ICU and 52 % [Figure 2, relative risk (RR) 0.28 95 % CI (0.21 to 0.48)] in the clinics (Table 2). In addition, the high- level distance of the mean effect on heterogeneity test p-value greater than 0.05 and partition heterogeneity that it has been determined to abide by fixed effect model. In these meta- analysis results it is seen that care bundles reduce CRBSI, the high-level distance of the mean effect at the wide interval according to the Cohen (1992) classification system. As this meta- analysis includes only experiment control and RCT, it is possible to say that evidence for these results is strong.

Discussion

It is clear that CRBSI is a prevalent risk in critical care adjustments. Our findings indicate the success rate of the care bundles in preventing CRBSI is 52 % in clinic settings and 68 % in ICU contexts, which is consistent with similar study findings and suggests that the issue of healthcare-related infections in the ICU and clinics is substantial (5,28).

Identifying the incidence of serious issues caused by CRBSI is important in improving patient safety. The importance of care bundles in the prevention of CRBSI was found thanks to the results of previous studies (22-27).

CRBSI, it should be noted, is not only affected by care bundles. System-associated parameters also contribute to CRBSI. These parameters rank clinical nurses according to their work style, attitudes, behaviors, level of information and level of education by "a mixer variable", which influences the success of care bundles. Furthermore, the experimental group's compliance with care bundles was determined to be high. O'Neil et al. (26) found that the rate of CRBSI have lowed both control group and experimental group after the intervention. Both groups were affected from care bundles, this is an application mistake. Also, the control group was monitored three times longer than the experimental group. In the study by Hebbar et al. (24), the rate of CRBSI carried similar characteristics in both the experimental and control groups at the beginning. After training, however, sample groups were observed over a period of two years and it was determined that the rate of CRBSI decreased by 95 % in the experimental group and increased by 26 % in the control group. In Gerceker et al. (27), similar care bundle practices were used in both the experimental and control groups and they were observed for an average period of 7-8 months. In the experimental group, Tegaderm with chlorhexidine was used. It was determined that the rate of CRBSI was zero in the experimental group and 1.7 in the control group for 1000 catheter days. Undoubtedly, patient-related factors are influential in the development of CRBSI. The compliance rate of care bundles changed according to the presence of chronic diseases (29). Kaya et al. (25) found that the sample group features were created to resemble APACHE II scores. Thus, the researchers attempted to control for mixer variables. Additionally, Gerceker et al. (27) performed their research with single group patients in a pediatric hematology unit.

The literature shows that the number of practices in the care bundle is limited by several interventions. For this reason, the patient related, and organizational parameters are not got a grip and CRBSI cannot become hard to avoid deal with. The literature review revealed that both RCT and experimental-control study designs are less frequent and generally conducted in the single center. CVC is inserted by the physicians and generally used by the nurses. The researchers should inquire into the opinions of the involved physicians and nurses. By doing so, a sense of autonomy might improve among the healthcare professionals, and the quality and safety of healthcare might increase. The limitations of this meta-analysis are that it covers only six studies, that the experimental and control groups had no similar characteristics at the beginning of the study, and that the studies differ from one another in terms of their sample sizes. Furthermore, methodological differences among the studies (differences in care bundle practices, low-quality scores, etc.) were accepted as a limiting principle in the interpretation of the results.

CRBSI is affected by patient-related factors. In this context, in Kaya et al. study, experience and control groups similar in APACHE II scores that so researchers have struggled to under control mixer variables. Accordingly, in Gerceker et al. study, the patients in a pediatric hematology unit was researched. In the literature reviews show that care bundles contain a few practices. Previously studies generally measured healthcare professionals have loyalties about these practices. However, success of care bundles is affected patient related factors as well as the rate of organizational structure and workstyle success. Despite of previously studies experience-control or RCT, some important details did not consider such as CVC has inserted by the physicians but used by the nurses. Practices about care bundles contents should above all applied nurses' views and experiences. Thus, it may improve autonomy of health care professionals which increased quality and safety of health care. The limitations of this meta- analysis are containing only six studies, that the experimental and control groups had no similar characteristics at the beginning of the study, and that the studies differ from one another in terms of their sample sizes. Furthermore, methodological differences among the studies (differences in care bundle practices, low-quality scores, etc.) were accepted as a limiting principle in the interpretation of the results.

Conclusion

Most common infections in the intensive care unit frequently catheter related. CRBSI cause of increasing complication risk, is required extra time and labor. Besides, care bundles are reduced morbidity, mortality, costs and prolonged on hospital stay that are required new interventions and plans. Care bundles preventive of CRBSI are healed quality of healthcare. However, it is under controlled mixer variables that is important.

As is frequently encountered with CRBSI, the most common infections are catheter related. CRBSI are increased complication risk, required extra time and labor requirement. However, care bundles reduce morbidity, mortality, costs and prolonged on hospital stay that are required new interventions and plans. Care bundles preventive of CRBSI are effective in improving the quality of healthcare and reducing the instance of CRBSI but mixer variables affect the success rate of central line bundles.

References

1. Salama, M. F., Jamal, W., Al Mousa, H., & Rotimi, V. (2016). Implementation of central venous catheter bundle in an intensive care unit in Kuwait: Effect on central line-associated bloodstream infections. *Journal of Infection and Public Health, 9*(1), 34-41. doi:10.1016/j.jiph.2015.05.001

2. Furuya, E. Y., Dick, A. W., Herzig, C. T., Pogorzelska-Maziarz, M., Larson, E. L., & Stone, P. W. (2016). Central line-associated bloodstream infections reduction and bundle compliance in ICUs: A national study. *Infection Control and Hospital Epidemiology, 37*(7), 805-810. doi:10.1017/ice.2016.67

3. Devrim, İ., Yaşar, N., İşgüder, R., Ceylan, G., Bayram, N., Özdamar, N., ... Ağın, H. (2016). Clinical impact and cost-effectiveness of a central line bundle including split-septum and single-use prefilled flushing devices on central line–associated bloodstream infection rates in a pediatric intensive care unit. *American Journal of Infection Control, 44*(8), e125-e128. doi:10.1016/j.ajic.2016.01.038

4. Ista, E., van der Hoven, B., Kornelisse, R. F., van der Starre, C., Vos, M. C., Boersma, E., & Helder, O. K. (2016). Effectiveness of insertion and maintenance bundles to prevent central-line-associated bloodstream infections in critically ill patients of all ages: A systematic review and meta-analysis. *The Lancet Infectious Diseases, 16*(6), 724-734. doi:10.1016/S1473-3099(15)00409-0

5. Marang-van de Mheen, P. J., & van Bodegom-Vos, L. (2016). Meta-analysis of the central line bundle for preventing catheter-related infections: A case study in appraising the evidence in quality improvement. *BMJ Quality & Safety, 25*(2), 118-129. doi:10.1136/bmjqs-2014-003787

6. Dudeck, M. A., Edwards, J. R., Allen-Bridson, K., Gross, C., Malpiedi, P. J., Peterson, K. D., ... Sievert, D. M. (2015). National healthcare safety network report, data summary for 2013, device-associated module. *American Journal of Infection Control, 43*(3), 206-221. doi:10.1016/j.ajic.2014.11.014

7. Grigonis, A. M., Dawson, A. M., Burkett, M., Dylag, A., Sears, M., Helber, B., & Snyder, L. K. (2016). Use of a central catheter maintenance bundle in long-term acute care hospitals. *American Journal of Critical Care, 25*(2), 165-172. doi:10.4037/ajcc2016894

8. O'grady, N. P., Alexander, M., Burns, L. A., Dellinger, E. P., Garland, J., Heard, S. O., ... Raad, I. I. (2011). Guidelines for the prevention of intravascular catheter-related infections. *Clinical Infectious Diseases, 52*(9), e162-e193. doi:10.1093/cid/cir257

9. Institute for Healthcare Improvement. (n.d.) What is a bundle. Retrieved from http://www.ihi.org/resources/Pages/ImprovementStories/WhatIsaBundle.aspx

10. Chen, Y. M., Dai, A. P., Shi, Y., Liu, Z. J., Gong, M. F., & Yin, X. B. (2014). Effectiveness of silver-impregnated central venous catheters for preventing catheter-related blood stream infections: A meta-analysis. *International Journal of Infectious Diseases, 29*, 279-286. doi:10.1016/j.ijid.2014.09.018

11. Ramritu, P., Halton, K., Collignon, P., Cook, D., Fraenkel, D., Battistutta, D., ... Graves, N. (2008). A systematic review comparing the relative effectiveness of antimicrobial-coated catheters in intensive care units. *American Journal of Infection Control, 36*(2), 104-117. doi:10.1016/j.ajic.2007.02.012

12. Donelli, G., & Francolini, I. (2001). Efficacy of antiadhesive, antibiotic and antiseptic coatings in preventing catheter-related infections. *Journal of chemotherapy*, *13*(6), 595-606. doi:10.1179/joc.2001.13.6.595

13. Yücel, N., Lefering, R., Maegele, M., Max, M., Rossaint, R., Koch, A., ... Schierholz, J. (2004). Reduced colonization and infection with miconazole-rifampicin modified central venous catheters: A randomized controlled clinical trial. *Journal of Antimicrobial Chemotherapy*, *54*(6), 1109-1115. doi:10.1093/jac/dkh483

14. Walz, J. M., Avelar, R. L., Longtine, K. J., Carter, K. L., Mermel, L. A., Heard, S. O., & 5-FU Catheter Study Group. (2010). Anti-infective external coating of central venous catheters: A randomized, noninferiority trial comparing 5-fluorouracil with chlorhexidine/silver sulfadiazine in preventing catheter colonization. *Critical Care Medicine*, *38*(11), 2095-2102. doi:10.1097/CCM.0b013e3181f265ba

15. Theaker, C., Juste, R., Lucas, N., Tallboys, C., Azadian, B., & Soni, N. (2002). Comparison of bacterial colonization rates of antiseptic impregnated and pure polymer central venous catheters in the critically ill. *Journal of Hospital Infection*, *52*(4), 310-312. doi:10.1053/jhin.2002.1310

16. Wang, H., Tong, H., Liu, H., Wang, Y., Wang, R., Gao, H., ... Liu, M. (2018). Effectiveness of antimicrobial-coated central venous catheters for preventing catheter-related blood-stream infections with the implementation of bundles: A systematic review and network meta-analysis. *Annals of Intensive Care*, *8*(1), 71. doi:10.1186/s13613-018-0416-4

17. Moher, D., Liberati, A., Tetzlaff, J., Altman, D. G., & Prisma Group. (2009). Preferred reporting items for systematic reviews and meta-analyses: The PRISMA statement. *PLoS Medicine*, *6*(7), e1000097. doi:10.1371/journal.pmed.1000097

18. O'Grady, N. P., Alexander, M., Burns, L. A., Dellinger, E. P., Garland, J., Heard, S. O., ... Healthcare Infection Control Practices Advisory Committee (HICPAC). (2011) Summary of recommendations: Guidelines for the prevention of intravascular catheter-related infections. *Clinical Infectious Diseases*, *52*(9), 1087-1099. doi:10.1016/j.ajic.2011.01.003

19. Cohen, J. (1992). Statistical power analysis. *Current Directions in Psychological Science*, *1*(3), 98-101. doi:10.1111/1467-8721.ep10768783

20. Thalheimer, W., & Cook, S. (2002). How to calculate effect sizes from published research: A simplified methodology. *Work-Learning Research*, 1-9.

21. Ferguson, C. J. (2007). Evidence for publication bias in video game violence effects literature: A meta-analytic review. *Aggression and Violent Behavior*, *12*(4), 470-482. doi:10.1016/j.avb.2007.01.001

22. Marsteller, J. A., Sexton, J. B., Hsu, Y. J., Hsiao, C. J., Holzmueller, C. G., Pronovost, P. J., & Thompson, D. A. (2012). A multicenter, phased, cluster-randomized controlled trial to reduce central line-associated bloodstream infections in intensive care units. *Critical Care Medicine, 40*(11), 2933-2939. doi:10.1097/CCM.0b013e31825fd4d8

23. Sacks, G. D., Diggs, B. S., Hadjizacharia, P., Green, D., Salim, A., & Malinoski, D. J. (2014). Reducing the rate of catheter-associated bloodstream infections in a surgical intensive care unit using the institute for healthcare improvement central line bundle. *The American Journal of Surgery, 207*(6), 817-823. doi:10.1016/j.amjsurg.2013.08.041

24. Hebbar, K. B., Cunningham, C., McCracken, C., Kamat, P., & Fortenberry, J. D. (2015). Simulation-based paediatric intensive care unit central venous line maintenance bundle training. *Intensive and Critical Care Nursing, 31*(1), 44-50. doi:10.1016/j.iccn.2014.10.003

25. Kaya, H., Turan, Y., Akbal, S., Tosun, K., Aksoy, E., Tunalı, Y., & Aydın, G. Ö. (2016). The effect of nursing care protocol on the prevention of central venous catheter-related infections in neurosurgery intensive care unit. *Applied Nursing Research, 32*, 257-261. doi:10.1016/j.apnr.2016.08.006

26. O'Neil, C., Ball, K., Wood, H., McMullen, K., Kremer, P., Jafarzadeh, S. R., ... Warren, D. (2016). A central line care maintenance bundle for the prevention of catheter-associated bloodstream infection in non-ICU settings. *Infection Control and Hospital Epidemiology, 37*(6), 692-698. doi:10.1017/ice.2016.32

27. Gerçeker, G. Ö., Yardımcı, F., & Aydınok, Y. (2017). Randomized controlled trial of care bundles with chlorhexidine dressing and advanced dressings to prevent catheter-related bloodstream infections in pediatric hematology-oncology patients. *European Journal of Oncology Nursing, 28*, 14-20. doi:10.1016/j.ejon.2017.02.008

28. Holzmann-Pazgal, G., Kubanda, A., Davis, K., Khan, A. M., Brumley, K., & Denson, S. E. (2012). Utilizing a line maintenance team to reduce central-line-associated bloodstream infections in a neonatal intensive care unit. *Journal of Perinatology, 32*(4), 281-286. doi:10.1038/jp.2011.91

29. de Wet, C., McKay, J., & Bowie, P. (2012). Combining QOF data with the care bundle approach may provide a more meaningful measure of quality in general practice. *BMC Health Services Research, 12*(1), 351. doi:10.1186/1472-6963-12-351

Gamze Zengin and Hayat Yalın

Quality of Life in Individuals with Stroke

Abstract

Objective: Stroke can often have a negative impact on the entire life of individuals, especially in individual, social and economic terms. This study will prepare a favorable ground for expanding studies on the quality of life of individuals with stroke in the field of nursing, evaluating whether there are similar results in different time intervals and different groups, and will also guide the decisions to be taken on how to improve the quality of care service provided.

Materials and Methods: The sample of the study includes 202 patients. In this study, which was carried out with quantitative technique, the Patient-Disease Description Form containing information about sociodemographic characteristics and diseases, London Handicap Scale and Barthel Index were used as data collection tools.

Results: 100 female and 102 male patients participated in the study and the mean age was calculated as 61.7 years. Patients According to the Barthel Index, 43 (21.3 %) were fully dependent, 63 (31.2 %) were highly dependent, 61 (30.2 %) were moderately dependent, 17 (8 %) were mildly dependent, 18 (8.9 %) are fully independent. However, a positive correlation was found between London Handicap Scale scores and Barthel Index scores.

Conclusion: The quality of life in individuals with stroke is affected not only by the consequences of the disease and disease, but also by many other variables such as social, physical environment, mental status, pre-stroke disability and socioeconomic status.

Keywords: Quality of Life, Stroke, London Handicap Scale, Barthel Index

Introduction

It is seen that when the total disease burden in Turkey evaluated at national level, the primary cause is cardiovascular disease, the second degree is caused by cerebrovascular diseases. The presence of chronic diseases not only changes the lives of affected individuals, but also affects many aspects of the care they receive. Especially, stroke is considered as a reason that causes disability and reduces the quality of life (1).

Stroke is the third major health problem in the world that can cause death and various disabilities (2). Considering at the studies in recent years, studies intended to examine other factors related to quality of life and quality of life occurred in individuals after stroke have increased in importance. The most important reason of this is that quality of life in individuals with stroke is also a representation of the individual's perception and interpretation of the effects an individual encountered after a stroke (3,4).

While 30 % of patients in the acute phase of stroke die within about a year, approximately one-third of those who continue their lives become dependent on others in order to perform daily life activities in later periods (5). The role of nursing care in individuals with stroke is undeniably important. Assuming that especially, individuals with stroke are in a group of patients who need direct nursing care both in terms of medical and care service (6), the significance level of nursing services and studies on this subject is also increasing. In the light of the notional basis and study findings, it is aimed to determine the quality of life of patients with stroke in this study.

Materials and Methods

The population of study consists of 2400 patients who applied to the Stroke polyclinic of Neurology Department of Dr Sadi Konuk Training and Research Hospital in the last year. The sample of the study consists of 202 patients who came to control to the Stroke polyclinic of Neurology Department of Dr Sadi Konuk Training and Research Hospital had a previous stroke (ischemic and hemorrhagic) and met the sample selection criteria.

Inclusion and Exclusion Criteria

- Primarily, whether the patients meet the condition of "voluntarily agreeing to participate in the study"
- Whether the patients had a stroke at least three months ago
- Participants are 18 years or older
- The absence of severe perception disorder and not having any disability before stroke was searched

Data Acquisition Method and Tools

In this study performed with quantitative technique the data collection technique is the survey practice. After obtaining necessary permissions in order to conduct the study, the Patient-Disease Identification Form containing information about sociodemographic characteristics and diseases, London Handicap Scale and Barthel Index were applied to the patients included in the study.

Tab. 1: Cronbach's Alpha Values

	Cronbach's Alpha	Number of Items
London Handicap Scale	0.863	6
Barthel Index	0.947	10

The Patient-Disease Identification Form is a questionary form developed to determine the profiles of the patients using the current literature information. The form consists of two part, "Sociodemographic Characteristics Form" and "Disease Description Form".

London Handicap Scale (LHS)) is the most widely used measurement tool that evaluates disability in stroke patients. It is a general quality of life scale related the health published by Harwood and Ebrahim in 1994 (7). The Turkish validity and reliability study were carried out by Yalın and Sabuncu (8).

The scale, consisting of six parts, measures a disability profile and general disability severity in six different dimensions (movement, physical independence, occupation, social relations, adaptation, and economic competence). The maximum score obtained from the scoring scale is 30, by giving "5" points to the one showing the best situation and "0" to the worst situation among the answer options.

The Barthel Index was developed by Mahoney and Barthel (1965) and is used especially in patients who experience loss of sensory and motor functions. The scoring level of this index, which consists of ten sub-dimensions including daily life activities such as eating, washing, daily care, dressing, defecation, micturition, getting out of bed, going to the toilet, walking around, climbing stairs is between "0" points and "100" points. In order to the individual to be evaluated independently, he / she must get at least "60" score (9).

Statistical Analysis of Data

SPSS 21.0 Statistical package was used for statistical analysis. Kolmogorov - Smirnov distribution test was used to examine the normal distribution. The general reliability of the London Handicap Scale was found 0.863 and The Barthel Index general reliability was found 0.947 (Table 1). Pearson chi-square test was used to compare qualitative data. Spearman Correlation Analysis was used for relationships between scales. The results were evaluated at 95 % confidence interval and p<0.05 significance level.

Results

The demographic characteristics of 202 stroke patients included in the study are shown in Table 1. The age average of the patients was 61.680±15.891 (21-96), 50.5 % (n=102) of the patients were male. It was determined that 88.1 % of patients (n=178) were married, 58.9 % (n=119) were primary school graduates, 85.1 % (n=172) were not working, and 95 % had a social security. The average body mass ratio of the patients was calculated as 26.361±4.630 (15.43-44.08).

The stroke type variable of the patients is shown in Table 2. According to the stroke type variable, it was determined that 74.8 % (n=151) had ischemia and 25.2 % had hemorrhage. It is distributed as 49 % (n=25) is intracerebral lobar according to the location of hemorrhage, 55.3 % (n=83) is lacunar infarcts (LACI) according to the ischemic stroke clinical classification, 55.6 % (n=84) is veinlet occlusion according to the ischemic stroke etiological classification. It was determined that the speech of 96.5 % of the patients was normal.

According to the neurological deficit variable of the patients shown in Table 3, 68.3 % (n=138) of the patients were found to have loss of strength in the right arm and 52.2 % (n=105) of the patients in the right leg. It was found that 97.5 % (n=195) of the patients obeyed orders, 97.5 % (n=195) did not have a place orientation problem, and 98 % (n=196) did not have time orientation problems. It was found that the total mean score of the patients on the London Handicap Scale was 19.936 (±6.262) and the total mean score of the patients on the Barthel Index was 56.630 (±32.320).

As a result of the correlation analysis conducted to determine the relationship between the total score of the Barthel Index and the London Handicap Scale, a positive significant relationship was found between the scores at the level of 88.9 % (r=0.889; p=0.000) (Table 4). According to this, as the Barthel Index score increases, the total score of the London Handicap Scale increases.

When London Handicap Scale and Barthel Index were compared in terms of group variables, no statistically significant relationship was found between marital status, location of hemorrhage, etiological and clinical classification of ischemic stroke, obedience to orders, time orientation, problem of place orientation, speech and social security.

The difference between the group averages was found to be significant according to the results of the Kruskal Wallis Test, which was conducted to determine whether the mean scores of the London Handicap Scale total scores of the patients differ significantly in terms of the educational status variable (KW=29.617; p=0.000). Mann Whitney U test was applied to determine

Tab. 2: Distribution of Socio-demographic Characteristics (n=202)

	Variables	Frequency	Percentage
Age	49 and below	47	23.3
	50-59	35	17.3
	60-69	55	27.2
	70-79	35	17.3
	80 and above	30	14.9
	Total	202	100.0
Gender	Female	100	49.5
	Male	102	50.5
	Total	202	100.0
Body Mass Ratio	Weak	8	4.0
	Normal Weight	76	37.6
	Slightly fat	82	40.6
	Obese	36	17.8
	Total	202	100.0
Marital Status	Married	178	88.1
	Bachelor	24	11.9
	Total	202	100.0
Educational Status	Illiterate	24	11.9
	Literate	14	6.9
	Primary Education	119	58.9
	High School	30	14.9
	University	9	4.5
	Others	6	3.0
	Total	202	100.0
Employment Status	Employment	30	14.9
	Unemployment	172	85.1
	Total	202	100.0
Social Security	Have social security	192	95.0
	No social security	10	5.0
	Total	202	100.0

which group caused the difference. Accordingly, the total score of the London Handicap Scale (23.222±3.114) was found to be higher in university graduates (Table 5). The difference between the group averages in terms of the educational status variable of the Barthel Index total scores was also found significant (KW=29.019; p=0.000<0.05). According to this, the Barthel Index total

Tab. 3: Disease (Stroke) Diagnosis (n=202)

	Variables	Frequency	Percentage
Stroke Type	Hemorrhage	51	25.2
	Ischemia	151	74.8
	Total	202	100.0
Hemorrhage Localization	Intracerebral lobar	25	49.0
	Subcortical	14	27.5
	Subarachnoid	12	23.5
	Total	51	100.0
Ischemic stroke clinical classification	Total anterior circulation infarcts (TACI)	25	16.7
	Partial anterior circulation infarcts (PACI)	26	17.3
	Lacunar Infarcts (LACI)	83	55.3
	Posterior Circulation Infarcts (POCI)	16	10.7
	Total	150	100.0
Ischemic stroke etiological classification	Large artery atherothrombosis	27	17.9
	Cardio embolism	28	18.5
	Veinlet occlusion	84	55.6
	Rare etiologies of stroke	4	2.6
	Not classified etiology	8	5.3
	Total	151	100.0
Speech	Normal	195	96.5
	Mild aphasia	7	3.5
	Total	202	100.0

Tab. 4: Spearman Correlation Analysis of the Relationship Between London Handicap Scale and Barthel Index

	Variables	London Handicap Scale Total Score
Barthel Index	r	0.889
Total Score	P	**0.000**
	N	202

score (69.000±33.151) was found to be higher in high school graduates. It was found that the higher the education level, the higher the quality of life.

The difference between the group averages was not found significant according to the results of the Kruskal Wallis H-Test, which was conducted to determine whether the mean scores of the London Handicap Scale and Barthel Index show a significant difference in terms of body mass ratio variable (p>0.05) (Table 6).

The difference between the group averages was found to be statistically significant according to the results of the Kruskal Wallis H Test , which was conducted to determine whether the mean scores of the London Handicap Scale total scores of the patients differ significantly in terms of the employment status (Mann Whitney U=1 466.000; p=0.000). According to this both the London Handicap Scale total scores (23.833) and the Barthel Index total scores (77.333) were found to be high in the working group (Table 7).

The Mann Whitney-U test was used to determine whether the mean scores of the London Handicap Scale total scores of the patients differed significantly according to the stroke type variable (Table 8). As a result of the test, the difference between the group averages was found to be statistically significant (Mann Whitney U=2 960.000; p=0.013 <0.05). Both the London Handicap Scale total scores (20.510) and the Barthel Index total scores (59.934) were found to be high in patients with stroke type ischemia (Mann Whitney U=2 901.000; p=0.008 <0.05).

Discussion

In line with the literature, the findings of the study conducted to determine the quality of life of patients after stroke were discussed under three headings: comparison of the sociodemographic findings with the literature, comparison of the findings regarding the disease with the literature, comparison of

Tab. 5: Comparison of London Handicap Scale and Barthel Index with Education Status Variable

		n	Mean	SD	KW	p
London Handicap Scale Total Score	Illiterate	24	14.000	5.150	29.617	**0.000**
	Literate	14	18.286	6.462		
	Primary Education	119	20.872	5.919		
	High School	30	21.633	6.568		
	University	9	23.222	3.114		
	Others	6	17.333	3.830		
Barthel Index Total Score	Illiterate	24	26.458	25.302	29.019	**0.000**
	Literate	14	57.143	26.509		
	Primary Education	119	59.160	31.207		
	High School	30	69.000	33.151		
	University	9	68.33	25.249		
	Others	6	46.667	32.197		

Tab. 6: Comparison of London Handicap Scale and Barthel Index with Body Mass Ratio Variable

		n	Mean	SD	KW	p
London Handicap Scale Total Score	Weak	8	20.000	9.024	1.233	**0.745**
	Normal Weight	76	19.816	6.334		
	Slightly Fat	82	19.585	6.130		
	Obese	36	20.972	5.877		
Barthel Index Total Score	Weak	8	54.375	41.095	1.157	**0.763**
	Normal Weight	76	58.290	31.692		
	Slightly Fat	82	54.024	32.102		
	Obese	36	59.583	33.045		

Tab. 7: Comparison of London Handicap Scale and Barthel Index with Employment Status Variable

		n	Mean	SD	KW	p
London Handicap Scale Total Score	Employment	30	23.833	4.942	1 466.000	0.000
	Unemployment	172	19.256	6.231		
Barthel Index Total Score	Employment	30	77.333	24.059	1 423.000	0.000
	Unemployment	172	53.023	32.271		

Tab. 8: Comparison of London Handicap Scale and Barthel Index with Stroke Type Variable

		n	Mean	SD	KW	p
London Handicap Scale Total Score	Hemorrhage	51	18.235	5.694	2 960.000	0.013
	Ischemia	151	20.510	6.358		
Barthel Index Total Score	Hemorrhage	51	46.863	30.773	2 901.000	0.008
	Ischemia	151	59.934	32.259		

the results of the Barthel Index and London Handicap Scale in stroke assessment with the literature.

Comparison of Sociodemographic Findings with the Literature

The sociodemographic status of the patients participating in the study was examined and it was found that the patients included not only 65 years and older, but also those under 49 years old. In addition, the average age was calculated as 61.7 years. In many studies on stroke and quality of life, the age range in question is generally 65 years and older. In a study conducted by Akinpelu et al., The average age of the participants was reported as 63 years (10).

It was found to be 71 in Denmark and America and 73 in Australia (11). We think that this difference is low due to the fact that the young population in our country is higher compared to western countries.

In previous studies, it has been seen that the quality of life of individuals with a stroke was associated with age (11), gender (8), education level (12), depression (2), length of hospital stay (9), functional status (3), and social participation (13). The findings are parallel with the literature.

Comparison of Findings Regarding the Disease with the Literature

As a result of the analysis of the stroke subtypes of the patients participating in the study, it was found that predominantly ischemic stroke (74.8 %). In the study conducted by Eskiyurt et al. (14), 66.3 % of the patients were found to have ischemic stroke, and in the study conducted by Kumral et al. 77 % of the patients were found to have ischemic stroke. While our results are similar to those of Kumral et al. They are different from other literature findings (15).

When the motor and sensory losses of the cases were investigated, motor and sensory losses were found in the right arm of 68.3 %, the left arm of 66 %, the right leg of 52.2 %, and the left leg of 70.4 %. According to the study conducted by Kolapu and Oluwotitofunmi, it was stated that 40 % of the patients had a loss of strength on the left side of their body and 60 % on the right side (2). Our study is parallel with the literature.

Comparison of the Results of the Barthel Index and London Handicap Scale in Stroke Assessment with the Literature

In this study, as a result of the analysis of the relationship between the London Handicap Scale and the total scores of the Barthel Index, it was seen that both scales had a positive significant relationship with each other and as the quality of life increased according to the London Handicap Scale, addiction decreased. This situation is directly proportional to assumed predictions.

Various results have been reached regarding the link between the London Handicap Scale and the Barthel Index. In the study, it was seen that the total score of the London Handicap Scale was similar in all participants, the average was 57, and the Barthel Index scores varied between 5 and 20 points and remained below the high score limit. Nevertheless, there are results that there is a significant relationship between the scores of both scales. Our study is parallel with the work of Harwood and Ebrahim, who prepared LHO (8). The mean of the LHO was found as 72 (16) in the study conducted by Sturm et al. The study is lower than the results of Sturm et al. It is also necessary to take into account the differences between the social structures in which studies are carried out and, in this case, it can be said that the scale scores are also consistent.

It was found that the total scores of both the London Handicap Scale and the Barthel Index Scale (74.894±27.336) were the highest in patients aged 49 and under, and that the total scores of both scales decreased as the age got older. Gündüz and Erhan stated that there is no significance between age and the Barthel Index (17). Sharma et al. stated that the quality of life of patients 75 years and older decreased (18). Our study is parallel to the study of Sharma et al. and different from Gündüz and Erhan's study. It can be said that the reason for the difference is chronic diseases in advanced ages (17,18).

The total scores of the London Handicap Scale (23.222±3.114) of those with a university education level were found to be higher than other educational status. The Barthel Index total scores (69.000±33.151) of those with high school education were found to be high. Topçu and Bölüktaş stated that the lower the education level, the lower the quality of life (19). Our result is coherent with the literature. It is detected that both the London Handicap Scale total scores (23.833) and the Barthel Index total scores (77.333) were found to be higher in the employment group. In the study conducted by Topçu and Bölüktaş, it was stated that the economic situation affects the quality of life, and the quality of life of individuals with a good economic situation is high in all areas of life (19). The literature supports our results.

The difference between the total scores of the findings London Handicap Scale and Barthel Index and the group averages of body mass ratio was not significant (p>0.05). It was determined that the findings in the obese group had higher scores in the total scores of both scales. Obesity is known to cause the formation of many diseases today.

Conclusion

In this study, analyzes were conducted to evaluate the quality of life of individuals with stroke from a nursing perspective. Although there is a relationship between the Barthel Index and the London Handicap Scale at the stage of findings, it should be considered that there may be many other dimensions affecting the quality of life after stroke. In addition to all these, the development of tools used in measuring the quality of life and the evaluation of the usability of existing tools on the society is another important factor. In this study, it was aimed to test the widespread use of the London Handicap Scale, whose Turkish validity and reliability study was recently conducted, in individuals with stroke and the scale was found to be applicable in the study findings.

In this study, it was attempted to mainly focus on the effect of loss of function after stroke. In future studies, considering other factors affecting the quality of life will be useful for understanding and improving the quality of life. But more specifically, the quality of life in individuals with stroke, and in terms of practice, it will help healthcare providers to form a comprehensive understanding of patients.

Recommendations for further studies can be summarized as follows:

- Considering other environmental and medical factors that affect the relationship between stroke and quality of life will be beneficial for practices and regulations aimed at improving the quality of life.
- Increase in addiction levels of individuals with stroke after stroke will affect the extent of care they will receive, for this reason, the nursing service to be provided should have a comprehensive feature, individual-centered implementation and regulations should be made to eliminate obstacles in this regard.
- It is necessary to increase descriptive studies using measurement tools on the quality of life and disability levels of persons with disabilities. In this way, more reliable data will be obtained and the reliability of applications to be made in repetitive results will increase.
- Assessment of the knowledge levels and approaches of nurses and other health care providers in providing care to individuals with stroke will create awareness not only for the patient but also for the service provider and will contribute to the improvement of the quality of care and the quality of life that can be associated with it.

References

1. Lima, M. L., Santas, J. L., Sawada, N. O., & Lima, L. A. (2014). Quality of life of individuals with stroke and their caregivers in a city of Triângulo Mineiro. *Revista Brasileira de Epidemiologia, 17*(2), 453-464. doi:10.1590/1809-4503201400020013eng

2. Kolapu, H. T., & Oluwotitofunmi, P. G. (2009). The London handicap scale: Validation of a Yoruba (Nigerian) version among stroke survivors. *African Journal of Neurological Sciences, 28*(1). doi:10.4314/ajns.v28i1.55140

3. Jaracz, K., & Kozubski, W. (2003). Quality of life in stroke patients. *Acta Neurologica Scandinavica, 107*(5), 324-329. doi:10.1034/j.1600-0404.2003.02078.x

4. Patel, M. T., Tilling, K., Lawrence, E., Rudd, A. G., Wolfe, C. D., & McKewitt, C. (2006). Relationships between long-term stroke disability, handicap and health-related quality of life. *Age and Ageing, 35*(3), 273-279. doi:10.1093/ageing/afj074

5. Çelik, A. (2014). *İnmeli hastalarda fonksiyonel durumun bakım verenlerin bakım yüküne ve yaşam kalitesine etkisi.* (Unpublished master's thesis). Gülhane Military Medical Academy, Ankara, Turkey.

6. Türk, G., Hakverdioğlu, G., Eşer, İ., & Korshid, L. (2010). İnmeli hastaların hemşire kayıtlarının incelenmesi. *Dokuz Eylül University School of Nursing Electronic Journal, 3*(4), 171-174.

7. Harwood, R. H., Gompertz, P., & Ebrahim, S. (1994). Handicap one year after a stroke: Validity of a new scale. *Journal of Neurology, Neurosurgery, and Psychiatry, 57*(7), 825-829. doi:10.1136/jnnp.57.7.825

8. Yalın, H., & Sabuncu, N. (2019). Handicap and quality of life of the patients after stroke. In F. Eti Aslan (Ed.), *Scientific researches in health sciences* (pp. 115-135). Berlin: Peter Lang.

9. Mahoney, F. I., & Barthel, D. (1965). Functional evaluation: The barthel index. *Maryland State Medical Journal, 14*, 61-65.

10. Akinpelu, A. O., & Gbiri, C. A. (2009). Quality of life of stroke survivors and apparently healthy individuals in southwestern Nigeria. *Physiotherapy Theory and Practice, 25*(1), 14-20. doi:10.1080/09593980802622669

11. Gorelick, P. B. (1995). Stroke prevention. *Archives of Neurology, 52*(4), 347-355. doi:10.1001/archneur.1995.00540280029015

12. Aprile, I., Piazzini, D. B., Bertolini, C., Caliandro, P., Pazzaglia, C., Tonali, P., & Padua, L. (2006). Predictive variables on disability and quality of life in stroke outpatients undergoing rehabilitation. *Neurological Sciences, 27*(1), 40-46. doi:10.1007/s10072-006-0563-5

13. Kauhanen, M. L., Korpelainen, J. T., Hiltunen, P., Nieminen, P., Sotaniemi, K. A., & Myllyla, V. V. (2000). Domains and determinants of quality of life after stroke caused by brain infarction. *Archives of Physical Medicine and Rehabilitation, 81*(12), 1541-1546. doi:10.1053/apmr.2000.9391

14. Eskiyurt, N., Yalıman, A., Vural, M., Kızıltaş, H., Bölükbaş, N., & Çeşme, F. (2005). İnmeli olguların özellikleri ve fonksiyonel durum sonuçları. *İstanbul Tıp Fakültesi Dergisi, 68*(3), 71-77.

15. Kumral, E., Özkaya, B., Sagduyu, A., Şirin, H., Vardarli, E., & Pehlivan, M. (1998). The Ege stroke registry: A hospital-based study in the Aegean region, Izmir, Turkey. Analysis of 2,000 stroke patients. *Cerebrovascular Diseases, 8*(5), 278-288. doi:10.1159/000015866

16. Sturm, J. W., Dewey, H. M., Donnan, G. A., Macdonell, R. A. L., McNeil, J. J., & Thrift, A. G. (2002). Handicap after stroke: How does it relate to disability, perception of recovery, and stroke subtype?: The North East Melbourne Stroke Incidence Study (NEMESIS). *Stroke, 33*(3), 762-768. doi:10.1161/hs0302.103815

17. Gündüz, B., & Erhan, B. (2008). Quality of life of stroke patients' spouses living in the community in Turkey: Controlled study with short form-36 questionnaire. *Journal of Neurological Sciences [Turkish], 25*(4), 226-234.

18. Sharma, J. S., Fletcher, S., & Vassalo, M. (1999). Strokes in the elderly - higher acute and 3-month mortality - an explanation. *Cerebrovascular Diseases, 9*(1), 2-9. doi:10.1159/000015889

19. Topçu, S., & Bölüktaş, R. P. (2012). İnmeli hastalarda yaşam kalitesi ve sosyal desteğin yaşam kalitesine etkisinin incelenmesi. *Yeni Tıp Dergisi, 29*(3), 159-164.

İbrahim Elmas and Hayat Yalın

Life Quality of Nurses: Mardin Province Sample

Abstract

Objective: The study has been carried out to define the quality of life of nurses working in Mardin.

Materials and Methods: This descriptive study has been carried out with 225 nurses working in public hospitals in Mardin. The data has been collected by using personal information sheet and The World Health Organization Quality of Life (WHOQOL) questionary. For the analysis of the obtained data SPSS 22.0 packaged software has been used.

Results: It has been defined that 60 % of the nurses taking part in the study are female (n=153), 41.6 % of them (n=106) are between 26 and 30 years old, 51.4 % of them (n=131) are high school graduate, and 55.3 % of them (n=141) are married. The average scores of the WHOQOL-BREF sub-dimension of the nurses were calculated respectively as "physical quality of life" for 13.313 (±2.222); 13.271 (±2.292) for "psychological quality of life";13.197 (±3.190) for "social quality of life" and 11.855 (±2.229) for "environmental quality of life". A statistical significance was determined among workload, the way of work, choosing the profession, suitability to the profession, communication with colleagues, economic problem, vacationing, physical activity variables and quality of life, especially the sub-dimension of "environmental quality of life".

Conclusion: Among nurses' quality of life sub-dimensions, it was determined that the highest scores were for physical quality of life and the lowest were for environmental quality of life.

Keywords: Nursing, Scales, Life Quality, Mardin

Introduction

The concept of quality of life was considered as the state of excellence of man in ancient and medieval ages, the highest level of virtue, and having the highest level of beauty. Psychologists brought up the life satisfaction dimension of the quality of life in the 1970s. The concept of life quality entered the field of medicine after the 1970s and nursing after 1980s. The concept of life quality is difficult to describe since it is versatile, changing and developing constantly, differing from one person to another, what is enjoyable, describing what to be and how to live, and being affected by social, psychological, economic, and cultural factors (1). World Health Organization Quality of Life (WHOQOL) group described the life quality as "The cultural structure and values system that the patient lives in, as well as in terms of their own purposes, expectations, standards and concerns personal perception of their situation in life."

World Health Organization stated that its healthcare personnel were exposed to psychological, physical, and psychological risks in their workplace (2). In the studies conducted it was stated that there is a relationship between job satisfaction and health and quality of life, and that nurses provide their services in difficult working environment and conditions which affect their job satisfaction, health and life quality.

Serving many citizens at the same time within period of busy working time, increases the stress level of nurses. From this and similar situations nurses' quality of life is negatively affected. The life quality of nurses affects the service and others all. Safe and healthy working environment is an essential right for nurses and other workers, and it plays an important role in increasing the life quality. Working environment and conditions dramatically affect nurses' physical, psychological, social, environmental, and general life quality (3). For this reason, the study was carried out to determine the nurses' life quality.

Materials and Methods

Data of the nurses working in Mardin public hospitals between September 2017 and November 2017 were collected with permission of Dicle University Medical Faculty Ethics Committee and Mardin Public Hospital Association. Nurses who volunteer to participate in the study are informed and their consents has been taken.

The study is descriptive and analytical. In order to do Universe (n=750) generalization and representation the sample size was determined by the following formula.

In the research, the data were obtained by the researcher through face-to-face interview method, personal information form and World Health Organization Quality of Life. Personal information form created by the researcher consists of 28 questions in total including socio-demographic characteristics of nurses, their health behavior and job satisfaction. World Health Organization Quality of Life Scale-WHOQOL BREF is a form Created by the World Health Organization consisting of 26 questions. In the Turkish adaptation of the WHOQOL BREF Scale, there is another question regarding the environment, and it consists of 27 questions in total (4). While evaluating the findings of the study, SPSS 22.0 Statistical package for statistical analysis program has been used. In the case of two groups in the comparison of quantitative data independent samples t test was used for comparisons between groups. In the case of more than two groups in comparison of quantitative data Turkey test was used in One-way (Anova) test and the detection of the group causing the difference. The results were evaluated at a 95 % confidence interval and a significance level of $p<0.05$. World Health Organization Quality of Life Scale Cronbach's Alpha coefficient was found to be 0.900.

Results

Of the 255 nurses participating in the study it was determined that 153 were women, 141 were married, 63 were in the 26-30 age group, 131 of them were undergraduate, 75 of them had no children, 187 of them lived with their families, 153 of them had normal body mass index, 164 of them did not smoke and 225 of them did not use alcohol. It was determined that 147 of the nurses participating in the research have been working for five years or less, 142 of them by profession and 177 of them voluntarily chose the unit they worked in, 147 of them were less than five years, 72 of them were from 6 to 10, 19 of them were between 11 and 15, 10 of them were between 16 and 20, and 7 of them were more than 21 years.

When income, social life and daily activities of the nurses were questioned it was reported that 114 of them had more expenses than income, 169 of them had economic problems, 108 of them could not afford to go on holiday, 69 of them never went to the theater or cinema, 87 of them slept an average of six hours a day, and 63 of them did 30-60 minutes of physical activity three days a week.

The general quality of life of the nurses participating in the study was found to be moderate, and as stated in Table 1 the highest rank was in the field of the physical quality of life and the lowest rank was in the field of environmental quality of life.

Tab. 1: Quality of Life Scale Scores

	Mean	SD	Min.	Max.
Physical Quality of Life	13.313	2.222	7.430	18.290
Psychological Quality of Life	13.271	2.292	6.000	19.330
Social Quality of Life	13.197	3.190	4.000	20.000
Environmental Quality of Life	11.855	2.229	5.780	18.220
Overall Quality of Life	12.909	2.003	6.300	18.600

In order to determine whether there is a significant difference of the nurses participating in the study in terms of their physical, psychological, social and environmental quality of life the statistical significance of the differences between group means conditions were shown by one-way variance analysis (Anova) and t test (Table 2).

When the mean scale scores of the nurses according to the gender variable are compared, male nurses' (13.703) physical quality of life mean scores compared to female nurses (13.053) high and statistically significant (p=0.022 <0.05). When the scores of the quality of life scale are compared according to the marital status variable, the physical, psychological, in social and environmental areas those who are married have higher mean scores and statistical significance was found in the area (t=2.520; p=0.012 <0.05). When the quality of life scale scores are compared according to alcohol consumption status it was detected that those who consume alcohol have lower average of the quality of life scores in physical, social, psychological and environmental areas compared to those who do not consume.

A statistical significance was found in the field of psychological quality of life that those who do not have a chronic psychiatric disorder have higher life quality in physical, psychological, social and environmental areas compared to those who have such disorder (p=0.036<0.05). It was found that the average score of the quality of life scale was higher in psychological, social and environmental areas, and those working in the physical field in the form of daytime and shifts according to the type of work. A statistical significance was found in the field of environmental quality of life (p=0.002 <0.05).

It has been found that those who consider the profession very suitable for themselves have higher life quality in physical, psychological, social and social areas and a statistical significance was found in the areas of environmental (p=0.041 <0.05) and psychological (p=0.002 <0.05) quality of life.

Discussion

Scores obtained from the World Health Organization Quality of Life Scale (WHOQOL-BREF) was calculated respectively as following: 13.313±2.222 from the physical domain, 13.271±2.292 from the psychological domain, 13.197±3.190 and 11.855±2.229 from the circumferential area. According to these results, nurse's overall quality of life is moderate, and the highest average score is the physical area, the lowest the average is seen to be in the environmental area.

Tab. 2: Comparison of Quality of Life Scores According to Some Variables

Variable		n	Physical Quality of Life			
			Mean	SD	t	p
Gender	Woman	153	13.05	2.225	-2.307	0.022
	Man	102	13.70	2.171		
Martial Status	Married	141	13.33	2.260	0.096	0.923
	Single	114	13.30	2.184		
Use of Alcohol	Yes	30	12.74	2.232	-1.500	0.135
	No	225	13.39	2.215		
Chronic Psychiatric Disease	Yes	6	11.81	1.286	-1.683	0.094
	No	249	13.35	2.229		
Way of Working	Day	65	13.27	2.091	0.567	0.568
	Night	9	12.57	2.339		
	24 Hours	181	13.37	2.267		
Suitable Occupation	Appropriate Partly	62	13.71	2.255	1.445	0.238
	Suitable	158	13.22	2.207		
	Not Available	35	13.03	2.204		

(continued on next page)

Tab. 2: Continued

Variable		n	Psychological Quality of Life			
			Mean	SD	t	p
Gender	Woman	153	13.19	2.226	-0.654	0.514
	Man	102	13.39	2.393		
Martial Status	Married	141	13.39	2.494	0.926	0.345
	Single	114	13.12	2.015		
Use of Alcohol	Yes	30	12.47	2.257	-2.058	0.041
	No	225	13.38	2.280		
Chronic Psychiatric Disease	Yes	6	11.33	1.033	-2.110	0.036
	No	249	13.32	2.295		
Way of Working	Day	65	13.58	2.210	1.088	0.339
	Night	9	12.59	2.952		
	24 Hours	181	13.19	2.286		
Suitable Occupation	Appropriate Partly	62	13.97	2.273	6.408	0.002
	Suitable	158	13.22	2.230		
	Not Available	35	12.29	2.230		

Variable		n	Social Quality of Life			
			Mean	SD	t	p
Gender	Woman	153	13.05	2.977	-0.929	0.354
	Man	102	13.43	3.488		
Martial Status	Married	141	13.65	3.242	2.520	0.012
	Single	114	12.64	3.048		
Use of Alcohol	Yes	30	12.67	3.336	-0.970	0.333
	No	225	13.27	3.171		
Chronic	Yes	6	10.89	3.519	-1.802	0.073
Psychiatric Disease	No	249	13.25	3.169		
Way of Working	Day	65	13.39	3.213	2.362	0.096
	Night	9	10.96	2.289		
	24 Hours	181	13.24	3.171		
Suitable Occupation	Appropriate Partly	62	13.51	3.538	1.008	0.366
	Suitable	158	13.22	2.973		
	Not Available	35	12.55	3.485		

(continued on next page)

Tab. 2: Continued

Variable		n	Environmental Quality of Life			
			Mean	SD	t	p
Gender	Woman	153	11.90	2.193	0.402	0.688
	Man	102	11.79	2.290		
Martial Status	Married	141	11.91	2.268	0.449	0.654
	Single	114	11.79	2.186		
Use of Alcohol	Yes	30	11.45	2.348	-1.056	0.292
	No	225	11.91	2.212		
Chronic Psychiatric Disease	Yes	6	10.52	1.836	-1.491	0.137
	No	249	11.89	2.230		
Way of Working	Day	65	12.68	2.020	6.283	0.002
	Night	9	11.51	2.238		
	24 Hours	181	11.58	2.236		
Suitable Occupation	Appropriate Partly	62	12.39	2.118	3.246	0.041
	Suitable	158	11.78	2.231		
	Not Available	35	11.24	2.268		

Variable		n	Public Quality of Life			
			Mean	SD	t	p
Gender	Woman	153	12.80	1.942	-1.080	0.281
	Man	102	13.08	2.090		
Martial Status	Married	141	13.07	2.133	1.413	0.159
	Single	114	12.71	1.818		
Use of Alcohol	Yes	30	12.33	2.065	-1.686	0.093
	No	225	12.99	1.986		
Chronic Psychiatric Disease	Yes	6	11.14	1.680	-2.209	0.028
	No	249	12.95	1.993		
Way of Working	Day	65	13.23	1.843	2.062	0.129
	Night	9	11.91	2.221		
	24 Hours	181	12.84	2.035		
Suitable Occupation	Appropriate Partly	62	13.39	2.049	3.688	0.026
	Suitable	158	12.86	1.927		
	Not Available	35	12.28	2.105		

In the study, the difference was found to be statistically significant that the average scores of the quality of life of male nurses are physical, psychological, and social higher than the average of female nurses in the physical fields. In the research of Topal et al., it was determined that the life quality of females is better psychologically and there is no significant difference in perceptions of physical, social, and environmental situation (5). Wang et al. reported in their study that there is no statistical significance between gender variables (6). It is thought to be caused by the variability of the groups that these differences in studies on the effect of gender on quality of life.

In the study, the life quality score average of those whose marital status is married is higher in all sub-dimensions. There is a statistically significant difference between the differences in social quality of life. Similarly, in the studies of Hacıhasanoğlu and Yıldırım and Kıvanç, the points of those married ones' statistical significance were found in the social quality of life area (7,8).

Physical, psychological, social, and environmental quality of life scores of non-smokers and non-drinkers is higher than those using the means, and statistical significance was found in the differences between them. Yalçınkaya and Kıvanç evaluated the quality of life scores of alcohol and cigarette consumers in their studies and found the mean more meaningful than non-users. This situation It is thought to be caused by the difference in perception (8,9).

Physical, psychological, social, and environmental life of those who do not have a chronic physical and psychiatric illness quality score averages were found to be significantly higher than those who have. Similarly, in his research, Kıvanç has found the average score high in psychological and environmental areas of those who do not have any chronic diseases. Being healthy affects the quality of life positively as it is seen (8). According to the variable of working style, only daytime employees work in psychological, social and environmental areas, It was determined that high mean score in physical quality of life sub-dimension in daytime and shift workers differs between the scores and scores is statistically significant in the field of environmental quality of life. In the study of Kıvanç, Ergen et al., the average scores of physical and psychological qualities of life compared to both daytime and shift workers found significantly higher (8-10). In his study, Yüksel determined that those who keep watch at night are unwilling, unable to concentrate and feel sleepy (11). It is thought that those who work with the watch method cannot spare enough time for their social environment and therefore their quality of life is negatively affected.

It was detected that there is no statistical significance between income status and quality of life mean scores in the study. There is a correlation in the same direction between the increase in the income level and the quality of life mean. Similarly, in the study conducted by Şahin and Ay et al., a positive relationship was found between the score's income status and quality of life in studies (12,13). In study of Güngör et al., those whose income is equivalent to their expense social domain scores of qualities of life were found to be higher than those with lower income and expenses (14).

Quality of life score for those who consider the nursing profession very suitable for themselves is higher, and statistical significance in the areas of psychological and environmental quality of life has been determined. Similar to the results of the research, according to Kıvanç's study those who do not see the proportions of those who see the profession suitable for themselves physically and psychologically have a high degree of significance in the areas of social and environmental quality of life (8). It is thought that those who choose their profession voluntarily are more eager to learn, are more determined in the work environment and more positive in communication.

In our study, although statistical significance was not determined between the duration of working in the profession and the quality of life sub-dimensions it was determined that the working year increases in the psychological, social and environmental sub-dimensions, the mean scores. Similarly, in study of Kıvanç, Raduan et al. with the increase in working time it was determined that the mean scores of the quality of life sub-dimensions also increased (8,15). In the study of Güngör et al. the quality of life of those whose tenure in the profession is five years or more was determined to be higher than the ones whose is under the four years (p<0.05) (14). It is thought that this situation roots in the development of feelings of belonging to the institution of the employees over the time.

Conclusion

As a result of the study, it was determined that the nurses scores average for quality of life, the maximum score was obtained only in the social quality of life sub-dimension of the highest score for "Physical quality of life" is (13.313±2.222), the lowest score is taken from the "environmental quality of life" is (11.855±2.229). And a statistical significance of workload, working style, choosing the profession, suitability for the profession, communication with colleagues, economic problem, vacationing and physical activity variables and quality of life was also determined.

Expectations from all professions in the world; employees to be meticulous in fulfilling their duties and being good at human relationships. Especially in the field of health, this situation is more Important. Because the fear, stress and concerns of healthy/sick individuals applying to health care organizations due to more interest requirements.

A quality life in both working and personal lives of nurses are expected to continue. In this study, the quality of life of nurses, property of the scale used physical, psychological, social, environmental, and general quality of life. According to this, physical life with the highest average of the lower dimensions of nurse's quality the lowest average was determined to be the environmental quality of life. Factors affecting the quality of life of nurses are communication with colleagues, the way of working, daily workload, suitability for profession, holiday status, frequency of going to theater and cinema, alcohol use, gender, economic problems, eating 3 main meals and 2 intermediate meals per day, doing 30-60 minutes exercise 3 days a week, chronic physical disorder, chronic psychiatric disorder, marital status, choosing the profession voluntarily and smoking.

The necessity of improving work conditions for nurses to work more efficiently is seen. The necessary regulations on the subject are provided by the relevant institutions and organizations preparation and implementation can be recommended.

References

1. Akdemir, N. (2003). Hemşirelik uygulamalarında temel kavramlar. In N. Akdemir & L. Birol (Eds). *İç hastalıkları ve hemşirelik bakımı.* İstanbul: Vehbi Koç Vakfı SANERC.

2. Yavuz, A. (2014). *Sağlık işletmelerinde iş sağlığı ve güvenliği kapsamında çalışanlara yönelik şiddet.* (Unpublished master's thesis). Beykent University, İstanbul, Turkey.

3. Çatak, T., & Bahçeçik, N. (2015). Hemşirelerin iş yaşamı kalitesi ve etkileyen faktörlerin belirlenmesi. *Marmara Üniversitesi Sağlık Bilimleri Enstitüsü Dergisi, 5*(2), 85-95.

4. Eser, E., Fidaner, H., Fidaner, C., Yalçın, E., Elbi, H., & Göker, E. (1999). WHOQOL-100 ve WHOQOL-BREF'in psikometrik özellikleri. *Psikiyatri Psikoloji Psikofarmakoloji (3P) Dergisi, 7*(Ek 2), 23-40.

5. Topal, K., Eser, E., Sanberk, İ., Bayliss, E., & Saatci, E. (2012). Challenges in access to health services and its impact on quality of life: A randomised populations based survey within Turkish speaking immigrants in London. *Health and Quality of Life Outcomes, 10,* 11-20. doi:10.1186/ 1477-7525-10-11

6. Wang, X., Matsuda, N., Ma, H., & Shinfuku, N. (2000). Comparative study of quality of life between the Chinese and Japanese adolescent populations. *Psychiatry and Clinical Neurosciences, 54*(2), 147-152. doi:10.1046/j.1440-1819.2000.00650.x

7. Yıldırım, A., & Hacıhasanoğlu, R. (2011). Sağlık çalışanlarında yaşam kalitesi ve etkileyen değişkenler. *Psikiyatri Hemşireleri Dergisi, 2*(2), 61-68.

8. Kıvanç, Ç. (2016). *Sağlık çalışanlarının yaşam kalitesi.* (Unpublished master's thesis). Haliç University, İstanbul, Turkey.

9. Yalçınkaya, M., Özer, F., & Karamanoğlu, A. (2007). Sağlık çalışanlarının sağlıklı yaşam biçimi davranışlarının değerlendirilmesi. *TSK Koruyucu Hekimler Bülteni, 6*(6), 409-420.

10. Ergen, A., Tanrıverdi, Ö., Kumbasar, A., Arslan, E., & Atmaca, D. (2011). Sağlık çalışanlarının yaşam kalitesi üzerine kesitsel bir çalışma. *Haseki Tıp Bülteni, 49*(1), 14-19.

11. Yüksel, İ. (2004). Çalışma yaşamı kalitesinin tipik ve atipik istihdam açısından incelenmesi. *Doğuş Üniversitesi Dergisi, 5*(1), 47-58.

12. Şahin, N. (2001). *Hastanelerde çalışan hemşirelerin öznel yaşam kalitelerinin değerlendirilmesi, Kırıkkale devlet ve sosyal sigortalar kurumu hastaneleri örneği.* (Unpublished master's thesis). Ankara University, Ankara, Turkey.

13. Ay, S., Güngör, N., & Özbaşaran, F. (2007). Celal Bayar üniversitesi tıp fakültesi araştırma ve uygulama hastanesinde çalışan hemşirelerin yaşam kalitesi ve bunu etkileyen sosyo-demografik faktörler. In *2. Sağlıkta Yaşam Kalitesi Kongresi Özet Kitabı*, İzmir.

14. Güngör, N., Çıray, N., Vatansever, Ş., & Akyol, A. D. (2007). Yoğun bakım hemşirelerinin yaşam kalitesi, iş doyumu ve tükenmişlik düzeylerinin saptanması. *Yoğun Bakım Hemşireliği Dergisi, 11*(1), 10-18.

15. Raduan, C. R., Beh, L. S., & Jegak, U., & Idris, K. (2006). Quality of work life: Implications of career dimensions. *Journal of Social Sciences, 2*(2), 61-67. doi:10.3844/jssp.2006.61.67

Merve Tarhan, Pınar Doğan, and Ahu Kürklü

Nursing's Public Image in İstanbul: Comparison Between Generations

Abstract

Objective: Currently, nurses representing Baby Boomer, X and Y generations provide health care services to individuals in their own or other generations. This point of the view, the study was conducted with the aim of comparing the nursing image perceptions of individuals from different generations.

Materials and Methods: The descriptive-cross-sectional study was completed with 2426 individuals attending as outpatients and relatives in a private hospital group between January and June 2017 in İstanbul. Data were collected with a survey form comprising Personal Characteristics Form and Nursing Image Scale. Analysis of data used descriptive statistics, Mann-Whitney U test and Kruskal-Wallis variance analysis.

Results: More than half of participants were in generation Y (55.2 %). The median was determined as 64 (47-71) for Nursing Image Scale. The subscale perceived most positively was professional and educational qualities with median of 34 (25-40). The mean rank for Nursing Image Scale and subscales for participants in Generation Y were determined to be significantly higher than Generation X and Baby Boomer Generation (p<0.05).

Conclusion: The results of the study showed that nursing image is positive at moderate levels and that individuals in Generation Y perceive nursing image more positively compared to other generations. In line with this, it is recommended that scientific and social studies be developed led by managers and educators in the profession for individuals in public to accurately perceive nurses and the nursing profession.

Keywords: Nursing, Nursing Image, Generation Differences, Social Image

Introduction

All professions become professional by integrating with the social values of public, meeting requirements and gaining trust to a degree. Prof. Perihan Velioğlu emphasized that professionalism is tightly bound to social roots and defined nursing as responding to social requirements (1). As a result, nursing's public image provides important clues about the level of professionalism in the nursing.

Nursing's public image is known to be an important factor affecting members and candidates of the profession. Previous studies have shown that nursing's negative public image causes lowers work performance and self-esteem, stress, disappointment, and work dissatisfaction in nurses, affecting the quality and safety of care (2-5). Most Greek nurses have positive perceptions about the social recognition, career opportunities and work safety of the nursing profession (6). Iranian nurses appeared to have negative perceptions in terms of prestige, economic and social status (7). Studies in different geographies around the world has emphasized that nurses perceive the image of themselves and their profession positively at moderate or low levels (4-9). In Turkey, studies about nursing image among public, nursing students and nurses appear like the international literature; however, the numbers are insufficient (10-14). In our country, there is a need for current studies about public's perception of nursing image in addition to determination of effective and related factors.

The nursing profession currently comprises members of the profession representing the baby boomer generation (BB Gen), generation X (gen X) and Y (gen Y). Each generation, shaped by global events, technological developments, communication, and cultural characteristics experienced in each period, has their own specific common characteristics, values, and expectations (15,16). Individuals in the BB Gen dominantly display features like being workaholic, loyal to their organization and profession, attaching importance to promotion and reward systems, having high work satisfaction, being distant from technology and lack of tolerance for younger generations. Among the general characteristics of individuals in Gen X are moderate sense of commitment, high motivation, respect for authority, and sensitivity to public, while Gen Y are known as a more individualistic generation who have low sense of commitment, difficulty accepting authority, and are fond of freedom (17). In nursing, as individuals from the BB Gen advance towards retirement, it is known that a new generation known as generation Z, with different traits again, are about to enter the profession. Considering all generations, it is concluded that nurses in each generation will have different traits from each other (15). As a result, when individuals in public think of nursing, it is not known whether they pay attention to which generation nurses come from, consider nurses in their own generation or think of a single picture with the same features for all generations. Based on all these questions, the study was completed with the aim of comparing the nursing image perception of individuals from different generations.

Materials and Methods

This descriptive-cross-sectional study was completed among outpatient individuals and their relatives attending a private hospital group located in İstanbul

Tab. 1: Distribution of Planned and Accessed Sample Size (n=2400-2426)

Regions	Baby Boomer Generation		Generation X		Generation Y		Total	
	P*	A**	P	A	P	A	P	A
First Region	125	94	345	154	394	370	864	618
Second Region	98	139	284	319	338	541	720	999
Third Region	107	88	323	294	386	427	816	809
Total	330	321	952	767	1118	1338	2400	2426

*Planned Sample **Accessed Sample*

between January and June 2017. The population of the study comprised the total of 14,657,434 people living in İstanbul according to 2015 Turkish Statistical Institute (TSI) data (18), with sample size determined as 2400 with 2 % deviation and 5 % error. For selection of participants to be included in the study, the stratified random sampling method was used. Participants were first stratified according to generation and then according to İstanbul election regions. Table 1 shows the distribution of planned and accessed sample size according to stratification. The study included 2426 individuals living in İstanbul center and counties, aged 18 years and older, with education to at least primary educational level, who could communicate and agreed to participate in the study. As there was limited access to participants in the BB Gen residing in İstanbul's first election region, the final form of the sample size for the study is shown in Table 1.

Data were collected using a self-report questionnaire form comprising 38 questions in two sections on the following: Personal Characteristics Form and Nursing Image Scale.

Personal Characteristics Form: This form was developed by the researchers after the literature review to collect participants' personal characteristics (9,12,13). Personal characteristics were explained as: age, gender, marital status, educational level, profession, county of residence, whether they know nurses, experience staying in an organization as patient or caregiver and experience of receiving service from a nurse.

Nursing Image Scale: The scale was developed by Çınar and Demir (2009) consists of 28 items that measure three subscales of perceptions towards nursing image: general appearance (7 items) communication (6 items) and professional and educational qualities (15 items). The items are scored using a Likert scale ranging from 1 (disagree) and 3 (agree). Three items (4, 6 and 27) are reverse scored. The total score is created by summing and ranged from 28 to 84. Higher scores indicate positive perceptions of nursing image. Cronbach's alpha coefficient of the original version is 0.81 (19).

Data were collected by third year students attending the nursing department of İstanbul Medipol University receiving Research in Nursing course and by the researchers. In this course students completed the practical data collection process as five students guided by a researcher after informing the organization about the topic of the study and data collection process. Individuals attending the hospital as outpatients and relatives were reached during morning shift hours and given information about the study. After receiving oral consent, survey forms were completed with the face-to-face interview technique. Mean duration for responses was determined as 7-10 minutes.

Statistical Package for Social Sciences SPSS Version 25.0. (IBM Corp. Released 2017. IBM SPSS Statistics for Windows, Version 25.0. Armonk, NY: IBM Corp.) was used to analyze data. Categorical variables are given as number and percentage, while continuous variables are given as median (Q1-Q3) and mean rank. The Kolmogorov-Smirnov test showed the scales had non-normal distribution (p<0.05). Two-way comparison of the scale mean rank with independent groups used the Mann-Whitney U test and comparison of more than two independent groups used the Kruskal-Wallis variance analysis. Reliability analysis calculated the Cronbach alpha reliability coefficient for the scales. Significance level was accepted as <0.05.

Each survey form included information about the aim and topic of the study, directions for completing the survey form and confidentiality of participants. At the same time, this information was verbally explained to participants and verbal consent was obtained. Ethics permission was granted by İstanbul Medipol University Ethics Committee (Date: 21.12.2016/Decision No: 545) and written permission was provided by the hospital's nursing services director. Permission to use the scales was given by the authors completing the validity and reliability study via electronic mail.

Results

Personal Characteristics

Of participants, more than half were in Gen Y (55.2 %), approximately one thirds were in Gen X (31.6 %) and a small percentage were in BB Gen (13.2 %). The mean age of participants was 36.1 years (range: 19-73 years, SD:12.9) whereas more than a quarter were 25 years and younger (28.9 %). The majority

Tab. 2: Descriptive Results of Nursing Image Scale

Scale and Subscales	Median (Q1-Q3)	Cronbach's Alpha
Nursing Image Scale (28-84) *	64 (47-71)	0.93
General appearance (7-21) *	15 (12-17)	0.70
Communication (6-18) *	13 (10-16)	0.88
Professional and Educational qualities (15-45) *	34 (25-40)	0.91

*: Score ranges of the scale and subscales

of participants were female (62.1 %) and married (54.4 %). Of participants graduated, 32.2 % from primary education, 37.8 % from secondary education and 30.0 % from higher education. The professions of the participants were distributed following: student (24.0 %), laborer (21.8 %), housewife (21.2 %), officer (14.8 %), self-employed (13.3 %) and unemployed (4.8 %). The dominantly place of residence was the second region of İstanbul (41.2 %). Among participants, 60.7 % had experience as patients and 64.8 % had experience as caregivers. Of participants, 70.8 % knew a nurse and 80.2 % had received services from a nurse.

Descriptive Results

Participants reported moderately positive perceptions of nursing image with median of 64 (47-71). Of nursing image subscales from highest to lowest points, the order was 34 (25-40) medians for professional and educational qualities, 13 (10-16) medians for communication and 15 (12-17) medians for general appearance. In the study, Cronbach's alpha reliability coefficient for the scale was 0.93, and was determined to vary from 0.70-0.91 for the subscales. Table 2 presents the descriptive results of Nursing Image Scale.

Comparative Results

The comparative results between personal characteristics and nursing image perceptions of participants are given Table 3.

A statistically significant difference between the professional image perceptions and generations (p<0.001), age groups (p<0.001), educational level (p<0.001), profession (p=0.003), regions of residence (p<0.001), experience as caregiver (p=0.006) and experience of receiving nursing services (p=0.019). The nursing image perception was found to be significantly lower in participants

Tab. 3: Comparative Results Between Personal Characteristics and Nursing Image Perceptions of Participants (n=2426)

Personal Characteristics	Nursing Image Scale	
	Mean Rank	Test and p
Generations		
Baby boomer generation[a]	1023.36	KW=34.294
Generation X[b]	1189.09	p<0.001
Generation Y[c]	1273.11	a<b.c b<c
Age groups		
25 years and younger[a]	1282.92	
26-35 years[b]	1252.76	KW=39.887
36-45 years[c]	1234.55	p<0.001
46-55 years[d]	1129.96	d.e<a.b.c
56 years and older[e]	960.34	
Gender		
Female	1212.33	Z=-0.106
Male	1215.42	p=0.916
Marital status		
Married	1171.17	Z=-3.253
Single	1264.03	p=0.001
Educational Level		
Primary level[a]	1144.98	KW=18.889
Secondary level[b]	1289.22	p<0.001
Higher education[c]	1191.77	a.c<b
Profession		
Student[a]	1290.14	
Laborer[b]	1180.51	KW=17.835
Housewife[c]	1175.05	p=0.003
Officer[d]	1256.24	f<a.d.e
Self-employed[e]	1204.03	b.<a.c
Unemployed[f]	1045.49	
Regions of residence		
First region[a]	1063.41	KW=39.046
Second region[b]	1250.38	p<0.001
Third region[c]	1282.62	a<b.c
Knows nurses		
Yes	1208.80	Z=-0.515
No	1224.91	p=0.606
Experience as inpatient		
Yes	1229.69	Z=-1.416
No	1188.47	p=0.157

Tab. 3: Continued

Personal Characteristics	Nursing Image Scale	
	Mean Rank	Test and p
Experience as caregiver		
Yes	1242.52	Z=-2.767
No	1160.17	p=0.006
Experience of receiving nursing services		
Yes	1196.90	Z=-2.349
No	1280.64	p=0.019

KW: Kruskal-Wallis variance analysis, Z: Mann Whitney-U test

Tab. 4: Comparative Results Between Generations and Nursing Image Perceptions of Participants (n=2426)

Subscales of Nursing Image Scale	Mean Rank				
	BB Gen	Gen X	Gen Y	Test*	p
General Appearance	1088.83	1213.04	1243.67	12.757	**0.002**
Communication	1072.94	1208.73	1249.95	16.709	**<0.001**
Professional and Educational Qualities	1007.99	1172.43	1286.35	44.820	**<0.001**

*: Kruskal-Wallis variance analysis

who were in BB Gen, aged 56 years and older, married and unemployed, living in the first region of İstanbul, without caregiver experience and with experience of nursing services. The nursing image perceptions for participants in the BB Gen were determined to be significantly lower (p<0.001) than Gen X and Gen Y. The nursing image perceptions for participants in Gen X were found to be significantly lower (p<0.05) than Gen Y. There was not statistically significance difference between the nursing image perceptions of participants with other personal characteristics (p>0.05).

Nursing image perceptions of participants in the BB Gen towards general appearance, communication and professional and educational qualities subscales were found to be significantly lower than Gen X (p<0.01) and Gen Y (p<0.001). The nursing image perceptions of participants in Gen X towards professional and educational qualities subscale were found to be significantly lower (p<0.01) than Gen Y (Table 4).

The comparative results between items of Nursing Image Scale and generations of participants are given Table 5. The mean ranks for items "Nurses

Tab. 5: Comparative Results Between Items of Nursing Image Scale and Generations of Participants (n=2426)

	BB Gen	Gen X	Gen Y	Test value*	p value
1 Nurses are presentable clean people	1076.47	1182.87	1263.93	24.100	**0.000**
2 Nurses are polite and respectful people	1105.85	1209.99	1241.34	11.167	**0.004**
3 Nurses are cheerful, smiling people	1118.85	1202.24	1242.67	9.790	**0.007**
4 Nurses are authoritarian and tough-looking people	1200.78	1227.50	1208.53	0.558	0.757
5 Nurses wear uniforms and caps	1131.82	1238.89	1218.54	6.152	0.046
6 Nurses are generally attractive women	1165.50	1225.26	1218.28	2.010	0.366
7 Nurses listen to people	1086.51	1215.73	1242.69	14.759	**0.001**
8 Nurses allow people to ask questions	1089.71	1181.61	1261.48	20.556	**0.000**
9 Nurses offer solutions to the problems of healthy individuals	1141.93	1214.16	1230.29	4.686	0.096
10 Nurses offer solutions to the problems of sick individuals	1093.84	1202.90	1248.28	14.732	**0.001**
11 Nurses keep secrets	1147.78	1221.32	1224.78	3.744	0.154
12 Nurses are guiding counselors	1084.86	1215.98	1242.94	15.045	**0.001**
13 Nurses have difficult working conditions	1086.22	1182.77	1261.65	21.151	**0.000**
14 Nurses may work in many organizations apart from hospitals (factories, schools)	1152.38	1201.37	1235.12	4.749	0.093
15 Nursing education should be at university level	1012.99	1168.20	1287.58	55.142	**0.000**
16 Nurses may be managers	1102.15	1181.95	1258.30	17.401	**0.000**
17 Nurses may be teachers	1116.06	1206.29	1241.01	9.701	**0.008**
18 Nurses may perform scientific studies	1072.57	1196.87	1256.84	21.429	**0.000**
19 Nurses may be associate professors and professors	1127.00	1219.25	1230.95	6.678	**0.035**
20 Nursing is a profession with independent practices	1181.20	1212.38	1221.89	0.999	0.607

21	Nursing care carries vital importance for patient healing	1010.34	1188.30	1276.69	46.647	**0.000**
22	Nursing is an information-based profession	1032.30	1168.66	1282.67	47.036	**0.000**
23	Nursing is a skills-based profession	1039.06	1184.02	1272.25	38.138	**0.000**
24	Nursing services are important for health education of individuals and society	1068.56	1178.25	1268.48	29.389	**0.000**
25	Men can be nurses	1043.00	1172.52	1277.90	40.137	**0.000**
26	Nurses defend patient rights	1123.48	1233.27	1223.76	7.037	**0.030**
27	The reflection of nurses in the media is consistent with reality	1182.30	1185.12	1237.25	3.913	0.141
28	Nurses have high prestige in society	1172.49	1218.02	1220.75	1.450	0.484

*: Kruskal-Wallis variance analysis

are authoritarian and tough-looking people", "Nurses are generally attractive women" and "The reflection of nurses in the media is consistent with reality" in the general appearance subscale were determined no statistically significance between the generations (p>0.05). For the communication subscale items of "Nurses offer solutions to the problems of healthy individuals" and "Nurses keep secrets", there was not statistically significance difference between the generations (p>0.05). For the professional and educational qualities subscale, the mean ranks for items "Nurses may work in many organizations apart from hospitals", "Nursing is a profession with independent practices" and "Nurses have high prestige in society" had no statistically significance differences between the generations (p>0.05).

Discussion

Since the perceptions about a profession forms the identity of the profession, one of the most important factors in development of the nursing profession is the public's nursing image perception. Public's nursing image perception displays variability according to social and cultural features. As a result, the study is thought to contribute to the global picture of nursing image.

One of the basic results the study is that public has moderately positive perceptions of nursing image. Five years ago, studies in the world showed that nursing had low professional image as a profession, with the following characteristics: predominantly female, low education and socioeconomic level, having stereotypes like sexual objects, handmaiden or angels, duty-focused, non-scientific, depend on medical discipline and invisible (3,6,7,11,14,20-25). Studies in the last five years indicated that nurses and nursing students had moderately positive perceptions of professional image (2,4,9,10,26-29). There are limited studies on public's perceptions of nursing image. A study from Saudi Arabia reported the majority of participants had positive perceptions about nursing and that nearly half perceived nursing as a job not a profession (30). Another study in Italy stated that the image of nursing was generally positive and that it was perceived more positively by public and nursing students (9). In addition to this situation, studies comparing professional image perceptions in nurses and non-nurses found that non-nurses had lower perceptions of nursing image and nursing image was determined as a profession predominantly female, being assistants to physicians and caring others (12,31,32). Also, in this study it is determined that the public's perception of the nursing image is more positive than the study of Sis Çelik et al. (13). In this context, it is concluded that public's nursing image perception has positively changed from low levels toward moderate levels over the years. It is thought that steps taken on the road toward professionalism by the nursing profession are effective on this positive change.

In the study, there were no large differences between the nursing image perceptions of participants towards the subscales, with ranking from highest to lowest of professional and educational qualities, communication, and general appearance. Studies with public and nursing students were determined to have similar ranking for the subscales as in this study (12,13,26). In study by Keçeci et al., the majority of individuals living in Düzce stated that nurses had positive communication skills and professional qualities (24). According to subscales, nurses' perceptions of public nursing image from highest to lowest were ranked as interpersonal relationships, personal abilities and professional subjects in a study in Pakistan (2) and as general appearance, professional and educational qualities and communication in a study in Egypt (4). At this point, nurses have more negative public image perception in terms of general appearance. A study in America showed a photograph of three nurses and questioned nursing students about their agreement level for eighteen statements related to professionalism. The results of the study showed that students perceived nurses who spent time on their external appearance as being more professional, reliable and hardworking, while those who did not spend time on appearance were identified as having less self-confidence and compassion (33). Based on the cliché of "first impressions count", all aspects of nursing from care management to communication skills are shaped according to general appearance and this is thought to be one of the basic components of nursing image perception.

Comparative results between personal characteristics and nursing image perceptions showed that participants who were 56 years and older, married and resided in first region of İstanbul have more negative nursing image. The first region comprises counties on the Anatolian side of İstanbul including one of the counties with higher rates in terms of elderly population and educational level in İstanbul of Kadıköy (18). As a result, it is thought that the variability in nursing image perception according to age, marital status and region of residence are consistent results which support each other. Those with experience as caregivers and not receiving nursing services were observed to have more positive perception of nursing image. The study with public in Israel reported that individuals receiving nursing services had more positive attitudes towards nursing (25). Glerean et al. determined that positive and negative experiences were effective in selection of profession in study on nursing students (28). The qualitative study in Georgia stated that behavior of nurses during care processes and levels of independent decision-making ability affected public's nursing image perception (32). At this point, similar to the relevant literature, nursing service experience is an important element affecting image and as a result, it may be concluded that every nurse is responsible for public's nursing image perception.

Participants' perceptions of nursing image on both the scale and subscales according to generation are listed as Gen Y, Gen X and BB Gen from highest to lowest, which is another basic result in the study. Currently the nursing profession includes members representing these three generations with more from Gen Y and less from the BB Gen and Gen X (15). In the study, the generation of the nurses that participants in different generations considered while answering the questions is unknown. As a result, a definite conclusion cannot be reached about why nursing image perception differs between the generations. If participants considered nurses in their own generation when assessing nursing image, it is thought the result may be promising as the BB Gen and Gen X progress toward retirement. If participants in different generations considered Gen Y while assessing nursing image, the topic requires immediate focus due to the direct effects of Gen Y on nursing image and it is necessary to change the perception in line with the requirements of generations. In conclusion, perception of nursing image at different levels by individuals in different generations displays variation according to viewpoint.

Comparative results between items of Nursing Image Scale and generations showed that some items displayed variability in the order of Gen Y, Gen X and BB Gen. Participants in Gen X qualified nurses as less authoritarian, hard looking and attractive women, and more uniformed with cap and defending patient rights for the general appearance and professional and educational qualities subscale compared to other generations. At this point, it can be thought that participants in Gen Y and the BB Gen have negative opinions about general appearance.

Agreement levels for items that nurses are authoritarian and hard-looking, female, are individuals who recommend solutions for the problems of healthy individuals and keep secrets and that the image of nursing in the media reflects reality, have high independent professional practices and high prestige appeared to be similar between the generations. Studies in different geographies around the world agree on the opinion that today nursing is still perceived as a feminine and authoritarian profession (8,22,30,32) and that reflections in the media are distant from professional nursing (7,22,28). A study in Saudi Arabia showed that though the majority of individuals stated nursing was practiced in different organizations and was an esteemed profession, nearly two thirds were not aware about the topic of nurses' ability to make independent decisions (30). Another study in Nigeria reported that though individuals had positive nursing image perceptions, nearly half did not want their children to be a nurse (22). The studies in India and Indonesia stated that the majority of public perceived nurses as assistants to doctors performing technical work (8,30). Another study in Greece with nursing students and nurses found that 58 % stated their social environment did not give positive response when they chose their profession, while 64 % qualified nursing as lacking value and 58 % said it was an profession without autonomy (6). Media all around the world, similar to each other, portray nurses as lacking strength, education, with low skill levels and as assistants to doctors and devalue nursing (7,22,28). In addition to media portrayals in Turkey, instead of nurses performing professional practices where they can make independent decisions, they are dominantly dependent on clinicians and perform duty-focused work in line with the expectations and requirements of the health care system. In spite of steps taken toward professionalization in recent years like the popularization of postgraduate education in nursing, increased scientific study, and schools gaining faculty status, this is not reflected in the visible face of nursing (34). As a result, it is thought that the media in addition to internal dynamics in the nursing profession are effective on the basis of these negative stereotypes in public.

Conclusion

The results of the study show that nursing image is perceived positively at moderate levels, and that the order is Gen Y, Gen X and BB Gen for positive nursing image perception. General appearance in nursing is perceived more negatively and the generations have similar opinions about authoritarian appearance, female profession, ability to make independent decisions, ability to work in different sectors, prestige, and reflections in the media.

It is recommended that scientific studies be performed which describe the general appearance of professional nursing from the viewpoint of Turkish public, determine expectations from nursing and nurses in the generations and investigate which generation of nurse's individuals in public considered when forming nursing image perceptions. In order for public to understand nursing and nurses, it is recommended that development of general appearance-focused social studies be led by nurses who are managers and educators, that these be announced to public especially through social media and that these studies determine Gen Y and BB Gen, especially, as target audiences.

References

1. Velioğlu, P. (1985). *Hemşirelikte bilimselleşmeye doğru.* İstanbul: Bozak Matbaası.

2. Masih, S., & Gulzar, L. (2016). Association of nurses' self perception about their public image and their job satisfaction in tertiary care hospitals, Karachi, Pakistan. *International Journal of Advanced Nursing Studies, 7* (1), 55-61. doi:10.14419/ijans.v7i1.8407

3. Takase, M., Maude, P., & Manias, E. (2006). Impact of the perceived image of nursing on nurses' work behavior. *Journal of Advanced Nursing, 53*(3), 333-343. doi:10.1111/j.1365-2648.2006.03729.x

4. Abdelrahman, S. M. (2018). Relationship among public nursing image, self image and self-esteem of nurses. *IOSR Journal of Nursing and Health Science, 7*(1), 10-16. doi:10.9790/1959-0701091016

5. Ha, D. T., & Nuntaboot, K. (2016). Perceptions of how negative nursing image impact on nursing care and nursing competency development. In *4th Asian Academic Society International Conference (AASIC) 2016 Abstract Book,* 254-262. Retrieved from http://aasic.org/proc/aasic/article/view/182/179

6. Bakalis, N. A., Mastrogianni, E., Melista, E., & Kiekkas, P. (2015). The image a profile of the nursing profession in Greece high school students, nursing students and nurses. *International Journal of Nursing and Clinical Practices, 2,* 125-129. doi:10.15344/2394-4978/2015/125

7. Varaei, S., Vaismoradi, M., Jasper, M., & Faghihzadeh, S. (2012). Iranian nurses self-perception-factors influencing nursing image. *Journal of Nursing Management, 20*(4), 551-60. doi:10.1111/j.1365-2834.2012.01397.x

8. Gunawan, J., Aungsuroch, Y., Sukarna, A., Nazliansyah, & Efendi, F. (2018). The image of nursing as perceived by nurses: A phenomenological study. *Nursing and Midwifery Studies, 7*(4), 180-185. doi:10.4103/nms.nms_24_18

9. Rubbi, I., Cremonini, V., Artioli, G., Lenzini, A., Talenti, I., Caponnetto, V., ... Lancia, L. (2017). The public perception of nurses. An Italian cross-sectional study. *Acta Biomed for Health Professions, 88*(5), 31-38. doi:10.23750/abm.v88i5-S.6884

10. Kızılcık Özkan, Z., Ünver, S., Avcıbaşı, İ. M., Semerci, R., & Yıldız Fındık, Ü. (2017). Bir grup hemşirelik öğrencisinin mesleğe yönelik imaj algısı. *Hemşirelikte Araştırma Geliştirme Dergisi, 19*(1), 38-47.

11. Özata, M., & Aslan, Ş. (2010). Hastanelerde çalışan hemşirelerin mesleki imaj algılamalarının araştırılması. *Sosyal ve Ekonomik Araştırmalar Dergisi, 10*(9), 251-268.

12. Özdelikara, A., Mumcu Boğa, N., & Çayan, N. (2015). Hemşirelik öğrencilerine ve sağlık alanı dışındaki öğrencilere göre hemşirelik imajı. *Düzce Üniversitesi Sağlık Bilimleri Enstitüsü Dergisi, 5*(2), 1-5.

13. Sis Çelik, A., Pasinlioğlu, T., Kocabeyoğlu, T., & Çetin, S. (2013). Hemşirelik mesleğinin toplumdaki imajının belirlenmesi. *Florence Nightingale Hemşirelik Dergisi, 21*(3), 147-153.

14. Özsoy, S. A. (2000). Toplumda hemşirelik imajının belirlenmesi. *Ege Üniversitesi Hemşirelik Yüksekokulu Dergisi, 16*(2-3), 1-19.

15. Finkelman, A. (2016). *Professional nursing concepts: Competencies for quality leadership.* USA: Jones & Bartlett Learning.

16. Hendricks, J. M., & Cope, V. C. (2013). Generational diversity: What nurse managers need to know. *Journal of Advanced Nursing, 69*(3), 717-725. doi:10.1111/j.1365-2648.2012.06079.x

17. Polat, Ş. (2018). Farklı kuşaklardan hemşirelerle çalışmak ve hemşireleri yönetmek için ipuçları. *Sağlık ve Hemşirelik Yönetimi Dergisi, 1*(5), 48-56. doi:10.5222/SHYD.2018.048

18. Türkiye İstatistik Kurumu. (2015). *İstatistiklerle Türkiye.* Ankara: Türkiye İstatistik Kurumu Matbaası.

19. Çınar, Ş., & Demir, Y. (2009). Toplumdaki hemşirelik imajı: bir ölçek geliştirme çalışması. *Anadolu Üniversitesi Hemşirelik Yüksekokulu Dergisi, 12*(2), 24-33.

20. Emeghebo, L. (2012). The image of nursing as perceived by nurses. *Nurse Education Today, 32*(6), e49-53. doi:10.1016/j.nedt.2011.10.015

21. Rezaei-Adaeyani, M., Salsali, M., & Mohammadi, E. (2012). Nursing image on evolutionary concept analysis. *Contemporary Nurse, 43*(1), 81-89. doi:10.5172/conu.2012.43.1.81

22. Meiring, A., & van Wyk, N. C. (2013). The image of nurses and nursing as perceived by South African public. *Africa Journal of Nursing and Midwifery, 15*(2), 3-15.

23. Hoeve, Y., Jansen, G., & Roodbol, P. (2014). The nursing profession public image, self-concept and professional identity: A discussion paper. *Journal of Advanced Nursing, 70*(2), 295-309. doi:10.1111/jan.12177

24. Keçeci, A., Çelik Durmuş, S., Oruç, D., & Öner Kapısız, Ö. (2014). The society's view of nursing in Turkey. *Hospital Topics, 92*(2), 36-43. doi:10.1080/00185868.2014.906838

25. Hadid, S., & Khatib, M. (2015). The public's perception of the status and image of the nursing profession. *Medicine and Law, 34*(1), 69-90.

26. Elibol, E., & Harmancı Seren, A. K. (2017). Reason nursing students choose the nursing profession and their nursing image perceptions: A survey study. *Nursing Practice Today, 4*(2), 67-78.

27. Hussein, H. S., & Fekry, N. E. (2018). Relationship between job satisfaction, professional image and nurses marketing of the nursing profession. *The Medical Journal of Cairo University, 86*(2), 965-973. doi:10.21608/mjcu.2018.55765

28. Glerean, N., Hupli, M., Talman, K., & Haavisto, E. (2019). Perception of nursing profession-focus group interview among applicants to nursing education. *Scandinavian Journal of Caring Sciences, 33*(2), 390-399. doi:10.1111/scs.12635

29. Rayan, H. N., Shazly, M., & Saad, N. F. (2018). Perception of junior nurse students and nurse interns regarding public image of nursing. *Egyptian Journal of Health Care, 9*(2), 34-47. doi:10.21608/ejhc.2018.10106

30. Saied, H., Al Beshi, H., Al Nafaie J., & Al Anazi, E. (2016). Saudi community perception of nursing as a profession. *IOSR Journal of Nursing and Health Sciences, 5*(2), 95-99. doi:10.9790/1959-05219599

31. Sommers, C. L., Tarihoran, D. E., Sembel, S., & Tzeng, H. M. (2018). Perceived images and expected roles of Indonesian nurses. *Nursing Open, 5*(4), 501-506. doi:10.1002/nop2.156

32. Squires, A., Ojemeni, M. T., Olson, E., & Uchanieshvili, M. (2019). Nursing's public image in the Republic of Georgia: a qualitative, exploratory study. *Nursing Injury, 26*(4), e12295. doi:10.1111/nin.12295

33. Wills, N. L., Wilson, B., Woodcock, E. B., Abraham, S. P., & Gillum, D. R. (2018). Appearance of nurses and perceived professionalism. *International Journal of Studies in Nursing, 3*(3), 30-40. doi:10.20849/ijsn.v3i3.466

34. Yıldırım, A. (2014). *Sağlık sistemi ve yönetim ilkeleri ışığında hemşirelik.* Ankara: Hedef Yayıncılık.

Neriman Özge Çalışkan and Hayat Yalın

Patients' Perception of Nursing Care

Abstract

Objective: The study was performed with a view to determining perceived nursing care of patients.

Materials and Methods: Planned as a descriptive study, the population is adult patients who received patient treatment at a private hospital minimum for 24 hours. Data were collected by way of face-to-face interview from 165 patients from November 2017 to February 2018 through "Patient Perception of Hospital Experience with Nursing (PPHEN)" on the day of discharge.

Results: The mean age of the patients who participated in the study is 46.61±16.89 and 52.7 % of them (n=87) are female. Days of staying in hospitals range between two and twelve and average period of staying in hospital is determined as 3.79±2.20 days. The mean PPHEN total score is calculated as 69.88±7.57. The highest "Agreed" response on the scale is 94.5 % for "I am sure nurses will be there for me when I need". The lowest "Agreed" response on the scale is 57 % for "Nurses provided me with information about the things I was not aware of regarding the hospital". Total score of PPHEN were found to be statistically meaningful for the patients diagnosed with a circulating system disorders whose experience shifted towards good/favorable for nursing care, who were clearly satisfied with their day and night care sessions, and expressed that the nursing care received would play a remarkable role in their choice of hospital in the future (p<0.05).

Conclusion: The mean PPHEN total score is 69.88±7.57, and the highest score that could be attained on the scale is 75. Hence it is concluded that the perceived nursing care of the patients who took part in the study is favorable.

Keywords: Nursing Care, Perceived Nursing Care, PPHEN, Perception

Introduction

Involving both sciences and arts, nursing, a discipline, is defined as "as dynamic power in making an individual getting back to health and not dependent on others" by Virginia Henderson (1,2). The existential purpose of nursing is to help, and nurses do help by way of care, which is, by character, an independent function (3). Care is fundamental for nursing (4,5). Nurses play significant roles in sustainability and improvement of health and in rehabilitation, also they are indispensable members to health teams and offer uninterrupted care services for 24 hours (6,7).

How the patients perceive the care service offered at the time of treatment is crucial. Perception is subjective concept in which an individual interprets received stimulus from his own being or from the surrounding environment, and it is influenced by many factors. In a study by Azar et al. on evaluation of interdisciplinary care perception, it is determined that nursing is a discipline that has the most powerful and favorable relationship with the patients' perception of care (8). Patients' perception of nursing is likely to be influenced by a set of factors and is therefore likely to vary. Although perceived nursing care varies by patient's age, educational background, social status and cultural structure (7,9), perceived nursing care of patients are greatly influenced by the respect nurses show, importance to individuality, support received from nurses, satisfaction of needs and requirements, support in coping with a health problem, providing information about the procedures, giving clear answers to questions asked (10-13).

In a study by Van der Elst et al. on perceived nursing of patients, it is underlined that it is important to understand how patients distinguish "a good nurse" in order to be able to offer high quality care services and to come up with better patient results in case (14). The relationship between the nursing care, patient satisfaction with it and health care services is positive (15). Decrease in service quality result in delayed recovery and increased costs (7). Patients' perception of the existing activities in offering the best nursing case as possible since day 1 of hospitalization affects quality of nursing care quality, and consequently quality of healthcare services (10,12,13,16). For this reason, this study was conducted to determine perceived nursing care of patients.

Materials and Methods

Type and Objective of Study

The study was planned to determine perceived nursing care of patients and performed as a descriptive study.

Place and Duration of Study

The study was conducted between November 2017 and February 2018 at all services of a private hospital where patients received inpatient treatment (intensive care units excluded).

Study Population and Sample

The study was performed at internal and surgical mixed services of a private hospital (cardiovascular surgery, plastic surgery, orthopedics, brain surgery, oncology, gynecology) involving patients who received inpatient treatment and met the sample criteria.

Considering the number of patients who received inpatient treatment for minimum 24 hours, it was seen that about 80 % of them were adult patients. With the number of patients who received inpatient treatment for minimum 24 hours in a month is 900, and bed occupancy rate is 85 %, it was found that minimum convenience sampling for statistical estimations was 161 with 95 % confidence interval and, ±5 % sampling error. In this sense, number of samples that are needed to be taken for population generalization and representation should have been 161. With reference to the likelihood of loss of data, the study was completed with 165 patients. For the avoidance of doubt, patients who are 18 and above, literate, and received inpatient treatment for minimum 24 hours, conscious, well-adjusted to communication and cooperation and diagnosed with no psychiatric diagnoses volunteered in taking part in the study were included in the study.

Data Collection

Data were collected by using Patient Information Sheet and Patient's Perception of Hospital Experience with Nursing (PPHEN) scale.

Patient Information Sheet prepared in light of updated literature. The sheet is composed of 15 questions seeking answers to socio-demographics of the patients and perceived nursing care.

Patient's Perception of Hospital Experience with Nursing (PPHEN) was developed by Dozier et al. in USA in 2001 (17). The scale was adapted to Turkish by Kaşıkçı and Çoban in 2006 (7). The 5-point Likert scale involves 15 statements for nursing care. For each statement on the scale, one of the choices of "Agree: 5", "Slightly Agree: 4", "Undecided: 3", "Disagree: 2", "Strongly Disagree: 1" must be ticked. Point per choice prevails. Minimum 15 and maximum 75 scores are allowed on the scale. Higher total scores on the scale mean that patient perception of experience with nursing tends to go more favorable.

Data Analysis

The NCSS (Number Cruncher Statistical System) 2007 (Kaysville, Utah, USA) software was used for statistical analysis of data. On evaluating the study data, the Mann Whitney U test, in addition to descriptive statistical methods (mean, standard deviation, median, frequency, ratio, minimum, maximum) was used to compare data of the two groups that are non-normal. Kruskal Wallis test was used to compare three and more groups that are non-normal, and Dunn's was used to compare two groups. Spearman's Correlation Analysis was used to evaluate the correlations between variables. Significance was set $p < 0.05$, minimum.

Study Ethics

Research Ethics Committee Approval: The approval was obtained Acıbadem University and Acıbadem Health Institutions Medical Research Ethics Committee (ATADEK)

Institution Consent: The consent was obtained from the place where the study was conducted.

Permission to Use Scale was obtained from the author who adapted the PPHEN scale to Turkish.

Patient Consents: Patients who meet to the study criteria were explained the intended purpose of the study. Both verbal and written consents were received from the patients who volunteered in taking part in the study.

Results

Results for Patient Information Sheet

52.7 % of the population are female and 47.3 % are male. Their age varies from 18 to 84, and age average is 46.61±16.89. 77.6 % of the population is married, 57.6 % (n=95) received college education. 30.3 % are self-employed, 40 % are housewives and do not work for various reasons such as being retired (n=30), being unemployed (n=9), studying (n=5) and medical conditions (n=9).

Days of staying in hospitals range between two and twelve and average period of staying in hospital is determined as 3.79±2.20 days. It was found that 13.3 % of the patients were hospitalized for cardiovascular surgery, 12.7 % for orthopedics, 12.1 % for oncology, 22.5 % for gynecology, and internal diseases, 10.9 % gynecology for surgery and mixed services. It was further found that 21.8 % of the patients received treatment for urogenital system, 18.2 % for digestive system, 16.4 % for neural/musculoskeletal system, 13.9 % for respiratory system, 12.7 % for circulating system, 11.5 % for endocrine system diagnosis, 5.5 % for other diagnosis and 82.4 underwent a surgical treatment.

Tab. 1: Distribution by Patients' Characteristics Regarding Hospitalization Experience (n=165)

Variables		n	%
Previous hospitalization	Yes	127	77.0
	No	38	23.0
Reason for hospitalization (n=127)	Surgical	89	70.1
	Non-surgical/medication	38	29.9
Presence of any chronic disease	Yes	67	40.6
	No	98	59.4
Chronic diseases observed (n=67)	Cardiac diseases	18	26.9
	High Blood Pressure	17	25.4
	Thyroid	14	20.9
	Diabetes	9	13.4
	Cancer	9	13.4
Hospital attendance	Yes	155	93.9
	No	10	6.1
Hospital attendant staying in (n=155)	Permanently	141	91.0
	At intervals	14	9.0
Experience of providing care to a sick relative	Yes	84	50.9
	No	81	49.1
Experience of receiving nursing care prior to hospitalization(n=127)	Good/favorable	116	91.3
	No change	11	8.7
Any change in experience for nursing care during hospitalization (n=127)	Good/favorable	86	67.7
	No change	35	27.6
	Negative	6	4.7

Detailed information about hospitalization experience show in Table 1 above that 77 % of the patients (n=127) formerly stayed in hospital for surgical (70.1 %) and non-surgical/medication (29.9) reasons. 40.6 % of them had (a) chronic diseases(es). 93.9 % of the patients had hospital attendance, and 91 % had permanent hospital attendance while 50.9 % (n=84) formerly experiences providing nursing care to a relative who is sick.

When questioning the process of receiving nursing care by 127 cases who formerly experienced hospitalization, it was found that 91.3 % of them had good/favorable experience. On questioning the nursing care process for that specific hospitalization in comparison to any previous experience, it was found that 67.7 % of the patients had good/favorable experience with this one.

Tab. 2: Patients' Level of Satisfaction with the Nursing Care

Variables		n	%
Level of satisfaction with the nursing care (day)	≤ 8points	28	17.0
	9 points	25	15.2
	10 points	112	67.9
Level of satisfaction with the nursing care (night)	≤ 8points	29	17.6
	9 points	20	12.1
	10 points	116	70.3
Experience of nursing care received affects my choice of the institution in the future	Yes	149	90.3
	No	16	9.7

As is given in Table 2, patients' experience of nursing care received during day shift (from 8 a.m. to 6 p.m.) ranges between 4 and 10, and it is characterized by a mean of 9.41±1.06. Correspondingly, the patients' experience of nursing care received during night shift (from 6 p.m. to 8 a.m.) ranges between 3 and 10, and it is characterized by a mean of 9.36±1.27.

PPHEN Findings

Cronbach's alpha coefficient for the scale is 0.983 and it is seen that the scale is highly reliable. The participating patients' PPHEN scores range between 30 and 75, and the mean scale point is 69.88±7.57.

As is shown in Table 3, it is clearly seen that patients' feedbacks for "Agree" response to the above-given statements are the highest in "9. I am sure nurses will be there for me when I need" (94.5 %), followed by "6. Nurses made me feel comfortable in the hospital." (92.7 %), "4. Nurses paid all their attention to me during my care." (90.9 %), "3. Nurses took care of my requests instantly." (90.3 %), "15. I felt I was being taken good care by the nurses." (90.3 %) respectively.

It was found that there was no statistically significant difference between the total PPHEN scores of the patients based on gender, marital status, education, employment, age, duration of hospitalization, and type of treatment received (p>0.05).

Total PPHEN score of the patients diagnosed with a circulating system condition was found significantly higher than those of the respiratory system, neural / musculoskeletal system, digestive system and others (p=0.009; p=0.004; p=0.004; p=0.004; p<0.01 respectively).

Tab. 3: Patients' Responses to PPHEN

	Strongly Disagree		Disagree		Undecided		Slightly Agree		Agree	
	n	%	n	%	n	%	n	%	n	%
1. Nurses helped me become more realistic.	2	1.2	11	6.7	10	6.1	21	12.7	121	73.3
2. Nurses generously thought for me.	0	0.0	15	9.1	12	7.3	33	20.0	105	63.6
3. Nurses took care of my requests instantly.	2	1.2	1	0.6	3	1.8	10	6.1	149	90.3
4. Nurses paid all their attention to me during my care.	1	0.6	3	1.8	3	1.8	8	4.8	150	90.9
5. Nurses checked with me about most things about my care.	1	0.6	8	4.8	9	5.5	23	13.9	124	75.2
6. Nurses made me feel comfortable in the hospital	1	0.6	4	2.4	2	1.2	5	3.0	153	92.7
7. Nurses provided me with information about the things I did not know about the hospital.	4	2.4	7	4.2	32	19.4	28	17.0	94	57.0
8. I am sure the nurses informed the related parties regarding my needs and wants.	0	0.0	2	1.2	8	4.8	13	7.9	142	86.1
9. I am sure nurses will be there for me when I need.	1	0.6	1	0.6	2	1.2	5	3.0	156	94.5
10. I feel that the nurses feel what this illness means to me.	4	2.4	4	2.4	13	7.9	20	12.1	124	75.2
11. I know that some troubles have been achieved thanks to good efforts of the nurses.	0	0.0	5	3.0	19	11.5	20	12.1	121	73.3
12. Nurses helped me cope with my fears about the illness.	3	1.8	3	1.8	16	9.7	31	18.8	112	67.9
13. Nurses' explanations comforted me.	2	1.2	1	0.6	7	4.2	19	11.5	136	82.4
14. Nurses comforted me when I was receiving treatment	2	1.2	1	0.6	3	1.8	14	8.5	145	87.9
15. I felt I was being taken good care by the nurses.	1	0.6	1	0.6	6	3.6	8	4.8	149	90.3

Likewise, patients' PPHEN scores and former hospitalization, reason for hospitalization, having hospital attendance, hospital attendant's stay, experience of providing care to a relative who is sick, experience of receiving nursing care prior to this particular hospitalization do not show statistical significance (p>0.05).

Patient's total PPHEN score was fund to be statically significant based on the change of nursing care experience specific to the hospitalization (p=0.003; p<0.01). Total PPHEN score for good/favorable change is significantly higher than the negative change (p=0.010; p<0.05).

Patient's total PPHEN score was fund to be statically significant based on the input that experience of nursing care received affects the choice of the institution in the future (p=0.001; p<0.01). The cases whose choice of institution is affected by the experience of nursing care received is significantly high for the total PPHEN score.

A positive correlation of 42.8 % was found to be statistically significant for patients' level of satisfaction with the day and night shifts of nursing care sessions and total PPHEN scores (the higher the PPHEN total score is the higher the level of satisfaction is) (r:0.428; p:0.001; p<0.01).

Discussion

Perception is complex by nature as it is under influence of many surrounding factors. When evaluating the nursing care, patients' perception is crucial. When delivering a nursing care service, nurses make use of scientific knowledge and technical skills, and the attitude and approach to the patient affects the perceptions. The PPHEN scores of the patients who took part in the study ranges between 30 and 75 and is 69.88 (±7.57) on average. The mean scores for the scale were found similarly high in other studies performed to this end. Mean scores extracted from other similar studies are 62.30 (±16.09) in a study performed by Kayrakcı and Özşaker (15); 54.44 (±12.31) by Çoban and Kaşıkçı (7); and 70.56(±6.80) by Yeşil et al. (18).

Patients' Perceived nursing care of patients vary by a set of factors. Patient's perception of the nursing care experience, gender, age, educational background, and socio-cultural particulars are amongst the variables. The mean PPHEN score is (70.26) for male patients, and it is (69.54) for female patients. In a study performed by Çoban and Kaşıkçı (7) on perceived nursing care, the PPHEN score was found to be 56.68 for females and 52.31 for males. On reviewing the body of literature, it was found that both similar to and different from these results were obtained for the gender variable in many other studies on perceived nursing care. In a study conducted by Rafii et al. (12), it was shown, similar to our findings, that male patients were more satisfied with the nursing care than the female patients. However, studies conducted by Akgöz et al. (16), Arslan et al. (19), Momani and Korashy (20) indicated, unlike our findings that female patients were more satisfied with the nursing care than male patients. The difference can be explained by female population being doubled by male population in other studies. There is no statistically significant difference between the patients' gender and total PPHEN score (p>0.05). Similarly, it is found out in the study performed by Akgöz et al. (16), Fındık and Yeşilyurt (10), Arslan et al. (19), Rafii et al. (12) that gender is not influential on the perception. In a study conducted by Momani and Korashy (20) on patient experience in nursing quality, the difference between female and male patients were found to be statistically significant (p=0.01). Mean score difference between female and male patients can be explained by different percentages of male and female patients taking part in the study.

No statistically significant correlation was found between the patients' age and total PPHEN score (p>0.05). Similarly, Köberich et al. (9), Kuzu et al. (2) found not statistically significant on perceived nursing care experience in their study.

Unlike results of this study, Demir et al. (21) found in their study that elderly patients' level of satisfaction was statistically significant when compared to that of the younger patients. It is considered that the difference results from higher tolerance that presumably increases by age. The reason for no statistical significance being found out between the age groups and perceived nursing care experience in this study can be explained that expectation of patients in all age groups have been quite high considering the institution the study took place.

PPHEN mean score of patients who have elementary education is (72.09±4.10), which is higher than those of a college degree (69.82±7.22) even though no statistical significance was found in between (p>0.05). Similarly, in a study conducted by Demir et al. (21), it was found that the score of satisfaction of patients who have elementary education is higher than those of a college degree, whereas in studies performed by Ciğerci and Özbayır (22), and by Demir et al. (21), no statistical difference was found between the educational background and patients' level of satisfaction. In light of this particular finding, it can be suggested that individual awareness increases in parallel to level of education, and they expect more from a service provision, and this, in turn, adversely affects the level of satisfaction from service provision. As a result of many other studies, it was found that individual expectation

increased in parallel to the level of education, pointing out to a negative correlation between educational background and level of satisfaction (2,7,9).

No statistical significance was found between patients' marital status and
total PPHEN score (p>0.05). The mean PPHEN score of married patients was
found as 69.63, and that of the same for single patients was found as 70.76. In
studies performed by Fındık and Yeşilyurt (10), Kayrakcı and Özşaker (15),
similarly determined that marital status of patients had no influence on perceived nursing care and level of sensitization. In a study performed by Şişe
(23), it was indicated that perceived nursing care was lower for single patients
than married patients and that the difference was statistically significant. The
difference can be explained that married patients would have their spouse in
attendance at the hospital most of the time while single patients would less
frequently have attendance at the hospital. The reason why no statistical significance was found between material status and PPHEN score in this study
can be explained that needs and requirements were satisfied for single patients
because number of patients per nurse was little.

No statistical significance was drawn between the employment & occupation of patients and the total PPHEN score (p>0.05). The mean PPHEN score
was found as 69.49 for the employed, and 70.45 for the unemployed. As in our
study, the studies performed by Vural (24) on level of satisfaction with nursing
care experience, and by Yeşil et al. (18) on perceived nursing care determined
no statistical significance between status of being employed or unemployed,
and perceived nursing care experience and level of satisfaction of the patients.
As shown in other similar studies, it can be explained in that patients from
different professional background perceive nursing care similarly.

Other factors that are influenced by the perceived nursing care can be cited
as follows: patients' status at the time of hospitalization, nurses' approach to
the patients, and past experience with the health institutions and services.
Statistical significance was found between the patients' diagnosis and total
PPHEN score (p=0.011; p<0.05). Binary comparisons were made in order to
identify the group from which the difference stemmed. Total PPHEN score
of the patients diagnosed with a circulating system diagnosis was significantly higher than that of the neural/musculoskeletal system, digestive system
and other system diagnosis (p=0.009; p=0.004; p=0.004;p=0.004;p<0.01
respectively).

No data were found with the diagnosis in other similar studies. It is evaluated that patients diagnosed with a circulating system diagnosis needed nurses
more frequently in their daily activities, hence they asked for and received help

from a nurse more frequently, and had more interactions with the nurse in his experience of evaluation.

PPHEN score of the patients that underwent a surgical treatment (69.96±7.36) and the core of the patients that received a medical treatment (69.48±8.60) was found approximately equal despite the different number of sampling. No statistical significance was found between the type of treatment the patients received and the total PPHEN score (p>0.05). In a study by Vural (24) on patients' level of satisfaction, no statistical significance was drawn, similarly to our findings, between the type of treatment received by patients and patients' level of satisfaction with the nursing care. Based on the study results, it is considered that type of treatment received is not a factor that determines patients' experience of nursing care.

No statistical significance was found between the total PPHEN score and whether patients had a chronic disease (p>0.05). It is specified in a study conducted by Kılıç (25) that presence of a chronic disease had no statistical significance with the perceived nursing care. Unlike a study performed by Çoban and Kaşıkçı (7), a statistical significance was drawn between the presence of a chronic diseases and mean PPHEN results. It is interpreted that patients with no chronic disease had a relatively favorable perception of and higher satisfaction with nursing care than those diagnosed with a chronic disease. It is considered that an individual with a chronic disease is more vulnerable because of longer hospitalization periods, fatigue, life-long condition, and fragile state of mind. The reason why this study found no statistical significance can be explained by the fact that patients were provided with nursing care in line with their needs and expectations, and were supported with private nursing service depending on their specific condition(s) during their stay.

No statistical significance was found between the number of days spent at the hospital and PPHEN score (p>0.05). Similarly, in studies performed by Akgöz et al. (16), Kılıç (25), Kayrakçı and Özşaker (15), Demir et al. (21), no statistical significance was drawn between the number of days spent at the hospital and level of satisfaction. In a study by Köberich et al. (9) on the adaptive care perception, and by Şişe (23) on patients' level of satisfaction, it is indicated that the number of days spent at the hospital affects the perception. According to Köberich et al. (9), it is considered that the longer the patients stay at a hospital the stronger relationship they establish with nurses, consequently the patients feel more comfortable in expressing these needs and requirements, and nurses evaluate such needs and requirements more properly; and that longer stay at a hospital affects the level of satisfaction positively.

Unlike this, a study performed by Şişe (23) demonstrates that longer stay at a hospital affects the level of satisfaction adversely.

It is considered that longer stay at a hospital allow patients to observe nurses' approach every time they receive nursing care. Patients who have a hospitalization story in the last five years were more satisfied with the nursing care experience (12). No statistical significance was found between any former hospitalization and reason for hospitalization and total PPHEN score (p>0.05). Similarly, in studies performed by Fındık and Yeşilyurt (10), and Çiğerci and Özbayır (22), it was determined that hospital experience did not affect perception and/or satisfaction. This can be interpreted that patients were not influenced by any past experience, and their expectation from nurses did not change in each incidence of hospitalization (7). A study performed by Arslan and Kelleci (26) on the level of satisfaction with the nursing care and the affecting factors shows that the level of satisfaction was found significantly low for the patients with hospitalization experience. This was interpreted that patients with experience possibly had higher expectations.

No statistical significance was drawn between patients who had attendance at the hospital and the total PPHEN score (p>0.05). In studies performed by Çiğerci and Özbayır (22), by Kayrakcı and Özşaker (15), by Şişe (23), and by Çoban and Kaşıkçı (7), it was determined that there is no statistically significant relationship between having attendance at the hospital and the mean PPHEN scores. It is considered that patients' relatives played an important role in meeting patients' needs and requirements, thus those patients had relatively less expectations from nurses, and this, in turn, would lead to higher satisfaction levels in favor of nurses.

No statistical significance was found between patient's experience in providing care to a sick relative and total PPHEN score (p>0.05). The reason why individuals who provided care as a hospital attendant did not make any significant difference with the perception of receiving professional care service can be interpreted and explained in that the individual evaluates the caring service differently when he is the receiver and when he is the provider.

Statistical significance was found between patients' experience with the nursing care specific to the hospitalization and the total PPHEN score (p=0.003; p<0.01). As a result of binary comparisons, total PPHEN score of good/favorable change (70.91) was significantly higher than that of negative change (54.50) (p=0.010; p<0.05). No significant difference was found between the total PPHEN score of other groups (p>0.05). It can be interpreted that the patients who had a favorable change with their experience of nursing care during hospitalization had a positive perception since they were no longer influenced by the negative experience of former hospitalization or quality of nursing care was better this time.

Statistical significance was found to be positive between the level of satisfaction with the day and night nursing care sessions and the total PPHEN score (the higher total PPHEN score was the higher level of satisfaction was). Also, in a study performed by Yeşil et al. (18), it was determined that perceived nursing care quality score was significantly higher with the patients who were satisfied with their experience than with the patients not. It is found out that there is a positive correlation between satisfaction and perception.

The expressions numerated by 3, 4, 6, 9, 15 -contemplated to make difference between night and day shifts of nursing care- were compared to the level of satisfaction with day and night nursing care sessions. The expressions "Nurses took care of my requests instantly", "Nurses paid all their attention to me during my care", "Nurses made me feel comfortable in the hospital", "I am sure nurses will be there for me when I need", "feel I am being taken good care by the nurses" were found to have statistically significant relationship with the scores of level of satisfaction with day and night shifts of nursing care. It is seen that nurses of day and night shifts created identical perception of care, and that positive perception of nursing care experience increased the level of satisfaction as anticipated.

It was found out that 90.3 % of the patients (n=149) would again choose this institution in the future for satisfactory nursing care service received. The mean score for those who would choose the institution again is 70.63. The total PPHEN score had a statistically significant difference in that the experience of nursing care received affects the choice of institution in the future (p=0.001; p<0.01). In a study performed by Şişe (23) on the level of satisfaction with the nursing care experience, it was found that the patients that would choose the hospital (regardless of the correlation with the nursing care) had a statistically significant PPHEN score. The mean PPHEN score of those that would choose the hospital again was found as 89.6 (out of the total score of 100). In a study by Arslan and Kelleci (26) on the level of satisfaction with the nursing care and the affecting factors, it was indicated that 84.7 % out of 320 patients would choose this hospital again in the future (regardless of the correlation with the nursing care). In practice, the patients expressed that physicians were the essential factor that determined the choice of preferring the hospital again in the future. On questioning the influence of nursing care experience in choosing this hospital again in the future, 149 individuals expressed it was influential while 16 expressed it was not. It is considered that the result is significance because of the difference of body count.

Conclusion

Decisions made by the patients regarding the nursing care service they received, and their perception of such service affects how nursing care quality is classified. Patient satisfaction plays a crucial role in determining quality of a nursing care service. This study was performed to determine patients' perception of nursing care, and the total PPHEN score was calculated as 69.88±7.57. It is therefore concluded that perceived nursing care of the patients who took part in this study was favorable and the level of satisfaction with the nursing care experience was high.

Amongst the facts that affect perceived nursing care experience of the patients are diagnosis, change of nursing care experience received during hospitalization, and nursing care service received during day and night shifts. It was further found out that nursing care thus received was also influential in choosing the hospital again in the future. Patient-nurse relationship plays an immense part in establishing patient satisfaction that relies on patients' perceived quality of service, and service provision being in compliance with the expectations. A nurse assumes responsibility for defining requirements for care, applying it, and evaluating the patients' feedbacks. For sustainability of nursing care quality and satisfaction, the followings are highly recommended:

- A well-structured nursing care that relies on patient participation,
- Patients' perceived nursing care experience being evaluated regularly,
- Providing training for perception management and affecting factors intended for nurses,
- Performing works to determine perceived nursing care of patients' relatives and of nurses,
- To expand and popularize such works at different institutions.

References

1. Ünsal, A. (2017). Hemşireliğin dört temel kavramı: insan, çevre, sağlık & hastalık, hemşirelik. *Ahi Evran Üniversitesi Sağlık Bilimleri Dergisi, 1*(1), 11-25.

2. Kuzu, C., & Ulus, B. (2014). Cerrahi kliniklerde tedavi gören hastaların aldıkları hemşirelik bakımından memnuniyet durumlarının belirlenmesi. *Acıbadem Üniversitesi Sağlık Bilimleri Dergisi, 5*(2), 129-134.

3. Pektekin, Ç. (2013). *Hemşirelik felsefesi.* İstanbul: Tıp Kitabevi.

4. Afaya, A., Hamza, S., Gross, J., Acquah, N. A., Aseku, P., & Doeyela, D. (2017). Assessing patient's perception of nursing care in medical-surgical ward in Ghana. *International Journal of Caring Sciences*, 10(3), 1329-1338.

5. Can, Ş., & Acaroğlu, R. (2015). Hemşirelerin mesleki değerlerinin bireyselleştirilmiş bakım algıları ile ilişkisi. *Florence Nightingale Hemşirelik Dergisi*, 23(1), 32-40. doi:10.17672/fnhd.93977.

6. Akbaş, E. (2014). *Sağlık hizmetlerinde hasta memnuniyeti ve hasta memnuniyetini etkileyen faktörler Manisa Merkezefendi devlet hastanesi örneği*. (Unpublished master's thesis). Beykent University, İstanbul, Turkey.

7. Çoban, G. İ., & Kaşıkçı, M. (2008). Hastaların hemşirelik bakımını algılayışları. *Florence Nightingale Hemşirelik Dergisi*, 16(63), 165-171.

8. Azar, J. M., Johnson, C., Frame, A., Perkins, A., Cottingham, A., & Litzelman, D. (2016). Evaluation of interprofessional relational coordination and patients' perception of care in outpatient oncology teams. *Journal of Interprofessional Care*, 31(2), 273-276. doi:10.1080/13561820.2016.1248815

9. Köberich, S., Feuchtinger, J., & Farin, E. (2016). Factors influencing hospitalized patients' perception of individualized nursing care: A cross-sectional study. *Journal of BioMed Central Nursing*, 15(14), 1-11. doi:10.1186/s12912-016-0137-7

10. Yıldız Fındık, Ü., & Soydaş Yeşilyurt, D. (2017). Cerrahi hastalarının ameliyat sonrası hemşirelik bakım kalitesi algısı. *Anadolu Hemşirelik ve Sağlık Bilimleri Dergisi*, 20(3), 195-200.

11. Charalambous, A., Katajisto, J., Välimäki, M., Leino-Kilpi, H., & Suhonen, R. (2010). Individualised care and the professional practice environment: Nurses' perceptions. *International Nursing Review*, 57(4), 500-507. doi:10.1111/j.1466-7657.2010.00831.x

12. Rafii, F., Hajinezhad, M. E., & Haghani, H. (2009). Nursing caring in Iran and its relationship with patient satisfaction. *Journal of Advanced Nursing*, 26(2), 75-84.

13. Suhonen, R., Berg, A., Idvall, E., Kalafati, M., Katajisto, J., Land, L., ... Leino-Kilpi, H. (2009). European orthopaedic and trauma patients' perceptions of nursing care: A comparative study. *Journal of Clinical Nursing*, 18(20), 2818-2829. doi:10.1111/j.1365-2702.2009.02833.x

14. Van der Elst, E., Dierckx de Casterlé, B., & Gastmans, C. (2012). Elderly patients' and residents' perceptions of 'the good nurse': A literature review. *Journal of Medical Ethics*, 38(2), 93-97. doi:10.1136/medethics-2011-100046

15. Kayrakçı, F., & Özşaker, E. (2014). Cerrahi hastalarının hemşirelik bakımından memnuniyet düzeylerinin belirlenmesi. *Florence Nightingale Hemşirelik Dergisi, 22*(2), 105-113. doi:10.17672/fnhd.64060

16. Akgöz, N., Aslan, A., & Özyürek, P. (2017). Nöroşirurji hastalarının hemşirelik bakımı ile ilgili memnuniyet ve beklenti düzeylerinin incelenmesi. *Uluslararası Hakemli Hemşirelik Araştırmaları Dergisi, 9*, 73-95.

17. Dozier, A., Kitzman, H., Ingersoll, G., Holmberg, S., & Schultz, A. (2001). Development of an instrument to measure patient perception of the quality of nursing care. *Research in Nursing & Health, 24*(6), 506-517. doi:10.1002/nur.10007

18. Yeşil, P., Öztunç, Ö., Eskimez, Z., Tanriverdi, G., & Köse, İ. (2015). An investigation of patients' perceptions of nursing care: Case of intensive care. *International Journal of Caring Sciences, 8*(2), 412-417.

19. Arslan, S., Nazik, E., Tanrıverdi, D., & Gürdil, S. (2012). Hastaların sağlık hizmetlerinden ve hemşirelik bakımından memnuniyetlerinin belirlenmesi. *Turkish Armed Forces Preventive Medicine Bulletin, 11*(6), 717-724. doi:10.5455/pmb.1328186255

20. Momani, M., & Korashy, H. (2012). Patient experience of nursing quality in a teaching hospital in Saudi Arabia. *Iranian Journal of Public Health, 41*(8), 42-49.

21. Demir, Y., Gürol Arslan, G., Eşer, İ., & Khorshid, L. (2011). Bir eğitim hastanesinde hastaların hemşirelik hizmetlerinden memnuniyet düzeylerinin incelenmesi. *Florence Nightingale Hemşirelik Dergisi, 19*(2), 68-76.

22. Ciğerci, Y., & Özbayır, T. (2016). Cerrahi ve dahili kliniklerinde yatan hastaların hemşirelik hizmetlerinden memnuniyetleri. *Ege Üniversitesi Hemşirelik Fakültesi Dergisi, 32*(2), 25-34.

23. Şişe, Ş. (2013). Hastaların hemşirelik hizmetlerinden memnuniyeti. *Kocatepe Tıp Dergisi, 14*(2), 69-75.

24. Vural, Ö., & Vural, G. (2013). Kemoterapi alan jinekolojik kanserli hastaların hemşirelik bakım memnuniyetlerinin belirlenmesi. *Dokuz Eylül Üniversitesi Hemşirelik Yüksekokulu Elektronik Dergisi, 6*(1), 17-25.

25. Kılıç, E. (2014). *Cerrahi girişim geçiren hastalar ile aynı hastalara bakım veren hemşirelerin hemşirelik bakımı algılarının karşılaştırılması.* (Unpublished master's thesis). Çukurova University, Adana, Turkey.

26. Arslan, Ç., & Kelleci, M. (2011). Bir üniversite hastanesinde yatan hastaların hemşirelik bakımından memnuniyet düzeyleri ve ilişkili bazı faktörler. *Anadolu Hemşirelik ve Sağlık Bilimleri Dergisi, 14*(1), 1-8.

Nilgün Altunbaş and Hayat Yalın

Identifying the Expectations of Parents of Children, Who Have Bone Marrow Transplantation, from Healthcare Professionals

Abstract

Objective: The research was carried out to determine the expectations of the parents of children who had bone marrow transplantation from healthcare professionals.

Materials and Methods: The type of study was qualitatively, descriptively, and phenomenologically and was conducted between January and May 2016 in the pediatric bone marrow transplantation clinic of a private health institution, with the parents of children who had bone marrow transplantation. The data were collected from parents via face-to-face interview technique using a semi-structured in-depth individual interview guide, personal information form and a voice recorder. Analyzes of the interview records were categorized according to the themes of the questions in the interview guide and deciphered and evaluated by the researcher in company with the consultant.

Results: It was determined that the most important expectation of the parents who had a bone marrow transplant for their children from the healthcare personnel was regular and detailed information at every stage of the treatment to be applied to their children.

Conclusion: In line with the findings of the study it is concluded that mothers were the primary caregiver for most of the children who had bone marrow transplantation and had a good communication with the transplantation team, were informed at every stage of the treatment as expected and got support from the team during post-transplantation period.

Keywords: Child, Bone Marrow Transplantation, Parents, Expectation

Introduction

The hematopoietic system depends on the long-term cell formation capacity, the self-renewal and differentiation of hematopoietic stem cells (HSCs) into more mature cells during the life of a person. The development, differentiation, homing, self-renewal, and mobilization into peripheral blood or return to the microenvironment after stem cell transplantation of HSCs are provided by their interaction with transcription factors and stroma cells (1). Currently, there are three different types of stem cell sources for hematopoietic stem cell transplantation. Besides the bone marrow, peripheral blood stem cells and cryopreserved umbilical cord blood are widely used (2).

Hematopoietic stem cell transplants (HSCT) are the only commonly used treatment method for patients with various life-threatening hematological disorders to restore functions of bone marrow affected and damaged by genetic mutations (2). Physicians, in the clinics where various types of transplantation are performed, must be well-trained in specific subjects (2,3).

These are hematopoietic stem cell transplant indications, preparation regimen according to disease, pre-transplantation patient evaluation, high-dose chemotherapy, pre-transplantation and post-transplantation G-CSF use, Neutropenia management, lung complications, veno-occlusive disease, fungal management of infections, thrombocytopenia and bleeding tendency, hemorrhagic cystitis, nausea, vomiting and pain, management of terminal stage patients, graft insufficiency, proper donor selection, selection of patients according to research protocols and transfer of patient data to protocols, human leukocyte antigen typing methods and what they refer to, blood transfusion policy in ABO incompatible KHN, treatment of cytomegalovirus and other viral infections in the immunocompromised patient, acute and chronic donor attack disease management, evaluation of chimerism, diagnosis and treatment of immunodeficiency after KHN; being experienced at stem cell collection via cell processing, freezing, apheresis, erythrocyte separation, T cell selection and volume reduction (4).

Nurses working in stem cell transplantation units were expected to be experienced in pancytopenia patient follow-up and be able to recognize transplantation complications. While one nurse per patient is required in complicated patients, one nurse can care for three to four patients in more problem-free patients. Nurses working in this unit should also be experienced in courses of high doses of chemotherapy and radiotherapy. Veno-occlusive disease (sinusoidal obstruction syndrome), interstitial pneumonitis, bleeding, cardiac arrhythmia, congestive heart failure, mucositis stomatitis, dermatitis, viral, bacterial, and invasive fungus infections are the complications which nursery care is essential.

Nurses should also be experienced in the care of donor attack diseases and immunocompromised patients. Especially in units where research assistants and specialists rotate frequently, a non-rotating, constant nurse team is important in maintaining order and minimizing the margin of error. Furthermore, the existence of standard request forms for blood and blood products transfusion, fever management, chemotherapy and hydration will minimize the margin of error (4).

Materials and Methods

Research Problem

The need to be informed is among the primary needs of the companion. Also, the need for training begins with the decision of hematopoietic stem cell transplantation (5). Stetz et al. (1996) determined that family caregivers need information on issues such as preparing for care, managing care, facing difficulties, developing supportive strategies, and discovering the positive aspects of caregiving (6). According to the literature, it is stated that giving both written and verbal information and giving sufficient time to the patient and her family for synthesis of these information and asking questions is beneficial (5). Also, in the literature, it is emphasized that health professionals (physicians, nurses) should consider not only how the caregiver will help the patient, but also how they will support the caregiver in this process (7,8).

It is very important for parents to be informed adequately and to monitor their children in this direction in obtaining successful results with bone marrow transplantation. Nurses working in bone marrow transplantation centers can learn about the experiences of caregivers with specific questions, evaluate their demands and plan necessary interventions to meet these needs before problems arise. However, it was observed that the expected behavioral and practice changes of parents did not occur to the desired extent, despite all the training and information provided for the parents accompanying the children in the bone marrow transplantation unit where the study was conducted. Based on the necessity of determining the reasons for why expected behavior and practice changes did not occur, the research was planned and carried out.

Objective of the Research

This study aims to determine the expectations of the parents whose children had bone marrow transplantation from healthcare professionals.

The sub-goals determined within the framework of the general purpose are as follows:

- How do parents of children who have bone marrow transplantation experience the period from diagnosis of the disease to bone marrow transplantation?
- What are the expectations of parents of children who have bone marrow transplantation from professionals before, during and after bone marrow transplantation?

Research Model

The research was planned in a qualitative (descriptive phenomenology) model. The qualitative research design was chosen due to its ability to reach deep, multi way (qualitative) data acquisition and the purpose of the research. Since the aim of qualitative research was to understand the phenomena in depth, there was no need to determine the universe. That is why the research is based on a phenomenological basis (9).

The phenomenological approach in qualitative research basically aims to find the answer to the following question: "How is the case determined for these individuals experienced?". One of the main contributions of the phenomenological approach in qualitative research is that it reveals the experiences of individuals and how they perceive and interpret the world (10). If the research problem is to reveal the experiences shared by people on a particular phenomenon, the phenomenological approach would be appropriate for such a study (11).

Determination of the Sample

The sample of this study consists of parents of children, who had bone marrow transplantation, who comply with the specified sample criteria. Sampling criteria:

- The child to be discharged after completion of at least one bone marrow transplantation
- Being in outpatient clinic follow-up period after bone marrow transplantation
- Being the companion of the child during the transplantation
- Voluntarily participating in the study
- Being literate in Turkish and having no communication barrier
- Being 18 years or older

In qualitative researches, it is difficult to determine the number of samples in advance. The researcher decides on the adequacy of the number of samples, during the interviews, when individuals use the same expressions/concepts and repetition of these concepts, non-presentation of any new information and concept. (12,13).

Data Collection

The data were collected in İstanbul Bahçelievler Medical Park Hospital Bone Marrow Transplantation Center, between the dates 19.01.2016 and 31.05.2016 with the parents who comply with the determined sample criteria and volunteer to participate in the study.

Participants were informed and consents were taken before the interview. Participants read the forms and the researchers answer any questions. Privacy and ethical issues were particularly emphasized. Data were collected by face-to-face interviews and recorders.

The data were collected through "In-depth Interview Method", which is used in qualitative research methods and is a mutual and interactive communication process based on a predetermined question and answer style carried out for a serious purpose.

In the study, the data were collected using the "Parent Information Form" for socio-demographic data for identifying the parents, the semi-structured "In-depth Interview Guide" prepared by the researcher based on the relevant literature and expert opinion and developed by the researcher for the purposes of the study, and the Olympus VN-741PC recorder.

Pre-application

The interview with the first parent was conducted as a preliminary trial. Necessary adjustments were made in the interview guide.

Ethical Consent

Ethical consent was obtained from Dr. Sadi Konuk Research and Training Hospital Clinical Research Ethics Committee and institutional permission from Bahçelievler Medical Park Hospital in order to apply the study. Verbal and written consents were obtained by informing the parents before the interview.

Analyzing of Data

In the descriptive analysis method, data arranged and interpreted according to predetermined conceptual framework and themes and then analyzed (12,13). The stages of the study according to the descriptive analysis method.

Step 1: The interviews were deciphered by the researcher. At this stage, the audio recordings were listened, and the words of the parents written literally the same as they spoke

Step 2: "Raw data texts" were corrected and turned into "Processed text". The processed text is an organized, super text that contains appropriate answers to the research question compared to the raw text.

Step 3: Along with the text, notes such as the person's gestures, tone of voice, and pauses were taken. Some sentences that were incomplete and meaningless were corrected. In addition, the notes taken during the interviews were added to the processed text.

Step 4: Each interview text was read over and over until it was thoroughly understood. Notes were taken to the edges.

Step 5: The list was created by giving a separate code (nickname) for each parent interviewed.

Step 6: When an idea or an event was encountered in the research, a label (name, number, etc.) was placed on it and coded, and when the same idea or event was encountered again, the same code was written next to it.

Step 7: The similarities, differences, and relationships between the codes, obtained through interviews of eight parents, were analyzed.

Step 8: The codes were combined within themselves to create sub-themes. The order was from sub-themes to main themes. After the main themes were identified, the data was reported. During the data analysis and reporting phase, themes related to the following topics are revealed based on the interview guide:

- History of disease and treatment
- Observation notes of anticipation history from professionals before, during and after treatment were also used as an aid in creating themes and an additional resource was created when interpreting the findings

Reliability

The criteria suggested by Lincoln and Gubba (1985) were taken into consideration for the validity and reliability of the study (14). In line with these criteria, data were collected until data saturation was achieved in the study. In addition, notes were taken regarding the observations and experiences. Opinions and suggestions of experts were taken at every stage of the study. For the verifiability of the research data, the advisor, who is a faculty member of Bahçeşehir University Institute of Health Sciences, analyzed the data again (13,15-17).

Results

Parents' Characteristics

The study was conducted with eight parents of children who had at least one bone marrow transplantation. The characteristics of the parents were detailed by giving a flower name to each parent interviewed.

In line with the information received from parents; the parents' age range was 21 and 62. Educational background varies between literate and secondary education. Marital status: Only one of the eight parents is widowed, and the others are married. Two of the eight families live at home with their parents, including children. The number of children parents have: five of the eight parents have two children; a family has four children, and the other two families have one child. All accompanying parents are housewives. Occupations of parents' spouses are private sector and self-employment. All families have social security. Six of the parents are resided in İstanbul, one in Zonguldak and one in Ardahan. Four of them rated their economic status as good and four as average. Years of marriage ranges from two to thirty. Of the eight parents, five consulted to a physician for diagnosis with symptoms, one a month after birth, one when the child was five years old, and the other when the child was eight. After the initial diagnosis, the parents applied for transplantation at different times, which two parents after diagnosis, three parents after diagnosis and chemotherapy, one under treatment, one after three years and one after four years.

History of Disease and Treatment

The times of parents' consultation to the physician vary from right after birth to the age of 18. It was determined that the application for transplantation was in directly proportional to the urgency of the disease. It has been determined that, while in some diseases, the patient can survive for years with only blood transfusion when necessary, in some diseases transplantation with an appropriate donor is applied as soon as possible.

Expectations from Health Professionals

Expectations of the Parents before the First Bone Marrow Transplantation

It was observed that the parents had intense concerns during the pre-transplantation period due to the urgency of their children's health problem and therefore had not any expectations. However, at every stage of treatment, hopes for the child's recovery were widely expressed. The expressions of Daisy, Violet and Narcissus can be given as the best example for this; "I was hoping he would get better. It gets better quickly, I wanted it to never happen again." (Daisy) "The only thing I need is my child to get well." (Narcissus)

A. Have you been informed before the transplantation? By whom?

"Before the transfer, our physician had told us what would happen. He said that they would medicate but there was no need for us to be afraid. Our previous physicians had also told us. Therefore, we came here informed." (Daisy)

"Our nurse and physician told us that the first 10 days, the medications would be heavy." (Lily)

"Yes, the physician explained everything, and we decided with his father." (Narcissus)

B. What did you do during the preparation phase? How did you prepare?

"Paper was given for preparation, we did shopping, and we bought everything on the list and waited ready." (Daisy)

"They sent a list. The preparations were made according to it." (Violet)

C. Could you afford the needs? Did you get any economic assistance?

"We couldn't afford all the things written on paper, we bought most of them. We are not in a good economic situation, but my family supports us sometimes." (Narcissus)

"There was no economic problem. There is nothing too expensive on the list. We didn't get help from anyone." (Tulip)

D. Have you done research or talked to the families, who have had transplantation, before hospitalization?

"We have neither searched the transplantation nor talked to people. I did not know what the transplantation was alike, we trusted, and had no questions in mind. We trusted everyone. I had no expectations." (Daisy)

"One of our friends had been hospitalized here, so I asked to her what I was wondering about." (Violet)

"We saw transplantation patients in the clinic. Although we did not know, we did not make any research, or we could not ask anyone." (Narcissus)

E. Who greeted you on the day of transplantation? How were you guided? Did it meet your expectations?

"The first attempt was weird. Of course, I was expecting gowns, overshoes, but psychologically, it is bad. You explained the rules. I asked myself where I were. But it took a very short time for me to adapt, it was just that night." (Violet)

"The nurse met us. We went to our room. We placed our belongings. The rules were explained. The kitchen and the other places were shown. The emergency button was explained. They told me how to take care of the child. Our beds were shown. We took a bath. Catheter dressing was done. And it went just like that." (Honeysuckle)

F. Did you informed about the treatment?
"Physicians' explanations were satisfying enough. Nurses told anything before asking." (Violet)
  "We knew only what the physician told us. We do not know any medications. How could we know?" (Narcissus)

G. Did you have any expectations from the staff? If yes, what?
"Everyone is doing his best for children. There is no need to expect more. They even do not eat but are working really happy and make children happy. I thank everyone." (Tulip)

H. How did you dream of transplantation unit? And what did you find?
"I knew it was a closed place. But it is beautiful. I am not bored. But no visits. It is a little bad." (Tulip)
  "Very nice, clean, spacious, beautiful view; like a hotel" (Narcissus)

Expectations during Bone Marrow Transplantation

A. Can you tell us about the transplantation day? What did you expect?
For you, how should transplantation be like?
"I wasn't excited at all on the day of the transplantation. I waited patiently. Then the nurse and the physician came. Just as they told. Red blood. Only the bag was a little big. They calculated. They started giving it slowly through the catheter. They hid half of them. There was no problem. It was over after a few hours." (Tulip)
  "I thought they were going to take my child to a separate room like an operation. We were together. They pretended to give blood through the catheter. The nurses and physicians watched him. I was a little stressed that day. I thought they would do something to my child. But it was very nice. They stopped, continued and it went that way." (Lilac)

B. What did you experience? What did the staff do? How would you evaluate?

"Weeks continued, but then I got used to it. I started to like everyone. I said to myself that there was nothing to be afraid because they all were working for our good, supported and no need to be afraid, excitement was all over. We left ourselves to them." (Daisy)

"It is very difficult for the team. Sometimes they watch the patient till morning. They are dealing with the family at the same time. Both sides experience different stress. It is easier for parents, more difficult for them. May my Lord help them! I mean really heartfelt." (Honeysuckle)

C. What did you expect after the transplantation?

"I was expecting it to get better quickly, but it just didn't happen. It happened gradually with the treatment." (Lilac)

"Everything was not over; it was the beginning of the end. It seemed like miles to me. We always waited for the physician to say something. My only expectation was to be informed which was also happening. The nurses were telling everything about treatment and care. They were also psychologically relaxing." (Violet)

Expectations after Bone Marrow Transplantation

"We believed everything would be okay. We were going to have some trouble, of course. There was no crying after the transplantation, we always had dreams with my daughter." (Honeysuckle)

A. What kind of problems did you experience during the remaining period?

"My son had trouble taking the drugs. He vomited a lot. They fed him through vein. He used to have a problem with his stomach. Some foods were forbidden. He wanted burgers, but it was forbidden. He got well after a week or two. He started to drink his medicines and eat a little." (Tulip)

"I had a hard time finding blood. My husband was not here. I called everyone. They were looking for me too. You cannot go out either. Well, you didn't have many choices." (Narcissus)

B. Did you have any expectations?

"All our demands were met, there was nothing missing." (Lilac)

C. What did you observe?

"In any case, they came up and pleased me. They never upset me. Their approach was very nice." (Lilac)

"They know how to make children happy. Even the medication time was fun." (Honeysuckle)

"Everybody was so friendly and lovely. They were so equally treated to everyone that nobody could offense. They had nothing short of them but more. Always." (Daisy)

D. Have you been notified for discharge?

"Nurses told us everything, food, restrictions, cleaning, medication. And they gave the paper." (Lilac)

"We had given a paper for discharge and made our home ready. We obeyed the rules at home and got support for medications after the transplantation." (Daisy)

"We were fully informed therefor I was relaxed at home." (Violet)

"They told the medications, showed how injection used and said time came for discharge. We felt on top of the World. Daddy and brother came, and we discharged that night." (Narcissus)

E. Did you expect support / assistance from the team for follow-up and treatment at home?

"Yeah, I was confused about the drugs. There are so many medicines that I confused the hours. I was calling and asking the nurses, and then I was relieved." (Honeysuckle)

Discussion

Discussion of Findings Regarding the Characteristics of the Parents Whose Children Have Bone Marrow Transplantation, Time of Consultation to the Physician, and Time of the Application for Transplantation

With the data obtained in the study, it was determined that 87.5 % of the parents were between the ages of 21-56, 87.5 % were married and all of them were housewives. The educational status of the parents varies as 25 % primary education, 25 % secondary education and 50 % literate, and 5 % live at home with their parents, including children, and 75 % live with their spouses and children. The number of children parents have is as follows; 62.5 % is two, 25 %

is one and 12.5 % is four. Occupations of parents' spouses is as follows; 25 % is in private sector, 62.5 % is self-employed and 12.5 % is deceased.

In the study conducted by Taş (2009), it was detected that 78.5 % of the parents responsible for the care of the child were mothers and 40.9 % of the caregivers were between the ages of 36-40, 63.4 % of the mothers were primary school graduates and 82.8 % were housewives and 38.7 % were self-employed. It has been determined that 77.4 % of the families have a low income and 8.8 % have social security. In line with these results, the data obtained in our research and Taş's data, similarities were found between the caregivers, age groups, employment status and the professions of the parents' spouses (18).

Discussion of Findings Regarding the Determination of Expectations of the Parents Whose Children Have Bone Marrow Transplantation from Health Professionals Before, during and after the First Transplantation

The circular for the issues to be followed in the hospitals affiliated to the Ministry of Health in our country includes regulations for both correct diagnosis suitable for the patient, quality medical care, and friendly and tolerant behavior of the health professionals working in the treatment and being open to consultation and guidance (19).

Nurses are health professionals who provide the highest quality care in all stages of the disease, including informing patients and their families, treatment, rehabilitation, sustaining life with the disease, and terminal period care, and are responsible for improving the quality of life of patients.

Fife et al. identified five factors that may negatively affect caregiving family members in the early stages of hematopoietic stem cell transplantation. These are the pre-existing stress situation associated with the diagnosis of cancer, uncertainty about the transplantation process; fear that the disease cannot be treated after transplantation, the obligation to change the previous life of the caregiver and experiencing financial difficulties (20). Alike in our study, according to the interviews with the parents, there was no expectations before the transplantation due to intense stress and anxiety depending on uncertain outcomes of a treatment like transplantation; however psychological support and being informed were among expectations during and after the transplantation.

Discussion of the Expectations before the First Bone Marrow Transplantation

In the study conducted by Arıkan et al., it was found that as the companion experience increased, and the duration of the companionship decreased the level of coping with problems increased. However, it was found that the companionship experience and duration did not statistically significantly affect the coping with the problems of the companions included in the study (21). When the people who they consulted for their problems were examined, it was determined that the companions mostly consulted to nurses, but the group that consulted to the physicians solved their problems in the best way compared to the others. They determined that it is important for mothers to establish a good communication with healthcare professionals and those mothers make sacrifices. In the study, it is seen that the expectations are listed as good humor, tolerance, interest (31.2 %), cleaner clinic (9.7 %), meeting the demands and medicines of the child (3.7 %).

Kristjiansdottir identified the 43 needs of 34 parents in the pediatrics department and classified these needs as being honest of the healthcare professionals, being honest with them, providing information, support and guidance, personal needs, and needs related to other family members (22).

In the study of Yiu and Twinn, the expectations of mothers who are with their children in the hospital determined as understandability of their reactions, hospital fears, need for support and information and need for time allocation, and the need for help for parenting responsibilities (23). Bragadottir determined that expectations are listed as written information about the health status of children, economic assistance, and information about post-discharge (24).

In line with these results, our study showed similarities as the attendants mostly consulted to the nurse, good humor, tolerance, interest, cleaner clinic, meeting the demands and covering the medicines of the child, being honest of the health professionals, being honest with them, providing information, support and guidance, and information after discharge.

Discussion of the Expectations during the Bone Marrow Transplantation

Konukbay and Arslan found in their study that parents had dilemmas and problems about how to care for child during treatment. In these cases, they seek help and psychological support from the nurses, who are the closest source of information. It causes more anxiety, depression, fatigue, role conflict, social isolation, and distress in family members than patients during the illness. During this period, it was determined that children and their families experienced more fear, anxiety, and depression (25). According to these results, it was concluded that nurses provided support for demands and in coping with psychological problems.

Discussion of the Expectations after the Bone Marrow Transplantation

According to Callery, parents expect to take part in the care of their children during their hospitalization and think that this experience will be beneficial for them and their children. Even some parents want to participate in technical practices such as caring for the child's catheters. In addition, when they need to provide home care for the child, they feel more competent in performing these practices and providing emotional support to child (26). According to these results, our study is similar to this study that parents has support on parental information and requirements of care after discharge. According to the interviews with parents, it was determined that the post-transplantation process had no difference from the pre-transplantation process. The information obtained from the parents showed that actions and behaviors of health professionals did not change. The education process only differed in discharge period. The positive and negative results of the trainings were also managed by health professionals.

According to the results obtained toward the sociodemographic characteristics, the medical condition of the child is of primary importance when the expectations from health professionals before, during and after the bone marrow transplantation are examined. For this reason, it was determined that the expectation from the healthcare professionals in the transplantation unit was to inform the parents at every stage of the treatment. In this study, it was determined that the team working in the bone marrow transplantation unit had sufficient training in informing and well-practiced.

Conclusion

Bone marrow transplantation has been successfully applied in our country for years in parallel with the developments in the world. It is an indisputable fact that teamwork and team members should have sufficient knowledge and application skills to achieve successful results. It is known that the compliance of the parent or companion who constantly stays with the child, especially in pediatric patients during the transplantation process, has also an important role in the success of the treatment. Therefore;

- Establishing advanced and repeated training programs for health professionals working in the transportation team,
- Periodic evaluation and improvement of practices of newly appointed healthcare professionals,
- Creating written educational materials (brochures, booklets, etc.) together with information and education programs for the parents of the child hospitalized for treatment in the bone marrow transplantation unit and translation of these written materials into different languages,
- It is recommended to have interviews with parents regarding the practice and expectations before, during and after the bone marrow transplantation. These interviews are thought to be a guide in the periodic training program to be applied to healthcare professionals working in bone marrow transplantation.

For those who want to make a study in the bone marrow transplantation unit about parents; the following researches can be advised: the applications, recommendations, and healthcare professionals from the eyes of the parents in the unit.

In line with the data obtained from the research, for the realization of the parents' desired behavior and application skills.

- Ensuring that parents see the transplantation unit and are introduced to the health professionals (physicians, nurses) before the transplantation,
- Ensuring effective communication with healthcare professionals and informing the healthcare professionals about the specific situation and needs of the child, if any, at the information meeting held before the transportation
- During admission period, ensuring the parents make use of their spare time efficiently (reading books, solving puzzles, etc.),
- During the bone marrow transplantation, the primary observer of the child's treatment is the parents. Therefore, explaining the importance of reporting these negativities to the healthcare professionals, as they may be the first to notice any negative situations that may occur,
- Appropriate arrangement during the discharge period has a vital importance on preventing any problems. It is also recommended that even a slight problem of the child should be reported to healthcare professionals.

References

1. Ural, A. U. (2016). Hematopoetik kök hücre ve stroma biyolojisi. In *9. Ulusal Kemik İliği Transplantasyonu ve Kök Hücre Tedavileri Kongresi Bildiri Kitabı* (pp. 1-4) Antalya, Turkey: Türk Hematoloji Derneği.

2. Elmaaçlı, H. A. (2011). Uygun hematopoetik hücre kaynağı seçiminde dikkat edilecek hususlar. *Hematolog, 1*(1), 14-21.

3. Beksaç, M. (2011). HLA doku gruplarının değerlendirilmesindeki ana özellikler, akraba dışı verici taraması ve uygun verici seçiminde uyulması gereken hususlar. *Hematolog, 1*(1), 22-32.

4. Sucak, T. G. (2011). Türkiye'de kök hücre nakli ünitesi kurulması ile ilgili kriterler ve teknik ayrıntılar. *Hematolog, 1*(1), 286-300.

5. Yarbro, C. H., Wujcik, D., & Gobel, B. H. (2010). *Cancer nursing: Principles and practice.* U.S.A.: Jones and Barlett Publishers.

6. Stetz, K. M., McDonald, J. C., & Compton, K. (1996). Needs and experiences of family caregivers during marrow transplantation. *Oncology Nursing Forum, 23*(9). 1422-1427.

7. Yusuf, A. J., Adamu, A., & Nuhu, F. T. (2011). Caregiver burden among poor caregivers of patients with cancer in an urban African setting. *Psycho-Oncology, 20*(8), 902-905. doi:10.1002/pon.1814

8. Uğur, O., & Fadıllıoğlu, C. (2010). "Caregiver strain index" validity and reliability in Turkish society. *Asian Pacific Journal of Cancer Prevention, 11*(6). 1669-1675.

9. Erdoğan, S., Nahcivan, N., & Esin, N. (2015). *Hemşirelikte araştırma.* İstanbul. Nobel Tıp Kitapevleri.

10. Patton, M. Q. (1990). *Qualitative evaluation and research methods.* U.S.A.: Sage Publications.

11. Creswell, J. W. (2007). *Qualitative inquiry and research design: Choosing among five approaches.* U.S.A.: Sage Publications.

12. Kümbetoğlu, B. (2008). *Sosyolojide ve antropolojide niteliksel yöntem ve araştırma.* İstanbul: Bağlam Yayıncılık.

13. Yıldırım, A., & Şimşek, H. (2008). *Sosyal bilimlerde nitel araştırma yöntemleri.* Ankara: Seçkin Yayıncılık.

14. Lincoln, S. Y., & Guba, G. E. (1985), *Naturalistic inquiry.* U.S.A.: Sage Publications.

15. Rolfe, G. (2006). Validity, trustworthiness and rigour: Quality and the idea of qualitative research. *Journal of Advanced Nursing, 53*(3), 304-310. doi:10.1111/j.1365-2648.2006.03727.x

16. Shenton, A. K. (2004). Strategies for ensuring trustworthiness in qualitative research projects. *Education for Information, 22*(2), 63-75. doi:10.3233/EFI-2004-22201

17. Şencan, H. (2005). *Sosyal ve davranışsal ölçümlerde güvenilirlik ve geçerlilik.* Ankara: Seçkin Yayıncılık Sanayi ve Ticaret AŞ.

18. Taş, F. (2009). *Kemoterapi alan çocukların yaşadıkları semptomların yaşam kalitesine etkisi ve ebeveynlerin uygulamaları.* (Doctoral dissertation). Ege University, İzmir, Turkey.

19. T.C. Sağlık Bakanlığı Tedavi Hizmetleri Genel Müdürlüğü. (2001). *"Hastane Hizmetleri" konulu genelge.*

20. Fife, B. L., Monohan, P. O., Abonour, R., Wood, L. L., & Stump, T. E. (2009). Adaptation of family caregivers during acute phase of adult BMT. *Bone Marrow Transplantation, 43*(12), 959-966. doi:10.1038/bmt.2008.405

21. Arıkan, D., Saban, F., & Gürarslan, B., N. (2014). Çocuğu hastanede yatan ebeveynlerin hastaneye ve sağlık bakımına yönelik memnuniyet düzeyleri. *Dr. Behçet Uz Çocuk Hastanesi Dergisi, 4*(2), 109-116.

22. Kristjánsdóttir, G. (1995). Perceived importance of needs expressed by parents of hospitalized two- to six-year-olds. *Scandinavian Journal Caring Science, 9*(2), 95-103. doi:10.1111/j.1471-6712.1995.tb00394.x

23. Yiu, J. M., & Twinn, S. (2001). Determining the needs of Chinese parents during the hospitalization of their child diagnosed with cancer: An exploratory study. *Cancer Nursing.* December, *24*(6), 483-489. doi:10.1097/00002820-200112000-00011

24. Bragadottir, H. (1999). A descriptive study of the extent to which self-perceived needs of parents are met in paediatric units in Iceland. *Scandinavian Journal of Caring Science, 13*(3), 201-207.

25. Konukbay, D., & Arslan, F. (2011). Yenidoğan yoğunbakım ünitesinde yatan yenidoğan ailelerinin yaşadıkları güçlüklerin belirlenmesi. *Anadolu Hemşirelik ve Sağlık Bilimleri Dergisi, 14*(2), 16-22.

26. Callery, P. (1997). Caring for parents of hospitalized children: A hidden area of nursing work. *Journal of Advanced Nursing, 26*(5), 992-998.

Nurşah Büyükçamsarı Şanlıer, Fadime Çınar, and Fatma
Eti Aslan

Investigation of Risk Factors for Effective Pressure Ulcer Development Studies Have Been Made in Turkey: A Meta-analysis Study

Abstract

Objective: This meta-analysis was carried out to determine the risk factors affecting the development of pressure wounds.

Materials and Methods: In this study, Google Scholar, MEDLINE, Türk Medline, ULAKBİM and CINAHL data were collected between January 2010 and November 2019. The researches on their bases were scanned. 5.189 studies were reached as a result of the screening. Seven studies that met the inclusion criteria were included in the study. These studies were independently evaluated by three authors, and the kappa compliance rate was calculated in the SPSS 26 program. In the studies, the licensed CMA 3 (Comprehensive Meta-Analysis) version 3 (CMA 3) program of the CMA statistics package program and Kappa statistics were used for inter-rater agreement. In this study, "Risk Ratio=Odds Ratio" was used in the effect size calculation. Cochran's Q statistics were used to test heterogeneity in the studies. Classic Fail-Safe N and Tau coefficient calculation results to test publication bias was used. The study was recorded in the database "PROSPERO."

Results: Three of the studies included in the study were prospective, three were retrospective, one was descriptive, and one was descriptive retrospective. As a result of the examination, the sample size in the studies was between 46 and 1625, in almost all of the studies in patients who aimed to determine the pressure wound; It was determined that the Braden compression risk assessment scale and the Apache II score were used, and some studies used different scales in addition to the pressure wound assessment scales. In the studies, the risk factors effective in the development of pressure sores; demographic characteristics, the number of days with pressure wounds, days of hospitalization of patients with a pressure sore, Braden score, state of consciousness, the number of days on mechanical ventilation, disease and treatment characteristics, albumin level, hemoglobin level, muscle strength, acute physiology, and chronic health status, primary diagnoses, pressure wound development time, and comorbid diseases were determined. In this study, kappa values ranged between 0.843 and 0.881 on the basis of inter-rater reliability analysis articles. The general fit ratio kappa value was calculated as 0.849, and the reliability was found to be high.

Conclusion: In this meta-analysis conducted to determine the risks that affect the development of pressure sores; The number of days of hospitalization, Braden score, and albumin level was determined to be important risk factors.

Keywords: Pressure Sore, Decubitus, Nursing, Turkey

Introduction

Although pressure sores, which are frequently seen in bed-dependent patients, which are increasingly important in the world and in our country, are the service quality indicators of inpatient treatment institutions; It is a frequently encountered situation that decreases the quality of life of the patient, prolongs the duration of hospital stay, increases the risk of death and mortality, increases both the burden of caregivers and the cost of care. National programs have been established to prevent this situation. The National Pressure Ulcer Advisory Panel (NPIAP) pressure sore; It is defined as tissue damage caused by pressure and / or tearing. Pressure sore then gradually affects other tissue layers with the deterioration of tissue perfusion, causing partial loss of body cells. The duration of skin integrity deterioration varies from patient to patient, and this occurs in less than two hours. According to its severity, NIPAP (2009) defined pressure sores in four stages.

The stages of pressure injury are as follows:

Stage 1: Skin integrity is intact. Usually, there is non-blanchable erythema in the skin, mainly over a bony prominence or other regions.

Stage 2: There is partial-thickness skin loss in the dermis. The wound bed is pink or red, and there is a superficial wound without any slough.

Stage 3: There is full-thickness skin loss starting from the epidermis to the superior fascia. The adipose tissue is visible; however, the bone, tendon, or muscle are not exposed.

Stage 4: There is full-thickness tissue loss from the skin to the bone. There may be slough or eschar in some parts of the ulcer area. This stage mostly includes the sinuses and tunnels.

Unstageable Stage: It is the stage in which there is tissue loss in all layers of the skin or tissues. The loss of tissue in all layers is visible as the wound bed is obscured by yellow necrotic tissue.

Deep Tissue Pressure Injury: It is the non-intact tissue localized in an area in purple or maroon color or blood-filled bulla resulting from the injury of the subcutaneous soft tissue due to pressure or rubbing. Risk assessment scales are used in determining pressure wound risks and planning preventive interventions. To evaluate the risk of pressure sores, which is the most known in the literature; Braden, Norton, Knoll, Gosnell, and Waterlow Pressure Sore risk assessment scales are included. In addition to these, to evaluate the pressure wound during the surgical process, Revista Latino-Americana de Enfermagem (RLAE) created Elpo, Association of periOperative Registered Nurses (AORN), Munro and Scott Triggers scales are also available (1-3).

There are many risk factors that cause pressure sores to develop: Age, overweight, high risk according to the risk assessment scale, low hemoglobin, albumin level, malnutrition, drug use, chronic diseases, loss of neural function, immobilization, moisture, smoking, friction/shear forces, hospital stay, fecal and urinary Many factors such as incontinence, dehydration, the use of vasopressors such as norepinephrine in the treatment, the feeling of pain caused by pressure, the use of anesthetic agents, etc. (4-10).

In the literature, hospital-induced pressure sores are reported to develop in more than 1 million people in America every year (3). Pressure wound frequency in hospitalized patients is stated to be 10.2 % in total (11). European pressure on the wound to be included in a study of 25 hospitals in five countries, and the prevalence was 18.1 % prevalence in patients hospitalized in Turkey is approximately 10.4 % to 12.7 % (4). For the care and treatment of pressure sore, which is such a common and common problem; The economic cost of the pressure wound affecting 2.5 million patients a year in the USA is reported as 11 billion dollars annually, between 362 million dollars and 2.8 billion dollars in the Netherlands, 750 million pounds annually in the U.K. and 285 million USD annually in Australia (12). All these situations pose a high risk for patients. Therefore, intensive efforts are underway to identify risk factors that may cause pressure sores. Although these efforts are widespread, studies showing the results as a whole are quite limited.

In this study, it was aimed to systematically review national and international studies examining the risk factors causing pressure wounds and to evaluate the data obtained from the studies with meta-analysis method. It was thought that analyzing the risk factors of pressure wounds systematically and conducting a meta-analysis would contribute to the literature, with the aim of planning care with a holistic approach, would guide health professionals and guide other studies.

Research Questions

- Is the number of days of hospitalization effective in causing pressure sores?
- Is the Braden score effective in creating a pressure sore?
- Is albumin level effective in the formation of pressure sores?

Materials and Methods

Type, Place, and Duration of the Study

This research was conducted using the meta-analysis method, one of the quantitative research methods. The study was carried out in the Nursing Department of the Institute of Health Sciences of a foundation university between January 2010 and November 2019.

Ethical Requirements

Since the research is a meta-analysis study, the literature review model was used. Since the literature search does not directly affect animals or humans, ethics committee approval was not obtained for the research.

Application Steps of the Study

The application steps of the study were classified based on the PRISMA (Preferred Reporting Items for Systematic Reviews and Meta-Analyzes statement) (13) and MOOSE (Meta-analysis of Observational Studies in Epidemiology) criteria in the articles to be included in the meta-analysis. Articles that meet these criteria were determined and presented in Figure 1 and Table 1.

Detailed Literature Review

The keywords determined for this article calls where medical topics after determining the Turkey Science Terms (MeSH Browser) (14) called and then was determined "pressure ulcers, decubitus, decubitus, pressure sores, pressure sores, and Turkey, which is in return English of the word" pressure ulcer, pressure Articles on the subject were searched from databases using the keywords wound, decubitus, Turkey. Relevant research articles published between January 2010 and November 2019 on the subject were included in the evaluation in the searches from Google Scholar, MEDLINE, Türk Medline, ULAKBİM, and CINAHL databases. After the repetitions of the articles downloaded from separate databases were deleted, the titles, summary, and full-text stages of the articles were started, respectively. A total of 5,189 articles were reached in the searches made with the search strategy determined in five databases. The remaining articles were evaluated within the scope of the title and summary reading after eliminating the repetitive ones that did not fit the title and abstract. After the title and summary readings, the articles to be included in

Tab. 1: Moose (Meta-analysis of Observational Studies in Epidemiology)

The authors of the study and history	Country	Type of study	Sample size	Number of Hospitalization Days	Braden Score	Albumin Level	Quality evaluation score (A:9-12) (B:5-8) (C:1-4)
Gencer & Özkan, 2015	Turkey	Retrospective	569	✓	✗	✓	B
Efteli & Güneş, 2014	Turkey	Descriptive	70	✓	✓	✓	A
Gül et al., 2016	Turkey	Prospective	206	✓	✓	✓	B
Tokgöz & Demir, 2010	Turkey	Prospective	46	✗	✗	✗	B
Ersoy Ortaç et al., 2013	Turkey	Prospective	103	✓	✓	✓	B
Turgut et al., 2017	Turkey	Retrospective	1625	✓	✗	✗	B
Kıraner et al., 2016	Turkey	Retrospective	1074	✓	✓	✗	B

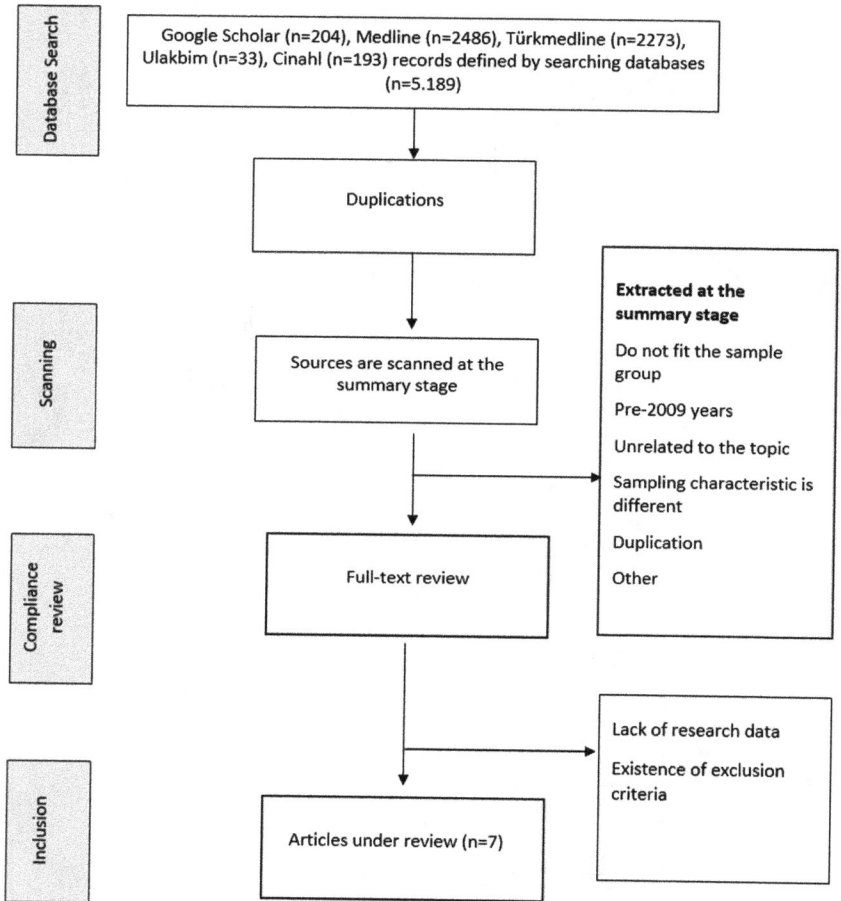

Fig. 1: PRISMA (Preferred Reporting Items for Systematic Reviews and Meta-Analyses Statement)

the full-text reading were determined. Articles found unrelated to the subject were classified in detail and excluded from the study. The data obtained from the studies include the name of the study, authors, year, country, type of study, sample size, number of days of admission, Braden score, albumin level, PRISMA (13) (Preferred Reporting Items for Systematic Reviews and Meta-Analyzes statement) and MOOSE (Meta-analysis of Observational Studies in Epidemiology) criteria.

Searching Articles and Inclusion Criteria in Meta-analysis

- Studies with original, quantitative articles,
- Articles are written only in English and Turkish in order to avoid linguistic bias on the relevant subject.
- Articles that are accessible within the university and published in a national/international peer-reviewed journal.
- Articles involving patients with pressure sores.
- Articles for the last 9 years (2010-2019).
- In the study, the articles that presented the total number of the groups and the changes in the main determining outcomes (frequency, number of pressure sore risk factors) were evaluated in full and quantitative terms.
- Full text of the works
- Lack of validity and reliability studies
- Thesis studies, systematic reviews, and oral or poster presentations presented in congresses on the subject were not included in the study.

Methodological Quality Assessment According to the Review, Coding, and Inclusion Criteria of Articles

Independent and detailed abstract and full-text readings of the articles were completed by two researchers/experts in order to prevent publication bias. The articles evaluated were coded according to their descriptive features. These defining features.

- Name of the study and its authors
- Publication year and country of the study
- Working types of study
- The sample size of studies
- Days of hospitalization
- Baden score and albumin level
- Quality evaluation score

Kappa statistics proposed by Polit and Beck and 12 of the research quality evaluation criteria were used in all of the studies. Each study was evaluated on all criteria and separately by the researchers, and if it did not meet each item, "1 point" was given a value of "0", and the studies that met the inclusion criteria were examined. A total of 0-4 points was evaluated as a weak article, 5-9 points moderate, and 9-12 points strong (15). As a result of the evaluation, the highest score was 12, and the lowest score was 7. A total score of 12 indicates the quality of the study. The graph showing the quality evaluation of the seven studies included in the meta-analysis and the distribution of the scores they got from each field is given in Table 1.

The consistency between the researchers for the article selection and bias scoring made independently by three authors was evaluated using Cohen kappa statistics. Kappa statistic between 0.41 and 0.60 was evaluated as moderate, between 0.61 and 0.80 significantly, and over 0.80 as a perfect fit.

The harmony between raters is calculated with the SPSS-26 program, and kappa values on the basis of articles are in Cohen's kappa 0.84 95 % confidence interval. [Confidence interval (CI) (CI: 0.843-0.881)]. The general fit rate kappa value in this study was calculated as 0.849, and reliability was found to be high.

Data Analysis

In the analysis of the data, "Comprehensive Meta-Analysis Academic / Non-profit Pricing (Version 3)," licensed software was used. The data of all the articles meeting the inclusion criteria and decided to be included in the study were entered into the CMA software, and Cochran's Q statistics were used to test the heterogeneity of the articles. None of the heterogeneity rate (I^2) in the heterogeneity assessment is below 25 %; If 25-50 % is low, 51-75 % is considered medium and above 75 % high (16). In the heterogeneity test, the random-effects model in the group, analyzes with p≤0.05, and in group analyzes with p>0.05, effect sizes, study weights, 95 % confidence intervals, and the overall effect size was calculated under the fixed effect model. "RR and OR" values were taken as a basis for evaluating the overall effect size in the analyzes performed for paired data. The statistical significance limit was accepted as p≤0.05 in the evaluation of the overall effect. In order to test the publication bias, the results of Classic Fail-Safe N and Tau coefficient calculation were used.

Results

Research Findings

As a result of scanning in the research, 5.189 studies were reached. Seven studies that met the inclusion criteria were included in the study. Three of the studies were prospective, three were retrospective, one was descriptive, and one was descriptive retrospective.

Evaluation of Methodological Quality

Sixteen of the studies (n=21) whose quality was evaluated by independent evaluators included in the study were evaluated as "medium," and 5 of them were evaluated as "strong."

Since studies evaluated medium and strong quality will be included in the meta-analysis, a total of seven studies met this criterion and were included in the meta-analysis. The graph showing the quality assessment of the seven studies included in the meta-analysis and the distribution of the scores they got from each field is given in Table 1. In this study, the agreement between coders was found to be 82 %. In the reliability analysis, Cohen's kappa is at 0.82 95 % confidence interval [Confidence Interval (CI) (CI: 0.724-0.921)]. Kappa value <0 worse fit than chance fit; 0.01-0.20 insignificant compliance; 0.21-0.40 poor compliance; 0.41-0.60 Moderate compliance; 0.61-0.80 good fit and 0.81-1.00 very good fit, or (17) 0.75 and above excellent, 0.40-0.75 medium-good and below 0.40 It is considered to be a poor fit (18).The kappa value (0.849) in this study shows that there is a very good level of agreement between encoders.

Effect Sizes and Heterogeneity

According to the findings obtained from the research studies, the sample of the research consists of 3,693 people. In the study, the heterogeneity test of the variables of the number of days of hospitalization, the Braden score, and the albumin level, which were considered as risk factors for pressure sores, was questioned.

With the analysis performed according to the random-effects model, it was determined that the overall effect size of the number of hospitalization days on the development of pressure wound was high and positive with a value of 0.090 (C.I.; 0.004-1.981; p<0.05) and it was statistically was determined to be (Table 2 and Figure 2).

As a result of the heterogeneity test, the p-value was found to be less than 0.05, and the Q (165.150) value was found to be greater than the value corresponding to the df value, and as a result of the individual studies included in the analysis, the studies examined according to the variable days of hospitalization considered as a risk factor for pressure wound in the meta-analysis application were found to be heterogeneous. I^2, the statistic value was calculated as 96.972. As a result of the calculations, the effect size distribution was evaluated according to the random-effects model.

With the analysis performed according to the random-effects model, it was determined that the overall effect size of the number of hospitalization days on

Tab. 2: Heterogeneity Test Results for the Number of Days of Hospitalization Variable

Model	Number Studies	Effect size and 95 % interval			Test of null (2-Tail)		Heterogeneity				Tau-squared			
		Point estimate	Lower limit	Upper limit	Z-value	P-value	Q-value	df (Q)	P-value	I-squared	Tau Squared	Standard Error	Variance	Tau
Fixed	6	0.803	0.642	1.004	1.928	0.054	165.150	5	0.000	96.972	13.831	13.890	192.936	3.719
Random	6	0.090	0.004	1.981	1.527	0.127								

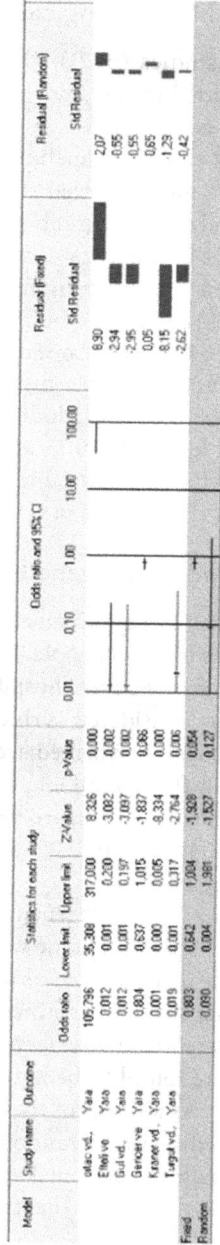

Fig. 2: Meta-analysis Diagram Showing the Impact Direction of the Research for the Number of Hospitalization Days

the development of pressure wound was high and positive with a value of 1.010 (C.I.; 0.156-6.532; p<0.05) and was statistically significant (Table 3 and Figure 3).

As a result of the heterogeneity test, the p-value was found to be less than 0.05, and the Q (42.984) value was found to be greater than the value corresponding to the df value, and as a result of the individual studies included in the analysis, it was determined that the studies examined according to the Braden score variable, which was considered as a risk factor for pressure wound in the meta-analysis application, were heterogeneous. I^2, the statistic value was calculated as 93.021. As a result of the calculations, the effect size distribution was evaluated according to the random-effects model. With the analysis performed according to the random-effects model, it was determined that the overall effect size of the albumin level on the development of pressure sores was high and positive with a value of 0.768 (C.I.; 0.522-1.130; p<0.05) and was statistically significant (Table 4 and Figure 4).

As a result of the heterogeneity test, the p-value was found to be less than 0.05, and the Q (6.640) value was found to be greater than the value corresponding to the df value, and as a result of the individual studies included in the analysis, it was determined that the studies examined according to the variable albumin level, which was considered as a risk factor for pressure sore in the meta-analysis application, were found to have a heterogeneous structure. I^2, the statistic value was calculated as 54.821. As a result of the calculations, the effect size distribution was evaluated according to the random-effects model.

In Figure 2, the meta-analysis results of seven studies examining the risk factors involved in the development of pressure sores and included in the study for the variables of hospitalization days, Braden score, and albumin level were shown with a forest plot. With the analysis performed according to the random-effects model, it was determined that the overall effect size of the number of hospitalization days on the development of pressure wound was high and positive with a value of 0.090 (C.I.; 0.004-1.981; p<0.05) and it was statistically significant. It was determined that this effect, which is an important risk factor in the development of pressure sores, plays a role in direct proportion to the increase in the number of hospitalization days. With the analysis performed according to the random-effects model, it was determined that the overall effect size of the Braden score on pressure wound development was high and positive with a value of 1.010 (C.I.; 0.156-6.532; p<0.05), and it was statistically significant. It was determined that this effect, which is an important risk factor in the development of pressure sores, has an inverse proportion, especially with the increase in the Braden score. It was determined

Tab. 3: Heterogeneity Test Results for Braden Score

Model	Number Studies	Effect size and 95% interval			Test of null (2-Tail)		Heterogeneity				Tau-squared			
		Point estimate	Lower limit	Upper limit	Z-value	P-value	Q-value	df (Q)	P-value	I-squared	Tau Squared	Standard Error	Variance	Tau
Fixed	4	0.640	0.405	1.009	1.920	0.055	42.984	3	0.000	93.021	3.233	3.223	10.389	1.798
Random	4	1.010	0.156	6.532	0.010	0.932								

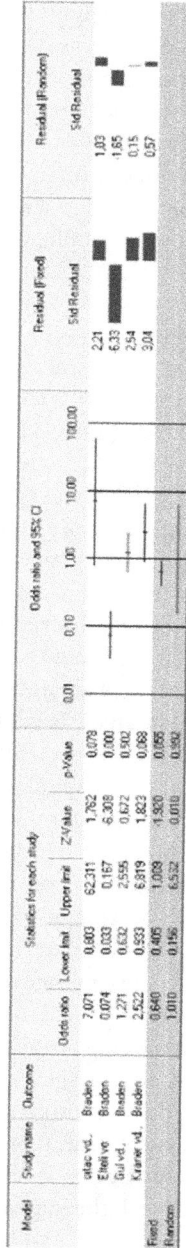

Fig. 3: Meta-analysis Diagram Showing the Impact Direction of the Research for Braden Score

Tab. 4: Heterogeneity Test Results for Albumin Level

Model	Number Studies	Effect size and 95 % interval			Test of null (2-Tail)		Heterogeneity				Tau Squared	Tau-squared		
		Point estimate	Lower limit	Upper limit	Z-value	P-value	Q-value	df (Q)	P-value	I-squared		Standard Error	Variance	Tau
Fixed	4	0.765	0.592	0.931	2.026	0.043	6.640	3	0.084	54.821	0.085	0.127	0.016	0.291
Random	4	0.768	0.522	1.130	1.340	0.180								

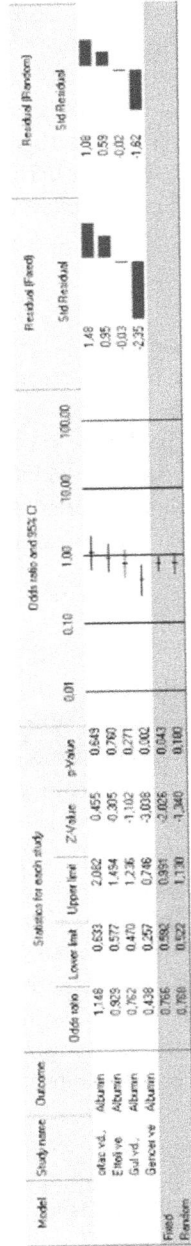

Fig. 4: Meta-analysis Diagram Showing the Impact Direction of the Research for Albumin Level

that patients with low Braden scores were at higher risk and the risk of pressure sores was higher than patients with high Braden scores.

With the analysis performed according to the random-effects model, it was determined that the overall effect size of the albumin level on the development of pressure wound was high with a value of 0.768 (C.I.; 0.522-1.1307; p<0.05) and was statistically significant. This effect was found to increase the risk of pressure sores in patients with low albumin levels, especially in patients with low albumin levels.

Broadcast Bias

Another way of determining the probability of publication bias, which is also considered as a summary of the meta-analysis data set, is to calculate Kendall's tau b coefficient. In the absence of publication bias, this coefficient is expected to be close to 1, and the double-tailed p-value does not make a significant difference; in other words, the p-value is expected to be greater than 0.05 (19). According to the values calculated in this statistic (Kendall's tau b=0.085; p=0.084), publication bias was not determined in the studies included in the meta-analysis.

Discussion

Pressure wound, which is one of the quality indicators of care, is increasing in importance all over the world. When the studies on this subject are examined; It is a frequently encountered situation that decreases the quality of life of the patient, increases the risk of death and mortality, increases both the burden of caregivers and the cost of care (5). The best approach to pressure sores is to try to prevent pressure sores before they occur. When the studies in the literature are examined, although there are many studies aimed at determining the pressure wound and preventing the associated risk factors, the studies showing the results as a whole are quite limited. The studies included in this meta-analysis included a total of 3,693 patients. The descriptors for determining the pressure wound in studies; age, gender, duration of hospitalization, pressure sore body area, pressure sores degree, duration of pressure sores, Apache II score, risk status of the patient according to the Braden risk assessment scale, in some studies different scales were used in addition to pressure sore rating scales, wound stage, The service before admission to the intensive care unit, state of consciousness, number of days of mechanical ventilation, disease and treatment characteristics, albumin level, weight, tissue perfusion, and oxygenation, medical diagnosis, drug therapy, nutritional status, hemoglobin level muscle strength, acute physiology and chronic It was determined that many risk factors such as health status, primary diagnoses, and comorbid diseases were evaluated (20-24) In studies conducted according to the results of this meta-analysis research, among the parameters considered in common, an increase in the number of days of hospitalization, a decrease in the Braden scurvy and albumin levels, and an increase in the post-surgical pressure wound were observed (20-24). While a decrease in the Braden score was observed to increase the development of pressure sores, some studies determined that pressure sore developed without using the Braden score to detect pressure sore (25).

According to the results of the study, it was determined that risk factors such as an increase in the number of days of hospitalization, a decrease in the Braden score, and a decrease in albumin level were effective in the development of pressure sores.

Conclusion

Based on the results of our research; in the development of pressure sores, it is recommended to evaluate patients in terms of pressure sores in the early period, to identify related risk factors and to establish prevention strategies, to conduct studies with high evidence level to accelerate the healing process by reducing the development of new pressure wounds.

References

1. Peixoto, C. D. A., Ferreira, M. B. G., Felix, M. M. D. S., Pires, P. D. S., Barichello, E., & Barbosa, M. H. (2019). Risk assessment for perioperative pressure injuries. *Revista Latino-Americana de Enfermagem, 27*, e3117. doi:10.1590/1518-8345.2677-3117

2. Munro, C. A. (2010). The development of a pressure ulcer risk-assessment scale for perioperative patients. *Association of Operating Room Nurses Journal, 92*(3), 272-287. doi:10.1016/j.aorn.2009.09.035

3. Adıbelli, Ş., & Korkmaz, F. (2018). Yetişkin hastalarda basınç yarası gelişme riskini değerlendirmede kullanılan ölçekler. *Süleyman Demirel Üniversitesi Sağlık Bilimleri Dergisi, 9*(2), 136-140. doi:10.22312/sdusbed.418289

4. Celik, B., Karayurt, Ö., & Ogce, F. (2019). The effect of selected risk factors on perioperative pressure injury development. *Association of Operating Room Nurses Journal, 110*(1), 29-38. doi:10.1002/aorn.12725

5. Alfonso, A. R., Kantar, R. S., Ramly, E. P., Daar, D. A., Rifkin, W. J., Levine, J. P., & Ceradini, D. J. (2019). Diabetes is associated with an increased risk of wound complications and readmission in patients with surgically managed pressure ulcers. *Wound Repair and Regeneration, 27*(3), 249-256. doi:10.1111/wrr.12694

6. Chen, Y., He, L., Qu, W., & Zhang, C. (2017). Predictors of intraoperative pressure injury in patients undergoing major hepatobiliary surgery. *Journal of Wound, Ostomy and Continence Nursing, 44*(5), 445-449. doi:10.1097/WON.0000000000000356

7. Ezeamuzie, O., Darian, V., Katiyar, U., & Siddiqui, A. (2019). Intraoperative use of low-profile alternating pressure mattress for prevention of hospital acquired pressure injury. *Perioperative Care and Operating Room Management, 17*, 100080. doi:10.1016/j.pcorm.2019.100080

8. Joseph, J., McLaughlin, D., Darian, V., Hayes, L., & Siddiqui, A. (2019). Alternating pressure overlay for prevention of intraoperative pressure injury. *Journal of Wound Ostomy & Continence Nursing, 46*(1), 13-17. doi:10.1097/WON.0000000000000497

9. Meehan, A. J., Beinlich, N. R., Bena, J. F., & Mangira, C. (2019). Revalidation of a perioperative risk assessment measure for skin. *Nursing Research, 68*(5), 398-404. doi:10.1097/NNR.0000000000000362

10. Shahin, E. S., Dassen, T., & Halfens, R. J. (2009). Incidence, prevention and treatment of pressure ulcers in intensive care patients: A longitudinal study. *International Journal of Nursing Studies, 46*(4), 413-421. doi:10.1016/j.ijnurstu.2008.02.011

11. Yeniçağ, R., & Rakıcıoğlu, N. (2012). Yaşlılarda bası yaraları ve beslenme tedavisi. *Sakarya Medical Journal, 9*(3), 387-397. doi:10.31832/smj.542000

12. National Pressure Ulcer Advisory Panel. (n.d.). Retrieved from https://npiap.com/

13. Moher, D., Liberati, A., Tetzlaff, J., Altman, D. G., & Prisma Group. (2009). Preferred reporting items for systematic reviews and meta-analyses: The PRISMA statement. *PLoS Medicine, 6*(7), e1000097. doi:10.1371/journal.pmed.1000097

14. U.S. National Library of Medicine. (n.d.). Medical subject headings 2020. Retrieved from https://meshb.nlm.nih.gov

15. Polit, D. F., & Beck, C. T. (2009). Literature reviews: Finding and reviewing research evidence. In *Essentials of nursing research appraising evidence for nursing practice* (pp. 169-193). China: Wolters Kluwer Health - Lippincott Williams & Wilkins.

16. Landis, J. R., & Koch, G. G. (1977). The measurement of observer agreement for categorical data. *Biometrics, 33*(1), 159-174. doi:10.2307/2529310

17. Fleiss, J. L., Levin, B., & Paik, M. C. (2013). *Statistical methods for rates and proportions.* John Wiley and Sons.

18. Higgins, J. P., Thompson, S. G., Deeks, J. J., & Altman, D. G. (2003). Measuring inconsistency in meta-analyses. *British Medical Journal, 327*(7414), 557-560. doi:10.1136/bmj.327.7414.557

19. Dinçer, S. (2014). *Eğitim bilimlerinde uygulamalı meta-analiz.* Ankara: Pegem Akademi.

20. Gencer, Z. E., & Özkan, Ö. (2015). Pressure ulcer surveillance report. *Journal of Turkish Intensive Care, 13*(1), 26-30. doi:10.4274/tybdd.81300

21. Ortaç Ersoy, E., Öcal, S., Oz, A., Yılmaz, P., Arsava, B., & Topeli, A. (2013). Evaluation of risk factors for decubitus ulcers in intensive care unit patients. *Journal of Medical and Surgical Intensive Care Medicine, 4*(1), 9-12. doi:10.5152/dcbybd.2013.03

22. Kıraner, E., Terzi, B., Uzun Ekinci, A., & Tunalı, B. (2016). Yoğun bakım ünitemizdeki basınç yarası insidansı ve risk faktörlerinin belirlenmesi. *Yoğun Bakım Hemşireliği Dergisi, 20*(2), 78-83.

23. Gül, Y. G., Köprülü, A. Ş., Haspolat, A., Uzman, S., Toptaş, M., & Kurtuluş, İ. (2016). Is braden scale reliable and sufficient to evaluate the risk of pressure ulcer occurrence in level 3 intensive care unit patients?. *Journal of Academic Research in Medicine, 6*(2), 98-104. doi:10.5152/jarem.2016.969

24. Ülker Efteli, E., & Güneş, Ü. (2014). Basınç yarası gelişiminde perfüzyon değerlerinin etkisi. *Anadolu Hemşirelik ve Sağlık Bilimleri Dergisi, 17*(3), 140-144.

25. Tokgöz, O. S. (2010). Nöroloji yoğun bakım ünitesinde bası yara insidansı ve risk faktörleri. *Selçuk Üniversitesi Tıp Dergisi, 26*(3), 95-98.

Selda Polat and Burcu Ceylan

Effect of Psychodrama on Self-Compassion Levels of University Students

Abstract

Objective: The aim of the study is to determine the effect of psychodrama on the self-compassion levels of university students.

Materials and Methods: The sample for this study, with a single group, pre-test-post-test pattern, comprised 45 university students attending different faculties in a foundation university who chose the psychodrama elective lesson. The students participated in purposefully planned psychodrama group studies for mean two hours per week over 11 weeks. Data were collected before and after the psychodrama group work with an information form, subjective self-compassion assessment tool and the Self-Compassion Scale (SCS).

Results: A statistically significantly high level of difference was identified between the students' self-compassion perception and SCS mean points before and after the psychodrama group study (p<0.001).

Conclusion: Students had increases in self-compassion perception and self-compassion points after psychodrama group study. In the study, psychodrama was shown to have supportive effect in terms of strengthening the self-compassion of students.

Keywords: Self-Compassion, Psychodrama, University Student, Effect

Introduction

Self-compassion is defined as an individual's awareness and acceptance of their own weaknesses and distressing situations and acting with understanding towards themselves and affectionate self-healing (1). The foundation of self-compassion is based on the Buddhist philosophy about the need for a person to show compassion for the self firstly in order to be compassionate towards others (2,3). Self-compassion does not mean that the individual needs of a person have priority over others. Situations like pain, failure and inadequacy are a part of being human and it is thought that each individual has the right to be accepted with compassion. Thus, people become aware that failure and mistakes are common to all humans, and instead of exaggerating the negative aspects of their experience, they accept the situation openly and in a balanced way (2-4). In the Turkish literature, self-compassion is used as a synonym of "self-sensitivity" (5,6) and "self-affection" (7,8).

Self-compassion is a strong marker of an individual's psychological well-being and mental health (3,9). Self-compassion transforms negative feelings into positive feelings through affection and awareness of the self, ensuring the individual can suitably adopt to situations changing themselves or those around them by more clearly conceptualizing emergency situations (3). Self-compassion increases positive feeling states and is a protective factor against anxiety, depression, and fear of failure. Individuals with high self-affection are happier, more optimistic, braver and have more courage to start again when they make mistakes (10). Those with high self-compassion are stated to be individuals who are aware of themselves, their problems and distresses and have positive attitudes toward themselves (11-14). Additionally, it is proposed that there are many positive correlations between self-compassion and well-being, and more importance is increasingly given to developing interventions to increase self-compassion (4).

Psychodrama, developed by J.L. Moreno, is an action-based psychotherapy method ensuring a person is brave and without anxiety. According to the psychodrama understanding, which rediscovers the truth through dramatization of reality, reliving problematic situations through action on the stage is more effective than talking-focused therapies (15,16). Psychodrama is an experiential encounter and experiential learning is the most permanent learning (17). As a result, in psychodrama sessions, the aim is catharsis, acquiring insight, testing reality, and developing logical thinking, learning, and inducing behavior changes (15,18,19). Psychodrama ensures individuals play roles bravely without anxiety (15). Leary et al. proposed that self-compassion reduced people's reactions to negative events (20). Studies related to self-compassion among university students have found positive correlations between self-compassion with wisdom, happiness, and optimism (21,22).

Psychodrama is an important technique in terms of personal awareness of university students. There are few and limited numbers of studies recommending the use of psychodrama techniques to strengthen self-compassion (23). In line with this information, this study aimed to determine the effect of psychodrama on the self-compassion status of university students. In line with this aim, the study sought to answer the following questions:

- Does psychodrama group study have an effect on the self-compassion perception levels of university students?
- Does psychodrama group study have an effect on the self-compassion levels of university students?

Materials and Methods

Research Type

This study is an interventional research with single group, pre-test-post-test pattern.

Population and Sample

The research was completed from November 2019 to January 2020 in a foundation university in İstanbul. The study group comprised 45 university students attending different faculties in the university who participated in an elective psychodrama lesson and who volunteered after being informed about the study.

Data Collection Tools

In the study, three data collection forms were used.

Information Form: This form contained 7 questions inquiring about the student's age, class, sex, place of residence, maternal and paternal educational level and whether they had any siblings.

Subjective self-compassion Assessment Tool: The self-compassion perceptions of students were determined with a subjective assessment device created by the researcher. Using this assessment device, the students were asked to give a value from 0 to 10 for their self-compassion perception. "0" points represented lowest self-compassion, while "10" points represented highest self-compassion. Subjective assessment devices are among assessment devices frequently used in psychodrama group studies.

Self-compassion Scale (SCS): Developed by Neff (2003), the original scale comprises 26 items in 6 subscales. The Turkish validity and reliability study were performed by Deniz, Kesici and Sümer (24). Different to the original, the Turkish Self-Compassion Scale (SCS) does not have six subscales but was determined to have a single-dimension structure. Additionally, two items were removed in item correlations, so the scale comprises 24 items. Those responding to the scale are requested to grade responses on a 5-point Likert type scale based on how frequently they act in relation to the stated situation as "nearly never=1" to "nearly always=5". Positive items on the scale are items 2, 4, 6, 8, 9, 11, 13, 14, 16, 18, 20, 21 and 24. Negative items on the scale are items 1, 3, 5, 7, 10, 12, 15, 17, 19, 22 and 23 and these require inverse grading. The Cronbach alpha coefficient of the scale was .89 and test-repeat test reliability was .83. In this study, the Cronbach alpha coefficient was found to be .77.

Implementation

The psychodrama elective lesson was opened in 2 groups. After the first meeting and assessment with participants, students who volunteered to participate in the study were given information about the targets, location, time, duration, and how the sessions will run in the psychodrama group. After the psychodrama session, they consented to providing information to the researcher after every session to create a written record of the process. Before beginning psychodrama sessions, data collection tools were completed by the students.

Each week planned group studies took two hours and continued for 11 sessions. Group studies were held in the university's psychodrama implementation laboratory. Participants determined their own nicknames in the first week and sessions were recorded in writing after each session using the nicknames the members gave themselves. After completing the 11 sessions, members assessed their group, and the data collection tools were administered again. As psychodrama is based on spontaneity and action, during group studies warm-up plays were led by the director to increase awareness of the self and feelings and self-compassion levels and protagonist-centered plays developed during the study were performed.

Group Process

The targets of the psychodrama group were structured around developing awareness and self-expression, spontaneity, creativity, empathy, and self-compassion levels in group sessions. The sessions were completed with 3 protagonist-centered plays and 8 warm-up plays. The first three sessions described psychodrama, and warm-up plays and sociometry implementations were performed about introductions to create group dynamics. Later, members performed warm-up plays and protagonist-centered plays in the remaining 8 sessions involving knowing themselves, developing self-compassion and change processes. Protagonist-centered plays were scenes about family, occupational, friend relationship and emotional situations. In the final session, feedback-based plays and implementations were performed to end the group. Participants shared their feelings, thoughts, and experiences during the psychodrama process with the group. After the final play, the group completed the self-compassion perception scale and self-compassion scale as post-tests and the group said goodbye.

Ethical Aspect of Research

Before the research, ethics committee permission was granted by Bahçeşehir University Scientific Research and Publications Ethics Committee Chair dated 27.11.2019 and numbered 2019/10 and official permission was obtained from the organization, scale permissions were granted and written consent was obtained from participants.

Analysis of Data:

The data obtained as a result of the research was analyzed in the computer environment. Assessment of findings related to descriptive characteristics of students used percentage and mean-standard deviation. The t test for dependent groups was used for in-group assessment to analyze the two measures of the self-compassion perception scale and self-compassion scale for students. The obtained results were tested at $p<0.05$ significance level.

Effect size was calculated with the "Cohen d" index. Accordingly

- $d \geq 1$ very large effect
- 0.8 large effect
- 0.5 moderate effect
- 0.2 small effect

Results

Descriptive Characteristics

The mean age of students was 21.51 ± 1.32 years, with 55.6 % in third year and 44.4 % in fourth year. Additionally, 88.9 % were female, 84.4 % lived in cities and metropolis, maternal education was high school for 42.2 %, paternal education was high school for 46.7 % and 80 % had at least one sibling (Table 1).

Comparison of Mean Points for Self-Compassion and Self-Compassion Perception and In-Group Variation before and after Psychodrama Group Studies

The mean self-compassion perception points were 6.93 ± 1.57 before the psychodrama group study and 7.30 ± 1.37 afterwards. The difference between mean self-compassion perception points of students before and after the psychodrama group study was identified to be significantly different at statistically high rate ($p<0.001$). The mean self-compassion points were 70.73 ± 8.64

Tab. 1: Distribution of Descriptive Characteristics of Students (n=45)

Descriptive characteristic	Mean±SD	
Age (Min-Max)	(20-25) 21.51±1.32	
	n	**%**
Class		
3	25	55.6
4	20	44.4
Gender		
Female	40	88.9
Male	5	11.1
Place of residence		
City + metropolis	38	84.4
Village + town	7	15.6
Mother's educational status		
Primary education	15	33.3
High school	19	42.2
University	11	24.4
Father's educational status		
Primary education	11	24.4
High school	21	46.7
University	13	28.9
Siblings		
No	9	20.0
Yes	36	80.0

before the psychodrama group study and 72.44±8.24 afterwards. The difference between mean self-compassion points of students before and after the psychodrama group study was identified to be significantly different at statistically high rate (p<0.001, Table 2). Power analysis with the G*Power (3.1.9.2) program found the effect size for self-compassion perception was 0.70 (moderate effect) with 95 % power by noting t=-4.045, while the effect size for self-compassion was 1.08 (very large effect) with 99 % power by noting t=-6.858.

Discussion

In this study assessing the effect of psychodrama for development of self-compassion status among university students, there were significant differences at statistically high rates between the mean points for self-compassion

Tab. 2: Comparison of Mean Points for Self-Compassion and Self-Compassion Perception and In-Group Variation Before and After Psychodrama Group Studies (n=45)

Scale Points	First Measurement			Final Measurement				
	Min	Max	Mean±SD	Min.	Max.	Mean±SD	t	p
Self-compassion perception	4	10	6.93±1.57	4	9	7.30±1.37	t=-4.054	**p<0.000**
Self-compassion	50	84	70.73±8.64	54	86	72.44±8.24	t=-6.858	**p<0.000**

perception and SCS points before and after the psychodrama group studies (p<0.001). The analyses showed that the psychodrama implementation was effective in increasing self-compassion status.

Psychodrama is "rediscovery of reality through action" and as a result, individuals relive events in their lives and gain different perspectives with psychodrama group experiences (25). Lawrence stated that psychodrama implementations positively affected the self-compassion and sensitivity levels of individuals (23). In studies investigating the effect of psychodrama group experiences on the self-sensitivity of university students, Bakalım et al. found the group experience positively affected the self-sensitivity levels of students (25). In the literature, the effect of psychodrama on self-compassion was investigated in different groups. İren Akbıyık et al. found psychodrama implementation had positive effect on strengthening self-affection among breast cancer patients. The study assessing the effect of psychodrama on self-affection and distressing situations among breast cancer patients by İren Akbıyık et al. showed that psychodrama had supportive effect in terms of lowering stress and strengthening self-affection (11). Studies with psychodrama implementations have revealed the positive effect of psychodrama on self-compassion occurs through positive effects on self-awareness, optimism, problem-solving skills, and ability to approach events logically. Self-compassion is stated to have the effect of increasing an individual's awareness levels, adjusted behavior when faced with situations like distress, failure and mistakes and easing the individual's ability to cope with negative experiences through positive routes (26).

Additionally, psychodrama implementations with university students are stated to be more effective in focusing on the problems of the protagonist person acting the problem on stage and in understanding themselves than talking (27). Kranz et al. found psychodrama techniques developed the students' communication skills and they gained awareness in recognizing themselves in psychodrama studies with university preparation students from different cultures (28). Şimşek found psychodrama had positive effect on optimism and logical thinking (29), while Hamamcı and Çoban (30) and Ulupınar (18) found it had positive effect on problem-solving perception. The results in this study show similarities to the studies performed with psychodrama implementations.

Conclusion

In this research, psychodrama was determined to increase the self-compassion perception and self-compassion levels of university students. Based on the findings obtained, it is recommended that.

- Psychodrama be applied to different variables due to being based on action, spontaneity, and creativity,
- The study be repeated with different groups and with a control group.

References

1. Özyeşil, Z. (2011). *Öz-anlayış ve bilinçli farkındalık.* İstanbul: Maya Akademik Yayıncılık.

2. Bennett Goleman, T. (2001). *Emotional alchemy: How the mind can heal the heart.* New York: Three Rivers Press.

3. Neff, K. D. (2003). The development and validation of a scale to measure self-compassion. *Self and Identity, 2*(3), 223-250. doi:10.1080/15298860309027

4. Yarnell, M. L., Stafford, E. R., Neff, K. D., Erin, D., Reilly, D. E., Marissa, C., ... Mullarkey, M. (2015). Meta-analysis of gender differences in self-compassion. *Self and Identity,* 14(5), 1-22. doi:10.1080/ 15298868.2015.1029966.

5. Akın, Ü., Akın, A., & Abacı, R. (2007). Öz-duyarlık ölçeği: geçerlik ve güvenirlik çalışması. *Hacettepe Üniversitesi Eğitim Fakültesi Dergisi, 33,* 1-10.

6. Öveç, Ü. (2007). *Öz-duyarlık ile öz-bilinç, depresyon, anksiyete ve stres arasındaki ilişkilerin yapısal eşitlik modeliyle incelenmesi.* (Unpublished master's thesis). Sakarya University, Sakarya, Turkey.

7. Bayramoğlu, A. (2011). *Self-compassion in relation to psychopathology.* (Doctoral dissertation). Middle East Technical University, Ankara, Turkey.

8. Andiç, S. (2013). *Ergenlik döneminde zihni meşgul eden konularla ilişkili değişkenler: bağlanma tarzları, öz-şefkat ve psikolojik belirtiler.* (Unpublished master's thesis). Ankara University, Ankara, Turkey.

9. İskender, M. (2009). The relationship between self-compassion, self-efficacy, and control belief about learning in Turkish university students. *Social Behavior and Personality an International Journal, 37*(5), 711-720. doi:10.2224/sbp.2009.37.5.711

10. Neff, K. D. (2009). Self-compassion. In M. R. Leary & R. H. Hoyle (Eds.), *Handbook of individual differences in social behavior* (pp. 561-573). New York: Guilford Press.

11. İren Akbıyık, D., Araparslan, B., & Yardımcı, Y. (2019). Meme kanseri hastalarında psikodrama gruplarının özşefkat ve distres üzerine etkisi. *Anadolu Psikiyatri Dergisi, 20*(6), 635-641.

12. Neff, K. D. (2003). Self-compassion: An alternative conceptualization of a healthy attitude toward oneself. *Self and Identity, 2*(2), 85-101. doi:10.1080/15298860309032

13. Bayar, Ö., & Dost, T. M. (2018). Üniversite öğrencilerinde öz-şefkatin yordayıcıları olarak bağlanma tarzı ve algılanan sosyal destek. *Hacettepe Üniversitesi Eğitim Fakültesi Dergisi (H. U. Journal of Education), 33*(3), 689-704. doi:10.16986/HUJE.2017029306

14. Deniz, M. E., Arslan, C., Özyeşil, Z., & İzmirli, M. (2012). Öz-anlayış, yaşam doyumu, negatif ve pozitif duygu: Türk ve diğer ülke üniversite öğrencileri arasında bir karşılaştırma. *Mehmet Akif Ersoy Üniversitesi Eğitim Fakültesi Dergisi, 1*(23), 428-446.

15. Altınay, D. (2015). *Psikodrama grup terapisi el kitabı.* İstanbul: Epsilon Yayıncılık.

16. Gimenez Hinkle, M. (2008). Psychodrama: A creative approach for addressing parallel process in group supervision. *Journal of Creativity in Mental Health, 3*(4), 401-415. doi:10.1080/15401380802527464

17. Ulupınar Alıcı, S. (2009). Psikodrama dersinin öğrenciler tarafından değerlendirilmesi. *Hemşirelikte Eğitim ve Araştırma Dergisi, 6*(2), 36-40.

18. Ulupınar, S. (2014). Psikodrama uygulamasının hemşirelik öğrencilerinin sorun çözme becerisine etkisi. *Anadolu Psikiyatri Dergisi, 15*, 55-62. doi:10.5455/apd.39822

19. Dökmen, Ü. (2005). *Sosyometri ve psikodrama.* İstanbul: Sistem Yayıncılık.

20. Leary, M. R., Tate, E. B., Adams, C. E., Allen, A. B., & Hancock, J. (2007). Self-compassion and reactions to unpleasant self-relevant events: The implications of treating oneself kindly. *Journal of Personality and Social Psychology, 92*(5), 887-904. doi:10.1037/0022-3514.92.5.887

21. Neff, K. D., Rude, S. S., & Kirkpatrick, K. L. (2007). An examination of self-compassion in relation to positive psychological functioning and personality traits. *Journal of Research in Personality, 41*(4), 908-916. doi:10.1016/j.jrp.2006.08.002

22. Kyeong, W. L. (2013). Self-compassion as a moderator of the relationship between academic burn-out and psychological health in Korean cyber university. *Personality and Individual Differences, 54*(8), 899-902. doi:10.1016/j.paid.2013.01.001

23. Lawrence, C. (2015). The caring observer: Creating self compassion through psychodrama. *The Journal of Psychodrama, Sociometry, and Group Psychotherapy, 63*(1), 65-72. doi:10.12926/0731-1273-63.1.65

24. Deniz, M. E., Kesici, Ş., & Sümer, A. S. (2008). The validity and reliability study of the Turkish version of self-compassion scale. *Social Behavior and Personality an International Journal, 36*(9), 1151-1160. doi:10.2224/sbp.2008.36.9.1151

25. Bakalım, O., Yörük, C., & Şensoy, G. (2018). Psikodrama grup yaşantısının rehberlik ve psikolojik danışmanlık öğrencilerinin öz-duyarlık düzeylerine etkisi. *Electronic Journal of Social Sciences, 17*(67), 949-968.

26. Sayın, M. (2017). *Üniversite öğrencilerinin öz-anlayış, kendini affetme ve başa çıkma stratejileri arasındaki ilişkiler örüntüsü: bir yol analizi çalışması.* (Unpublished master's thesis). Marmara University, İstanbul, Turkey.

27. Kim, K. W. (2003). The effects of being the protagonist in psychodrama. *Journal of Group Psychotherapy Psychodrama Sociometry, 55*(4), 115-127.

28. Kranz, P. L., Ramirez, S. Z., & Lund, N. L. (2007). The use of psychodrama action techniques in a race relations class. *College Student Journal, 41*(4), 1203-1209.

29. Şimşek, U. E. (2003). Bilişsel-davranışçı yaklaşımla ve rol değiştirme tekniğiyle bütünleştirilmiş film terapisi uygulamasının işlevsel olmayan düşüncelere ve iyimserliğe etkisi. (Unpublished master's thesis). Ankara University, Ankara, Turkey.

30. Hamamcı, Z., & Çoban, A. E. (2009). Psikodramanın psikolojik danışmanların problem çözme becerilerini algılama düzeyleri üzerine etkisi. *Ondokuz Mayıs Üniversitesi Eğitim Fakültesi Dergisi, 28*, 63-74.

Çiğdem Çelebi and Murat Dündar

Investigation of Circulation Areas Depending on Spatial Planning Criteria in Healthcare Facilities

Abstract

Objective: This paper aims to explore the circulation areas through spatial movement patterns of different sort of users. In the first chapter, the healthcare facility design has been investigated to define the basic design criteria through significant case studies conducted and published reports.

Materials and Methods: Studies on the planning of healthcare facilities reveal that the qualified spatial planning, which facilitates functional processes and ensures the integration of users, is based on particular design criteria. An important aspect of healthcare facility design, circulation areas allow the satisfied patient experience and the communication of staff. In order to examine the circulation areas of the healthcare facilities thoroughly, the healthcare facility design has been investigated to define the basic design criteria through significant case studies conducted and published reports. For this purpose, the medium-sized medical center has been examined using the case study method according to the criteria defined in the literature research.

Results: In the healthcare facility examined as a case study, it has been observed that spatial planning is determined according to user circulation, departments with special needs are separated from each other and common areas are correctly situated, although they are insufficient at some points. Within the scope of user frequency, it has been noticed that the density increases in front of the vertical circulation elements such as elevators and stairs, while horizontal circulation decreases as users walk to departments and in-department spaces. In this facility, which can be defined as a compact structure, users do not waste excessive time with circulation since the departments are connected both vertically and horizontally.

Conclusion: In order to have a more functional and efficient healthcare facility, there is a need for well-designed circulation areas where all users can integrate better and in-hospital process can realize easier.

Keywords: Healthcare Facilities, Circulation, Spatial Planning, Spatial Configuration, Time Consuming, Wayfinding

Introduction

Healthcare environments and their impact on patients has recently become a significant issue that concerns many fields in the design process. Regarding this process, physical and psychological environmental conditions to be provided for the healing of patient necessitate many design decisions to be made (1). Not only the patients' experience in hospital, but also how their families and staff are affected by hospital physical environment, gain importance to ensure the integrated quality of care. When the healthcare design is considered as an inclusive design for all user profiles, the circulation areas become the most important part of the design in terms of increasing hospital efficiency, ensuring patient satisfaction and supporting the treatment process with physical environment attributes.

The remarkable studies on hospital planning / design and its impact on user profiles have been brought together in a report by Ulrich and Zimring, in which they provided an opportunity to rethink the hospital design in the 21st century (2). In the same sense, the healthcare design has increasingly moving toward "evidence-based design" linking characteristics of the healthcare physical settings to patient and staff outcomes (3). In the context of architectural planning of healthcare design, "the structure of rooms and corridors impact the paths people take", so that the movement of users in healthcare buildings becomes important (4).

In studies focusing on circulation areas of healthcare facilities, Carthey has assessed such areas through optimization (minimization) of healthcare corridors (5). It is also important that Allison associate's circulation areas with wayfinding behavior (6). In essence, in the researches examining these areas through case studies, acoustical measures of noise, adverse events due to inadequate communication, patient and staff traffic etc. have been evaluated. Most of these studies that based on theoretical assumptions, quantitative measurements, and on-site observations, have not investigated the impacts of spatial planning of circulation areas and units in detail. Furthermore, no speculation has taken place concerning such areas in a holistic way through all facility users. So, the research has linked the quality of care, the wellbeing of the healthcare users with the circulation zones in terms of spatial planning of healthcare facility.

Many studies on the definition of circulation areas, which are important part of hospital design, have been approached from different perspectives. Circulation areas are also communication zones defined as "hospital streets, corridors, internal lobbies, and staircases that provide access between departments" (7).

Design of the circulation areas and the healthcare units attached to it, influences the users in many ways. The aim of this research is to investigate the circulation areas through the certain user profiles (patient, visitor, and staff) in terms of accessibility, time consuming and wayfinding that influence and shape spatial planning of such facilities.

Materials and Methods

In this paper, the circulation areas are examined on the basis of spatial planning. The physical aspects and its features of these spaces such as lighting, color, and signage are intentionally kept out of scope. The first point that requires clarification is the "circulation" space involves many functions and definitions for different types of users. This issue will be addressed as inclusive to all users by referring the featured arguments and researches in this field. After reviewing the main significant written resources on the subject, spatial planning criteria will be determined and evaluated depending on circulation maps revealing relations and the distance between units. Spatial planning criteria of healthcare facilities will be defined by analyzing certain healthcare design outcomes as case studies. In this study, intensity graphics, user-oriented cycle plans and abstracted architectural plans will be used to achieve substantial and understandable data.

In the first chapter, an overview of how healthcare facilities are evaluated in the architectural design process will be given. Under the same topic, firstly, the discourses on how this process affects the circulation areas and which parameters gain importance will be expressed. Secondly, the criteria affecting the circulation areas in spatial design will be determined in health buildings. Afterwards, the case study will be analyzed through the determined spatial design criteria and the outcomes will be summarized in conclusion.

Healthcare Facility Design

Today, healthcare facilities become a very comprehensive and complex type of structure realized by state or private institutions with large investments and thus, how architects design these investments have gained importance. For architects in this design process, new standards for patient and staff rooms, department unit layout and design for healing environments; all are the subject of architectural thinking. In order to improve patient experience and to make operations more efficient, rethinking patient flow is an important part of architectural planning (8). As the area of the healing and life-affirming, health facilities "have to be designed for improved performance and workflow, and with a high degree of flexibility and adaptability for constant change" (8).

The healing process in healthcare facilities is also integrated with "architecture and design's impact on patient outcomes, relatives and visitors' expectations, as well as of employees, and which seeks to minimize the negative effects of stress-inducing surroundings in healthcare facilities" (9). An effective and usable spatial planning of healthcare facility is structured through movement of users in space and the planning of space in which users comprehend, engage, and connect the function of the facility (10). Haron et al. argue that the effect of spatial configuration on the orientation of user behaviors is quite high and that the planning based on the spatial design principles provides a system in which empty spaces are turned into functional interiors and ensures user satisfaction (10).

Circulation Areas in Healthcare Facility

Circulation areas have different functional meanings than connecting different places together. The consistent design of the circulation offers us a communication space beyond people flow depending on the provision of many criteria. In particular, such areas have an impact on communication patterns of multidisciplinary teams in healthcare. Carthey highlights that the difficulties and system problems in treatment and adverse events are the result of inadequate interaction within a multidisciplinary care team (5). He exemplifies the study of Coeria et al. reported that inadequate communication between staff leads to a loss of time, disrupts patient care and can cause avoidable adverse events in clinical practice (11). The fact that the corridors are the setting for negotiation of medical and non-medical professionals has led to some researches on this issue. One of these conducted by Iedema and colleagues note that "...it may be that people regard corridor as back stages, or as spaces that are experienced as being less inscribed with conduct regulations and institutional prerequisites than the spaces that the corridors connect: front stages" (12). They point out that the corridors are place that doctors not only engage in juniors but also negotiate with families (12). Furthermore, Becker has stated the importance of sharing information and getting assistance by hospital staff. He also emphasizes that the corridor is a stage where team members from different disciplines share their knowledge, skills, and perspectives on the job. The corridor physical environments in hospitals provide an open medium for informal learning types in which unprepared encounters and chance (13).

Allison proposes that healthcare designers can apply to urban planning and design principles in the healthcare design for example Lynch's five elements on the image of city: paths, nodes, landmarks, edges and districts (6).

A systematic and hierarchical design of circulation zones as in urban planning supports way finding and users' experience (6). In a similar vein, Carthey argues that just as the streets and connection roads within a city are part of a hierarchical structure, each corridor within a hospital is a hierarchical part of the circulatory system of that hospital by supporting the argument of Allison (5). He also regards such areas as corridors that are "very important to the functioning of multidisciplinary clinical teams and quality of care delivery". Referring to the multifunctional features of the corridor zones of healthcare, Carthey proposes healthcare designers that such areas should be easily accessible and facilitate the interaction of different patient care teams (informal and formal), while reminding them not to ignore the functions and needs of all other healthcare facility users (5). He clarifies these needs as; "ensuring patient privacy, and preventing unwelcome noise from affecting patients, visitors and other staff" (5).

Pangrazio investigated the general circulation areas and their positive impacts on patients. According to him, these spaces provide users four different functionality.

- "collector spaces" as the entrance lobby and reception zones directing incoming person,
- "introspective spaces" including cafés and cafeterias,
- "movement spaces" involving corridors,
- "transition spaces" including passing between departments and elevator lobbies (14).

Carthey focused on the need of the movement of people and goods between units (5). In a healthcare facility, patient, staff, and visitors are part of the circulation area and described especially for the healthcare environment as "space for the movement of people and supplies in a department" (15). In this movement, each user profile has different circulation axes and intersects at many points and creates a traffic flow. Thus, circulation systems should not only provide clear and intuitive wayfinding for families, patients and accommodate the many staff members and services but also separate and control public, private, clean, and soiled traffic types (8). At this point, the designers are confronted with situations that multiple layers need to be separated and connected at the same time. The spatial planning of circulation "is made more complex by the many functions which needs specific adjacencies and short travel distances while at the same time controlling and directing traffic flow" (8). It is important for the visitor to find the right way and to support his/ her patient while the patient needs for emergency and privacy. Becker points out "the corridor is a neutral-zone, not owned by any particular professional discipline" (13). He focuses on especially the movement of staff by saying that "in this neutral zone, nurses, doctors, physical therapists, and other healthcare professionals interacted spontaneously and opportunistically" (13).

Circulation areas also play an important role as a part of public spaces and at some points can turn into waiting areas. In the architectural planning, the points where the circulation should expand or contract or make a turn vary depending on where the circulation is planned. As the corridor gains a waiting function in the entrance halls, it can expand, in the same way the corridor become narrower as it passes to wet areas. Planning quantities of space needed into healthcare starts with modular planning grid allowing flexible uses within a basic structural system (8). According to Sprow, to make a more efficient circulation, designers consider the basis of healthcare organization; accessibility to the healthcare facility at ground level, horizontal and vertical circulation routes between critical services, the separation of circulation types, effective distances between units without loss of time for patient, visitor and staff (8).

Spatial Planning Criteria for Circulation Areas

According to Bitgood, the circulation areas are basically divided into two types: horizontal and vertical circulation (16). The horizontal circulation areas define the circulation between units on the same floor. These areas include all walking areas that provide physical access to an area such as a corridor, waiting and entry. Vertical circulation refers to the access of the visitors to different levels by using the circulation elements. Stairs, ramps, and elevators are defined as circulation elements providing vertical circulation (16). Accurate planning of both types of circulation in a complex structure such as hospital is of great importance for the effective functioning of building. In horizontal circulation, access and waiting areas, access to vertical circulation elements, and to wet areas constitute the basis for efficient spatial planning. Research studies have shown that the effective spatial design can reduce stress and tension among the patients or staff and increase the overall efficiency and usability of the hospital design (17).

If the space does not have a clear spatial layout, it cannot be sensed, hence, it can cause especially workflow and way finding problems. At this point, the form of a circulation system should be visible and perceptible by the users within the spatial organization. The units around an open core can provide the users with more visual and audial functionality (18). Circulation system has a considered and designed architectural expression, which makes it easier to understand the structure. Therefore, the form of the building can be designed as a structural expression of spatial planning and the related circulatory system with it (19).

Distance Between Units - Time Consuming

Researchers state that the time required for users to move from one place to another is affected by the circulation design of the facility (20). The square meters of circulation areas are much more than other areas in the building planning. Although there is no standard value for the circulation areas in the literature, the design practice and the data collection of completed projects realized that 10-30 % of the total floor area is dedicated to the circulation for an efficient and cost-effective design (21). For this reason, the designers of healthcare facilities study to optimize the circulation areas (22).

In the report of Ulrich, the role of physical environment in the hospitals discussed, he mentions the studies investigating the effects of time consuming in the healthcare facilities (2). These studies show that "time saved walking was translated into more time spent on patient-care activities and interaction with family member" (23). The efficiency and the performance of staff can be particularly affected by the relationship between the spaces that is critical for the functionality of healthcare operations. In some cases, the drug may need to be injected into the patient within a certain period of time, and the drug preparation and injection spaces should be planned close together. It is also important that emergency parts are easily accessible and perceivable without loss of time in cases requiring emergency action. "Nurses are considered to be the users who spend the most of time providing direct care to the patients; therefore, it is natural to give their needs the higher priority when designing a hospital" (23).

The studies of Ozcan, comparing the intensive care unit examples in United States and Turkey, revealed that "Reducing walking distances between inpatient areas and support spaces will enable nurses to spend more with their patients" (24). His observation in the Turkish intensive units indicates the fact that the nurse support units are outside the intensive care units causes the nurse back and forth and therefore lose time, fatigue and expose them to the relatives of patients waiting outside. This may result in a decrease in the performance of the nurse, tension, and inefficiency. In the compact units, the interaction between the personnel and the family will not be effective, on the contrary the interaction within the staff will be effective so that the staff can handle his / her job more efficiently and the long distances do not lose time on foot (24). As similar examples in Turkey, in the United States, Ozcan argues that "ICU (intensive care unit), which is less compact and flexible, increased walking distances and charting time reduced staff time spent with patients" and ". . .increasing the unit size increases walking distances. . ." (24).

Bill Hiller argues, "buildings are fundamentally about movement and how it is generated and controlled" (25). The location and design of the stairs, corridors and ramps providing movement become the main determinants in the design process because they "affect the visitor's perception of space and level of visitor's satisfaction" (16). Bitgood also highlights that the conceptual orientation is one of the main aspects of circulation and he describes the conceptual orientation "consciousness and understanding of the circulation elements and arrangement of the facilities" (16). Any possible problem in this orientation causes the patient to lose time and become more nervous because of this time loss. In terms of disorientation of patients, time consuming results in a nervous situation that may have a serious impact especially on the patient's health condition (20).

Relations Between Units

Healthcare complexes are grifted structures where many different departments are planned in a whole, each department consists of different functional spaces and this whole is connected with an efficient circulation. Sprow focuses on the spatial needs of the healthcare facilities and argues that serving the different and demanding functional needs of hospital is possible by planning the units in detail from the inside to the outside rather than fixing the units into a complete form (8). The provision of functional health services in each room begins with the study of the relations between equipment and a space required for a room type. Then, this study is used as "functional planning modules" and departments are defined. Eventually, planning is carried out within the framework of functional flow, architectural balance, and holistic consistency (8). Sprow proposes "modular planning grid allowing flexible uses and shifting of function later, within a basic structural system" (8). He determines the basics of the hospital organization to provide more efficient circulation:

- Ground level access for public, outpatients and emergency,
- Horizontal and vertical circulation btw critical services,
- Distribution of support services and separation of traffic types,
- Efficient travel distances for patient, visitors and staff (8).

Relation between spaces also affects the social behaviors that are related to spaces created for the movement, activities and interaction (26). In order to regulate the spaces in the spatial layout, three key factors are identified. These are: visibility and interaction; sub-divisions; distance and proximity (26). Also, some studies focusing on the spatial configuration and its different interaction patterns examine "the degrees in which spatial integration influences movement and spatial behaviors" (27). The results of these studies showed that the more integrated spaces are allowing to more mobility and the spatial organization has a close relationship with the interaction patterns. Therefore, the proximity of space to other spaces and spaces allowing interaction with staff has become very essential for the hospitals where communication can save lives. The space organization requires a strategic thinking in the architectural planning process. In this planning process, it should be one of the most important targets to facilitate the workflow and establish a circulation pattern that strengthens the communication.

Wayfinding

According to Mollerup (17), the wayfinding problems in healthcare facilities are generally caused by four different reasons. One of these is that healthcare facilities have complex spatial planning. In this chapter, it is concentrated on the spatial organization of hospitals as a contributing factor of why people get lost in hospitals. Passini et al. (28) also point out that the concept of wayfinding is affected by two main physical factors: "the layout of the setting and the quality of the environmental information". Spatial planning refers to the organization and circulation of spaces, while "environmental information" defines to the quality of architecture and graphic to solve the wayfinding problem. It is important for healthcare facilities that the related units come together, the different functional units are separated from each other and overall system offer a spatial configuration with common areas and circulation system (4). Peponis et al. have noticed that people tend to pass through accessible corridors rather than a great number of spaces in their research (29). This research is based on observations of participants and measurements that objectively define spatial characteristics, and researchers also have realized that participants prefer more "integrated path" and choose accessible routes. "Integrated paths" refer to less turn able, easily traversable roads. They propose that it is significant to define such "integrated routes" in planning while fixing essential facilities and key points such as exit and entrance.

Passini associates the wayfinding features of physical space with the concept of "legibility" (28). According to Passini, the architecture of space should not only include a spatial configuration, but also a wayfinding system that can be understood and interpreted correctly (28). Passini calls this characteristic of space "legibility" and argues that a spatial planning that facilitates intuitive acquisition and understanding of environmental information has a "high legibility" factor (28). Furthermore, Arthur and Passini (18) state that if the space has a low legibility factor, it cannot help with wayfinding. The organization of space should cater the user who is trying to find its direction (18). The design criteria feeding the wayfinding system make the circulation areas a key force where people flow is directed, interrupted etc. Therefore, the circulation is "the space that we try to understand and in this space that we have to make our wayfinding decisions" (18).

Case Study: Neolife Medical Center

In this case study, the outcomes obtained by using architectural plans that have been analyzed by examination, study, and observation method. The observations have been made in order to determine the possible problems in the planning and current use of circulation areas within the healthcare facility, to find out whether the architectural plan objectives coincide with the operation of the healthcare and to question the architectural construct through user profiles. Since the hospital is a very comprehensive and large building type, a medium-sized medical center based on a specific treatment is selected as a case for observation. This study is also a know-how for hospital designers and reveals certain criteria to be considered prior to start the design process. In large hospitals, the circulation load is derived from the outpatient and inpatient areas, while the circulation load in the restricted medical centers is caused by different patient profiles and accompanying persons. Due to the lack of inpatient area and limited staff, an evaluation was made through different patient profiles.

The Neolife Medical Center, which is chosen as an example, has been established for the purpose of diagnosis and treatment of cancer and serves a monthly average of 1500 patients. These patients consist of new patient profiles coming for diagnosis and continuous patients coming to regular treatment. The patient profile, which is the first time to the center, firstly meet with the oncology doctor and then sent to the imaging area for diagnosis. The patient in the treatment process usually goes to the center for the treatment and also to the imaging area for interim checks. In the new patient, the relationship

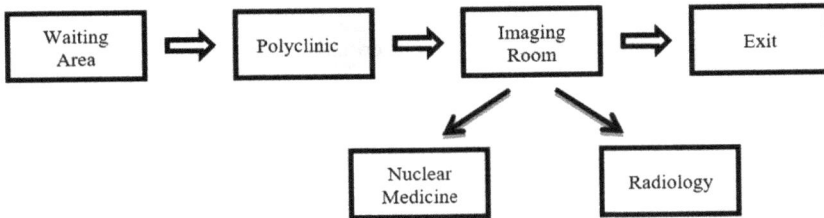

Fig. 1: Patient Scenario 1

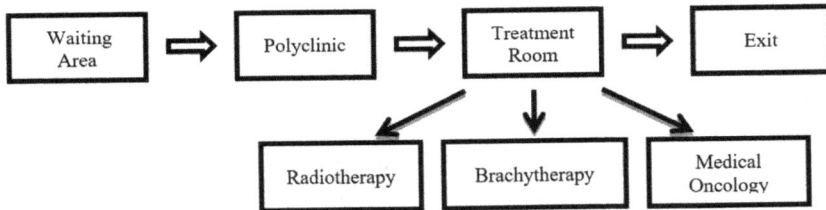

Fig. 2: Patient Scenario 2

and the circulation of areas that are intended for the purpose of diagnostic use were examined while in the patient under treatment, outcomes were based on the integrity of the units requiring treatment. In order to understand the relations of the units, the plans of the existing center were abstracted. In addition, different patient scenarios were defined schematically. In order to investigate the optimization of circulation, the distance and duration of the patients and the density of the circulation areas were observed, and the accessibility of vertical and horizontal circulation was questioned in terms of way finding.

Circulation Ways for User Profiles

Patient Scenarios

The patient, who came to the hospital for the first time and the patient coming regularly, has different circulation and perception within the hospital. The patient coming to healthcare facility for the first time, completes the registration process at the entrance info desk, meets with the doctor and then he/she is directed to the imaging area since imaging is required for diagnosis (Figure 1). If the patient came only for treatment, he/ she visits the info desk and then goes to the treatment area (Figure 2). The treatment areas are divided into medical oncology, radiotherapy, brachytherapy, and each treatment have its own specific area requirements. The medical oncology was planned on the first floor, radiotherapy, and brachytherapy on the basement. In addition, special treatment for international patients is defined on the second floor.

Circulation of Staff and Visitor

In this medium-sized healthcare facility, since the working capacity is low and there is no visitor profile visiting the inpatient, the circulation density is composed of patient and patient relatives. In addition, each floor has separate treatment areas and departments so that staff flow is carried out within the departments themselves. Only doctors and administrative staff use the overall healthcare facility for circulation. Since the number of staff and visitor as user profiles have not any critical effect on the circulation areas, the effects of patient flow have been taken into consideration. If the people come to the hospital for accompanying the patient, he/she moves in the waiting hall and the corridor of the treatment area. It has been observed that the waiting rooms and corridors of the hospital meet all this capacity.

Results

Unit Layout / Spatial Layout

Studying the physical accessibility pattern of a building through the spatial layout can imply how the potential user in that building is distributed and which parts of the layout are effective on this distribution. Movements of users within this medical center begin to gain meaning when it is embraced how the circulation areas providing movement flow are located between the interrelated spaces. For this reason, the medical center has been studied as a holistic structure, how the spaces are located within the whole, their accessibility and the way they joined the circulation have been observed and indicated on an abstracted image (Figure 3).

The circulation and waiting area on the ground floor are intertwined and the wet areas and vertical circulation elements are reached through this combined area. Since the location of wet areas and vertical circulation are perceived from the main waiting hall, the newcomer can find the areas without experiencing the wayfinding problem and getting lost. Because of the fact that the polyclinics are defined on the ground floor (Figure 4), doctor meetings can be easily carried out after the info desk. Also, as it is a medical center that includes cancer treatment, patients need to be treated regularly and this makes

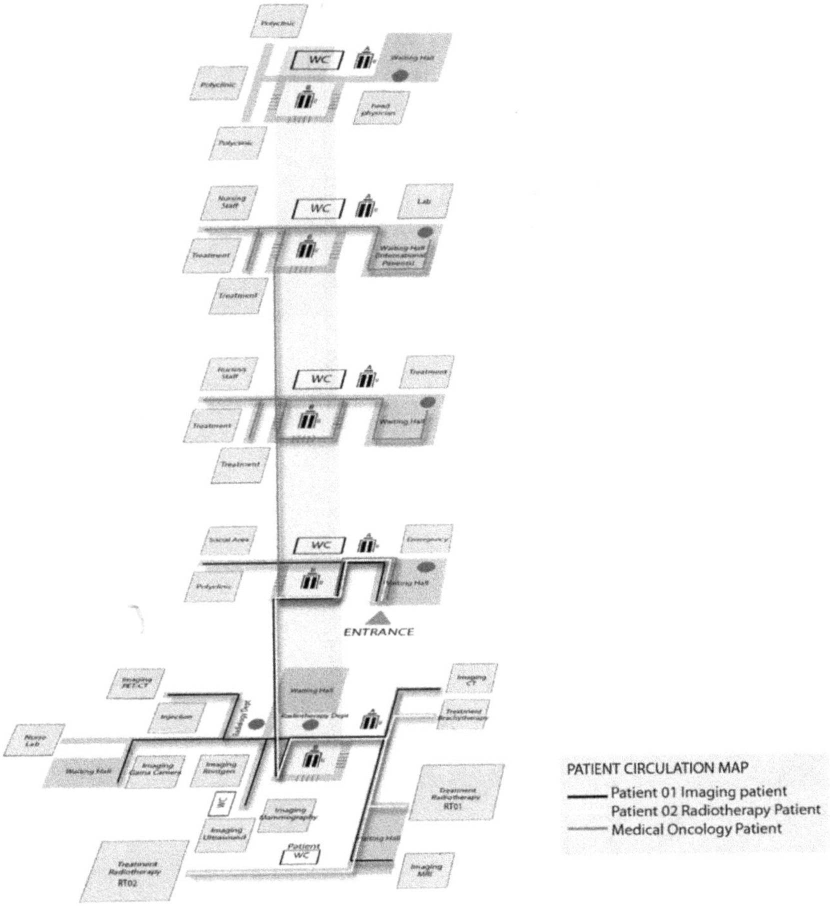

Fig. 3: Patient Circulation Map

the accessibility of treatment areas important. The patients can access to treatment areas by using stairs or elevators.

On the 1st and 2nd floors of the medical center (Figures 5 and 6), there are treatment areas of medical oncology. In these treatment areas, the patient is treated by injection. These areas have their own waiting areas, and these waiting areas are open to the main circulation zone where the staircase and elevator are connected to it. Therefore, it is intuitively felt that user will pass

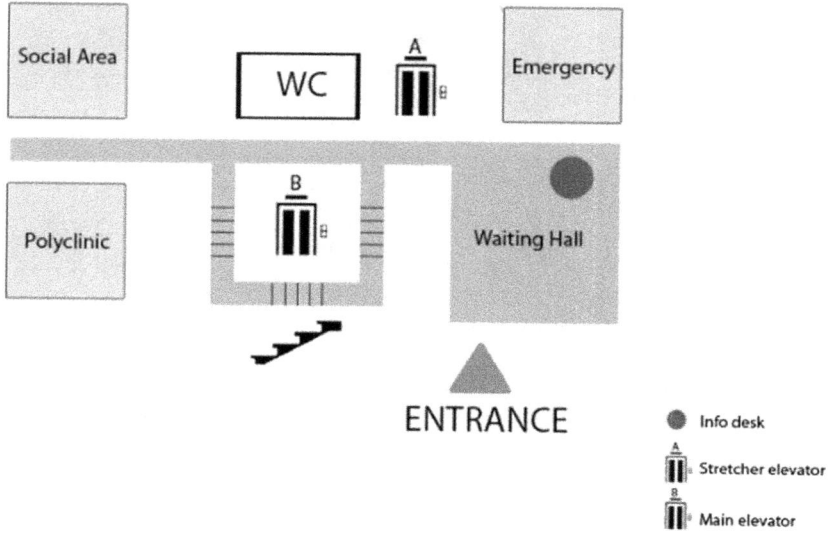

Fig. 4: Ground Floor Plan

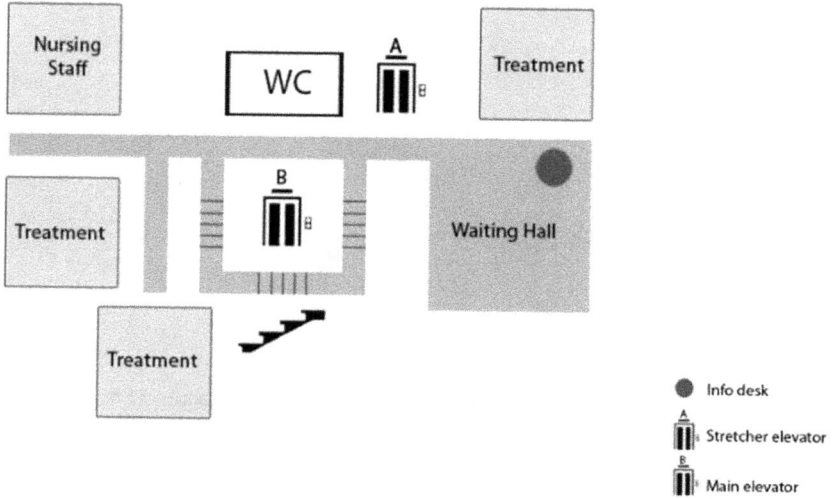

Fig. 5: First Floor Plan

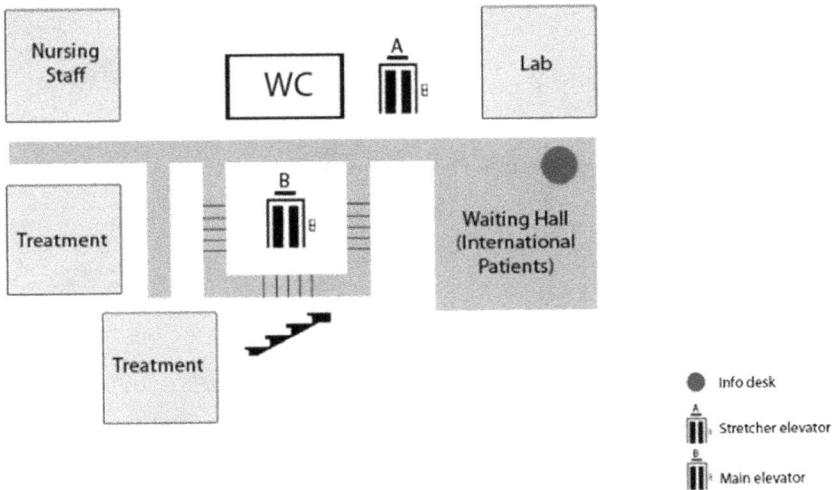

Fig. 6: Second Floor Plan

from the main corridor to the waiting hall. The treatment areas can be defined as the spaces where many injection seats are located and separated from each other by movable partition. The fact that the waiting area is close to the treatment areas and has a good permeability to communicate can make the patient and patient relatives feel safe and can facilitate the movement of the staff.

On the 3rd floor of the medical center, there are administrative offices and reserved doctor rooms to be used in case of need. Likewise, there is a waiting area that connects to the main circulation zone and a secondary corridor leading to doctor's rooms (Figure 7).

According to spatial relationship analysis of basement floor (Figure 8), it is significant that the radiotherapy areas are not related to the waiting area. Because the size of the waiting area defined for the whole floor and the perceptibility of the patient were not sufficient, it was noticed that the secondary corridors were used as a waiting area. The basement consists of radiotherapy and imaging units and each section consists of supporting units connected to the circulation line. The presence of MRI identified within the radiotherapy complicates the circulation of patients and staff within the department itself.

Because of that Radiotherapy02 is far from the core and has a long circulation route, the patient cannot easily reach the treatment and the staff have to walk long distance between the reception and the treatment area and hence

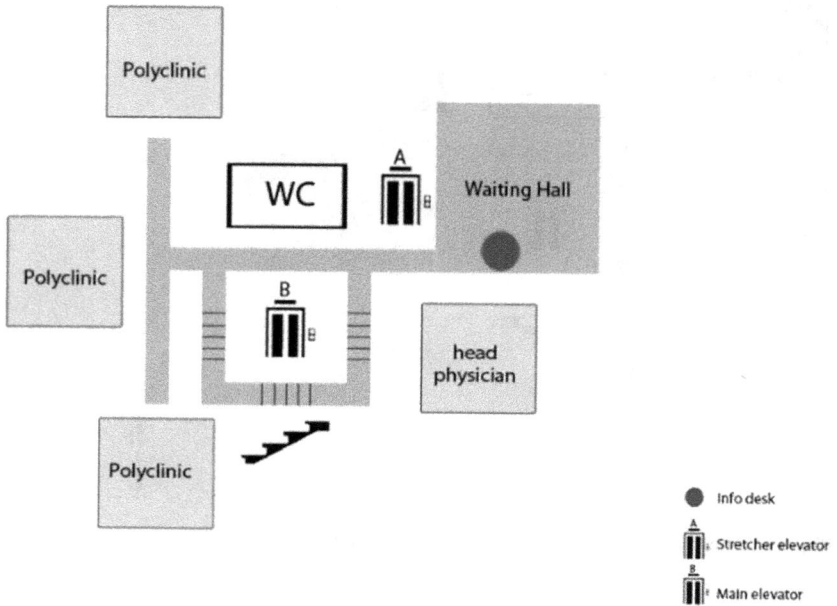

Fig. 7: Third Floor Plan

lose a lot of time (Figure 9). Both radiotherapy areas were planned separately due to the landform. Furthermore, the staff working in both of them is
common and the same group of staff carries out the planning for the treatment
of the patient. In this spatial organization, the fact that two treatment areas
are distant from each other creates difficulties in terms of staff circulation and
communication with each other.

Frequency of Users

Circulation density increases in certain main zones of the hospital and in the
areas connected to the main circulation and in the areas where the movements
of the users intersect. On the other hand, according to the number of patients
coming to the hospital for a specific treatment or only for the examination
and the number of staff working in the departments, the density of circulation
changes. The results of the observations made within one day were matched
with the number of monthly patients and an abstracted density graph was
derived according to the data obtained. Since the medical oncology treatment

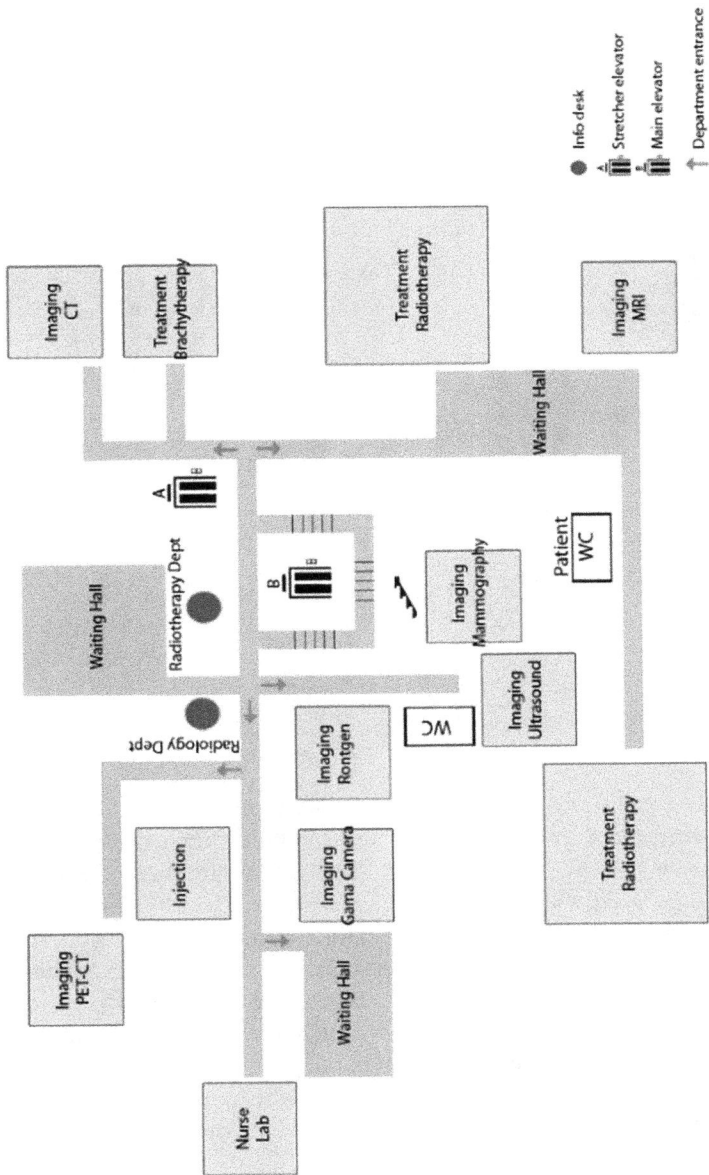

Fig. 8: Basement Floor Plan

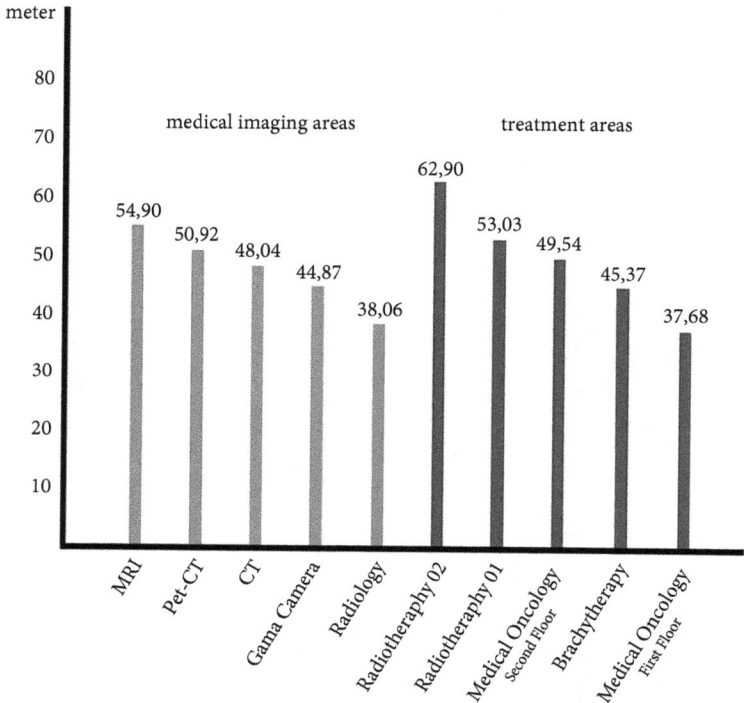

Fig. 9: Distance to The Entrance

areas on the 1st and 2nd floor are used very rarely, only the circulation density in the basement and the ground floor has been taken into consideration. The densest area is the circulation area in which vertical circulation elements are planned to be faced with wet areas and narrowed in width, and this density decreases towards treatment and examination units (Figures 10 and 11). The most widely used department is the nuclear medicine department in this medical center, but the patient and patient relatives use the corridors as a waiting area. Also, the corridors in nuclear medicine and radiology departments are not designed to wait and cause density. On the other hand, since radiotherapy department is not used frequently according to the number of patients in the second half of 2018, it is observed that the density of circulation areas decreases in this unit.

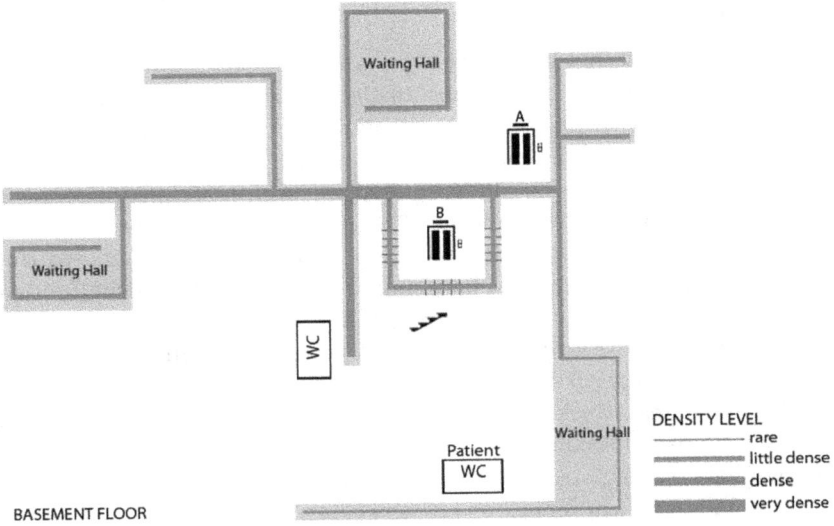

Fig. 10: Basement Floor Density

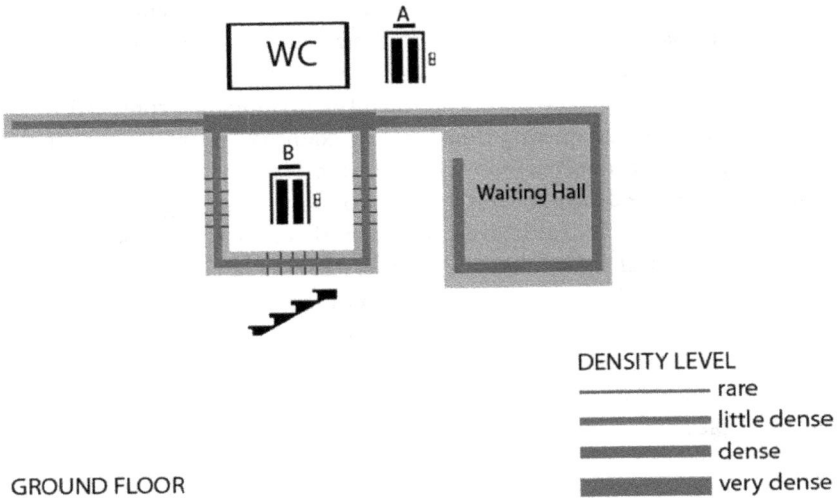

Fig. 11: Ground Floor Density

398 Çiğdem Çelebi and Murat Dündar

Discussion

This case study did not include visitors, which are significant user of large hospital complexes, but allowed examination of two specific patient profiles. The diagnosis and the treatment of patients need centralized vertical circulation and support services that are easily accessible to both types of patients. This type of healthcare program is required to considerably specific rooms in which specific services are conducted. Therefore, the planning of such spaces has more flexible and efficient circulation areas allowing specific patient-centered process. These services have similar program units: patient information desk, waiting area, dressing or preparation rooms, staff units, injection rooms, administrative units and a systematic pattern of patient and staff circulation. The pattern of circulation areas changes according to the treatment and the diagnosis areas which are self-sufficient units and have their own internal rooms in terms of functional and adjacency and circulation. In general, both of them have waiting areas need a close horizontal connection to diagnostic imaging and treatment rooms.

This study will provide the hospital authorities with the most convenient and hassle-free circulation in the healthcare facility and contribute to the establishment of the most appropriate spatial layout. Beside the necessity of planning for the functional processes of imaging and treatment departments emerged in this study, it is important to design polyclinics and other units in scientific ways and to ensure great ease in healthcare circulation especially for patients. The fact that healthcare facility corridors are confused at any time, that patients are wasting time for test, examinations and appointments by wasting time in unexpected ways, that staff loss time between unrelated units, that all these delays adversely affect workflows, that negative impacts of patient' delays on their health levels, are issues that need to be handled in both small and large-scale health facilities. Understanding how these problems can or cannot be solved in a medium sized health facility can be an example of designing the most suitable spatial organization for such medical centers. This study can be extended to an even larger scale, by examining the scope of all intended users at the introduction of the article and exposing the problems of more complex hospitals.

Conclusion

In terms of spatial planning criteria, circulation areas of healthcare facilities seem to have strong impact on patients move and staff functioning. While this study focuses on especially the circulation of cancer patients during their diagnosis and treatment process, it also emphasizes the importance of studying the movement of staff mostly using the same circulation areas of healthcare facilities.

The analysis of spatial organization of the oncology medical center where the circulation areas of that were stressed aimed to support the spatial accessibility of the patient, to strengthen her/ his adaptation to the place and to reduce the stress during the long and intensive treatment process. With this study, the importance of correctly associating medical units and defining patient/staff flow scenarios at the design process are revealed in terms of facilitating intuitive wayfinding and preventing time loss of users. Therefore, maximum effort should be put into providing efficiency and quality of circulation system in order to promote the recovery of patients, to support the patient feel confident and to improve the interaction between patient and staff.

References

1. Akalin-Baskaya, A., & Yildirim, K. (2007). Design of circulation axes in densely used polyclinic waiting halls. *Building and Environment, 42*(4), 1743-1751. doi:10.1016/j.buildenv.2006.02.010

2. Ulrich, R., & Zimring, C. (2004). The role of the physical environment in the hospital of 21st century: A once-in-a-lifetime opportunity. Report to The Center for Health Design for the Designing the 21st Century Hospital Project. 2-19. Retrieved from https://www.healthdesign.org/system/files/Ulrich_Role%20of%20Physical_2004.pdf

3. Hamilton, K. D. (2003). Four levels of evidence-based practice. *Healthcare Design, 3*(4), 18-26.

4. Haq, S., & Zimring, C. (2003). Just down the road a piece: The development of topological knowledge of building layouts. *Environment & Behavior, 35*(1), 132-160. doi:10.1177/0013916502238868

5. Carthey, J. (2008). Reinterpreting the hospital corridor: "wasted space" or essential for quality multidisciplinary clinical care?, *Health Environments Research & Design, 2*(1), 17-29. doi:10.1177/193758670800200103

6. Allison, D. (2007). Hospital as city: Employing urban strategies for effective wayfinding. *Health Facilities Management, 20*(6), 61-65.

7. Department of Health. (2013). DH health building notes. Retrieved from https://www.gov.uk/government/collections/health-building-notes-core-elements

8. Sprow, R. (2012). Planning hospitals of the future. In G. D. Kunders, *Designing hospitals of the future* (pp. 5-15). Bangalore, India: Prism Books Pvt Ltd.

9. Mullins, A. M. F., Folmer, M. B., & Fich, L. B. (2015). Evidence based knowledge: Towards architecture that supports the healing process in health-care buildings. In K. K. Roessler (Ed.), *Arkitektur og Psykologi* (pp. 13-26). Odense: Institut for Psykologi Syddansk Universitet.

10. Haron, S. N., Hamid, M. Y., & Talib, A. (2010). *Towards service quality: An understanding of the usability concept in healthcare design.* Paper presented at ASEAN Conference on Environment Behavior Studies, Riverside Majestik Hotel, Kuching, Sarawak, Malaysia.

11. Coiera, E. W., Jayasunya, R. A., Hardy, J., Bannon, A., & Thorpe, M. E. C. (2002). Communication loads on clinical staff in the emergency department. *The Medical Journal of Australia, 176*(9), 415-418.

12. Iedema, R., Long, D., Carroll, K., Stenglin, M., & Braithwaite, J. (2005). Corridor work: How liminal space becomes a resource for handling complexities of multi-disciplinary health care. In *APROS 11: Asia-Pacific Researchers in Organization Studies: 11th International Colloquium* (pp. 238-247). APROS.

13. Becker, F. (2007). Organizational ecology and knowledge networks. *California Management Review, 49*(2), 42-61. doi:10.2307/41166382

14. Pangrazio, J. R. (2013). Planning public spaces for healthcare facilities. *Health Facilities* Management. Retrieved from https://www.hfmmagazine. com/articles/418-all-access

15. McLagan, D. (1978). *A Glossary of building and planning terms in Australia.* Adelaide, Australia: Griffin Press Ltd.

16. Bitgood, S. (2010). An analysis of visitor circulation: Movement patterns and the general value principle. *Curator the Museum Journal, 49*(4), 463-475. doi:10.1111/j.2151-6952.2006.tb00237.x

17. Mollerup, P. (2009). Wayshowing in hospital. *Australasian Medical Journal, 2*(10), 112-114. doi:10.4066/AMJ.2009.85

18. Arthur, P., & Passini, R. (1992). *Wayfinding: People signs and architecture.* New York: McGraw Hill.

19. Doğu, F., & Erkıp, F. (2000). Spatial factors affecting wayfinding and orientation: A case study in a shopping mall. *Environment and Behavior, 32*(6), 731-755. doi:10.1177/00139160021972775

20. Elettol, R. M. A., & Bahauddin, A. (2011). A competitive study on the interior environment and the interior circulation design of Malaysian

museums and elderly satisfaction. *Journal of Sustainable Development,* 4(3), 216-217. doi:10.5539/jsd.v4n3p223

21. Kazanasmaz, Z. T., & Tayfur, G. (2012). Classifications for planimetric efficiency of nursing unit floors. *METU Journal of The Faculty of Architecture, 29*(1), 1-20. doi:10.4305/METU.JFA.2012.1.1

22. NHS Estates. (2005). *Ward layouts with single rooms and space for flexibility.* Norwich: The Stationery Office (TSO).

23. Nazarian, M., Price, A. D. F., & Demian, P. (2011). A review of different approaches to access and people circulation within healthcare facilities and the application of modeling, simulation and visualization. Loughborough University. Retrieved from https://dspace.lboro.ac.uk/2134/9196

24. Ozcan, H. (2006). Healing design: A holistic approach to social interaction in pediatric intensive care units in the united states and turkey. In *1st International CIB Endorsed METU Postgraduate Conference: Built Environment & Information Technologies* (pp. 243-260).

25. Hillier, B. (1996). *Space is the machine: A configurational theory of architecture.* London, England: Space Syntax.

26. Sailer, K., & Penn, A. (2007). The performance of space: Exploring social and spatial phenomena of interaction patterns in an organization. In *Architecture and Phenomenology Conference,* Haifa, Israel.

27. Kılıç-Çalğıcı, P., Czerkauer-Yamu, C., & Çil, E. (2013). Faculty office buildings as work environments: Spatial configuration, social interaction, collaboration and sense of community. *ITU Journal of the Faculty of the Architecture, 10*(2), 178-197.

28. Passini, R., Rainville, C., Marchand, N., & Joannette, Y. (1998). Wayfinding and dementia: Some research findings and new look of design. *Journal of Architectural and Planning Research, 15*(2), 133-151.

29. Peponis, J., Zimring, C., & Choi, Y. K. (1990). Finding the Building in Wayfinding. *Environment and Behavior, 22*(5), 555-590. doi:10.1177/0013916590225001

Gökay Kurtulan and İrem Sarıhan

Comparison of Health Literacy Levels of Bahçeşehir University Faculty of Health Sciences and Architecture and Design Students

Abstract

Objective: The aim of this study is to compare the health literacy levels between Bahçeşehir University Faculty of Health Sciences (FHS) and Faculty of Architecture and Design (FAD) students.

Materials and Methods: The research was conducted using quantitative research method. The universe of the research consists of Bahçeşehir University FHS and FAD students. Power analysis has been made for sample calculation. 100 students from both faculties were included in the study. Volunteers and students who do not have oral communication barriers were included in the study. Turkey Health Literacy Scale-32 (THL-32) was used as a data collection tool. Sociodemographic data of the participants were also collected. The THL-32 scale was found to be reliable and valid as a result of the study conducted by the Turkish Republic Ministry of Health. The scale creates a scientific framework in explaining the health literacy levels of students.

Results: As a result of the research, health literacy level of the students of the FHS was found to be higher than the students of the FAD.

Conclusion: With the advancement of technology and the increasing complexity of health systems, the concept of health literacy has gained importance. Inadequate health literacy is an issue that has both individual and social consequences. To improve health literacy, education programs and awareness-raising activities should be organized for individuals to understand the importance of health literacy. These programs should be initiated at an early age and the level of health literacy in all segments of the society should be increased with these programs.

Keywords: Health Literacy, Health Literacy Level

Introduction

With the developing technology, health systems, health policies and the delivery of health services are changing and becoming more complex every day. Efforts to increase health literacy gain importance in minimizing this complexity. In the information era, individuals are expected to understand their illnesses and make useful decisions for themselves. The term health literacy was first used in 1974. In the health literature, the definition of health literacy was found years later (1,2). The World Health Organization defines health literacy as people's access to and comprehension of health information and using this information in daily life to maintain health (3). Inadequate health literacy of the individual means not being able to access correct information in health-related decisions, not being able to benefit from the provided services effectively, having problems in managing the treatment process, having difficulties in following the warnings and instructions of the healthcare personnel during the treatment process or making wrong applications. In addition, the unnecessary examination of the people causes an increase in hospital costs and a deterioration in health at the same time (4-8).

The importance of health literacy has been recognized worldwide as the World Health Organization declared health literacy as a key factor in health promotion (9,10). Studies on health protection, effective and efficient maintenance of health services and development of health policies have gained importance with the increase of chronic diseases in the world. The health policies of countries on the protection of health and efforts to increase the health literacy levels of individuals have also gained momentum (11).

Health literacy is understood as a major public health problem and importance of health literacy have increased in modern societies. That is why, studies on this subject increased in Turkey. The European Health Literacy Scale (HLS-EU) that used in European countries adopted to Turkish and a new scale named Turkey Health Literacy Scale-32 (THL-32) has been developed (12).

There are many reasons for the low level of health literacy, and this situation causes many problems, both individual and social. Increasing chronic diseases, changing living conditions and consequently changing dietary habits, increased use of unnecessary emergency services and hospitals, errors in drug use, communication problems between healthcare professionals and patients due to information asymmetry are experienced due to insufficient health literacy. These problems have negative consequences on the health system (13). Research shows that health literacy level is not enough in Turkey (14). There are many studies related to health literacy by the Ministry of Health. The positive results of these studies can only be possible with the social awareness of health literacy (15-18).

Materials and Methods

This study was approved by the decision of Bahçeşehir University Scientific Research and Publication Ethics Board, dated 22.05.2020, numbered 20021704-604.01.02-E.2172, on "Project Application". All participants were

Tab. 1: 2 × 4 Matrix Components of the THL-32 Scale and Item Numbers of the Components

Health Literacy	Accessing Information	Understanding Information	Evaluating Information	Using Knowledge
Treatment and Service	1,4,5,7	2,8,11,13	3,9,12,15	6,10,14,16
Prevention from Diseases / Improving Health	18,20,22,27	19,21,23,25	24,26,28,32	17,29,30,31

informed about the study and their consents were obtained. In addition, to be able to apply the research in both faculties, institutional permissions were obtained from the relevant Dean's Offices.

The universe of the research consists of students of Faculty of Health Sciences (FHS) and Faculty of Architecture and Design (FAD), who are enrolled under-graduate education at Bahçeşehir University. Power analysis was used for sample calculation. At 95 % confidence level, the confidence interval was taken as 10 %, and the sample was calculated as 90 students for each faculty.

The questionnaire form used for data collection consists of 2 parts and a total of 42 questions. These sections are:

- Sociodemographic Information Part: In this section, students' age, gender, faculty of education, department, place of residence, family income, social security, etc. questions are included.
- THL-32: The scale was developed via "Health Literacy Turkey Reliability and Validity Research" in 2016 by the Turkish Republic Ministry of Health. THL-32 was developed in line with HLS-EU and consists of 32 questions in total. The reliability and validity study of the scale made by the Turkish Republic Ministry of Health and it has been implemented in Turkey. THL-32 was created in a 2x4 matrix structure. Accordingly, the scale consists of 8 components, 2 dimensions and 4 processes.

The sub-dimensions of the scale, the process and the related question numbers are given in Table 1 (15).

Thirty-two items were scored between 1 and 4 (1-very difficult, 2-difficult, 3-easy, 4-very easy). The indexes are calculated with the formula:

$Index=(average-1) \times (50/3)$

0 being the lowest and 50 the highest health literacy. Index, corresponds to the calculated individual index; average, corresponds to average of the item

answered for each person; 1, corresponds to the lowest possible value of the mean; 3, corresponds to the range of the mean; and 50, corresponds to the highest value determined for the new criterion.

According to the index results obtained, it was examined in four groups as 0-25 inadequate, 25-33 limited, 33-42 enough, 42-50 excellent health literacy. The overall internal consistency coefficient of the scale; it has been determined as 0.927 (15). The reliability level of this scale was tested using Cronbach's Alpha within the scope of this research and the general reliability level of the scale was found to be 0.925.

Because of the pandemic, the research was carried out in the form of an online questionnaire. A total of 240 students who are determined according to the sample selection criteria were reached. The data obtained were analyzed in the SPSS (Statistical Package for the Social Sciences) statistical program. The basic assumption of this study is that the students who participated in the study answered the questionnaire items correctly and sincerely. This research was carried out on Bahçeşehir University FHS and FAD bachelor's degree students and the information obtained from all students cannot generalize for Turkey.

Results

The age, gender, faculties and departments, place of residence, monthly income, and sociodemographic information of the students who are participating in the study is shown in Table 2.

75.4 % of the participants were women, 57.5 % enrolled in the FHS, and 78.8 % live in a metropolitan city. 47.5 % of the participants defined their monthly income as medium. The social security of 79.2 % is the Social Security Institution and the 41.7 % apply to private hospital as first health institution.

The percentages of the answers given by the students participating in the study to the THL-32 scale are shown in Table 3.

Most of the participants answered "Easy" to 23 questions, "Very Easy" to 8 questions, and "Difficult" to 1 question of the THL-32 scale. The general average of the answer "Very Easy" was 34.6 %, and it reached the highest value in the item 6 with 62.9 %. The general average of the answer "Easy" was 47.1 %, and it reached the highest value of 60.4 % in items 1 and 8. The general average of the answer "Difficult" was 15.1 %, and it reached the highest value in the 29th item with 35 %. The general average of the answer "Very Hard" was 3.1 %, and it reached the highest value with 14.6 in the 29th item. The general average of the answer "I have no idea" is 5.4 %, it reached the highest value in the 32nd item.

Tab. 2: Sociodemographic Characteristics of the Students Participating in the Study

Variables			n	%
Gender		Female	181	75.4
		Male	59	24.6
Age		18-20	46	19.2
		21-22	109	45.4
		23 and above	85	35.4
Faculty		Faculty of Architecture and Design	102	42.5
		Faculty of Health Sciences	138	57.5
Department	Faculty of Architecture and Design	Industry Products Design	16	6.7
		Interior Architecture and Envr. Design	28	11.6
		Architecture	58	24.2
	Faculty of Health Sciences	Nutrition and Dietetics	37	15.4
		Child Development	3	1.3
		Physical Therapy and Rehabilitation	40	16.6
		Nursing	6	2.5
		Audiology	11	4.6
		Healthcare Management	41	17.1
Residence		Village / Town	11	4.6
		City Center	40	16.6
		Metropolis	189	78.8
Monthly Income		Middle-Lower	10	4.1
		Middle	114	47.5
		High-Middle	88	36.7
		High	28	11.7
Social Security		No	35	14.6
		Social Insurance Institution	190	79.2
		Private Health Insurance	13	5.4
		Others	2	0.8
General Health Status		Bad	1	0.4
		Not bad	23	9.6
		Good	64	26.7
		Pretty good	124	51.6
		Excellent	28	11.7
First Applied Healthcare Institution		Family Health Center	71	29.6
		State Hospital	57	23.8
		University Hospital	7	2.9
		Private Hospital	100	41.7
		Private Practice	5	2.0

Tab. 3: Distribution of Participants' Responses to the Items of the Scale

Nu.	Items	Very Easy	Easy	Difficult	Very Difficult	I have no idea
1	To investigate whether it is a sign of illness or not when you have a complaint about your health.	26.2	**60.4**	7.5	1.3	4.6
2	To read and understand any article on this subject (such as brochure, booklet, poster) when you have a complaint about your health.	27.9	**56.7**	7.5	0.8	7.1
3	When you have a health complaint, assess whether the advice of your family or friends is reliable.	19.2	**53.3**	20.8	2.9	3.8
4	To find out which doctor you should consult when you want to go to a health facility.	**44.1**	38.3	14.2	1.7	1.7
5	To make research and find out how to make application (like making an appointment) when you want to go to a health facility.	**59.1**	32.9	6.3	1.3	0.4
6	To make an appointment via telephone or internet when you want to go to a health institution.	**62.9**	25.8	8.3	2.1	0.9
7	To search and find information about the treatments of the diseases that concern you.	26.3	**59.1**	10.4	1.3	2.9
8	To understand your doctor's explanations about your illness.	27.1	**60.4**	10.4	0.4	1.7
9	To evaluate the advantages and disadvantages of the different treatment options suggested by your doctor.	19.6	**51.2**	21.6	1.3	6.3
10	To use your medicines as recommended by healthcare professionals (such as doctor, pharmacist)	**49.1**	42.9	4.6	1.3	2.1
11	To understand the instructions for using the medicine in the medicine box.	**47.5**	45.0	3.3	2.1	2.1
12	To decide if you need a second opinion from a different doctor.	19.2	**46.6**	24.6	2.5	7.1
13	To understand information about pre-medical test preparations (such as dieting).	42.9	**46.3**	4.6	0.8	5.4

14	To search and find the location of the unit (laboratory, polyclinic) where you want to reach in the hospital.	28.3	**45.8**	20	4.2	1.7
15	To decide what to do in an emergency (such as accident, sudden health problem).	16.3	**41.2**	32.9	2.5	7.1
16	To call an ambulance when necessary.	35.4	**42.1**	9.6	2.1	10.8
17	To have health follow-ups and check-ups at regular intervals as your doctor recommended.	25.8	**45.0**	20.8	3.8	4.6
18	To research and find information about conditions that can be harmful to your health, such as being overweight and having high blood pressure.	40.0	**45.9**	3.3	0	10.8
19	To understand health warnings about conditions (such as being overweight and high blood pressure) that can be harmful to your health.	42.1	**46.3**	2.5	0.8	8.3
20	To research and find information on how to deal with unhealthy behaviors such as smoking and insufficient physical activity.	**48.8**	42.9	2.5	0.8	5.0
21	To understand health warnings about how to deal with unhealthy behaviors such as smoking and insufficient physical activity.	**45.8**	44.2	5.4	0.8	3.8
22	To research and find information about the health screenings you should have relation according to your age, gender, and health condition (such as breast screening for women and prostate-related diseases for men)	32.1	50.0	10.4	0	7.5
23	To understand the recommendations from resources such as the internet, newspapers, television, and radio for being healthier.	41.3	**52.0**	4.2	2.1	0.4
24	To decide whether the information suggested to be made for being healthier in resources such as internet, newspapers, television, and radio is reliable or not.	18.3	**35.0**	31.7	12.5	2.5
25	To understand information on food packaging that you think could affect your health.	20.4	**40.5**	28.3	7.5	3.3

(continued on next page)

Tab. 3: Continued

Nu.	Items	Very Easy	Easy	Difficult	Very Difficult	I have no idea
26	To evaluate the positive and negative characteristics of the environment you live in (such as house, street, neighborhood) that affect health.	27.1	**52.5**	14.6	0.8	5.0
27	To find information about what can be done to make the environment you live in (house, street, neighborhood) healthier.	22.9	**42.5**	22.9	1.7	10.0
28	To evaluate which of your daily behaviors (such as exercising, eating healthy, not smoking) affects your health.	**52.9**	41.3	3.3	0.8	1.7
29	To change your lifestyle (such as exercising, eating healthy, not smoking) for your health.	20.8	28.8	**35.0**	14.6	0.8
30	To be able to apply the written diet list given by the dietician.	19.2	**30.3**	27.9	11.3	11.3
31	To make suggestions to your family or friends about their health.	29.2	**49.6**	12.9	3.3	5.0
32	To interpret health-related policy changes.	12.5	**36.2**	26.7	5.8	18.8

"Very difficult" and "hard" response percentages is compared with the data from the study done in 2016 by Turkish Republic Ministry of Health on the individuals who are in 15 years and above by using THL-32 scale is shown in Table 4.

The percentages of "Difficult" and "Very difficult" responses given by the students of the FAD to the 4th, 15th, 25th and 32nd items are close to the THL-32 study. In the responses to items 27 and 29, it is seen that both faculties get close to the THL-32 study results. Especially in the 29th item, the students of the FAD defined the responses as "Difficult" or "Very difficult" with 50 % and the FHS with 49.3 %. This rate is also high in the THL-32 study (57.5 %). The THL-32 scale index scores according to the faculties of the students participating in the study are shown in Table 5.

The index scores of the 3rd, 9th, 12th, and 17th items show that both faculties have a limited level of health literacy. In the 30th and 32nd items, insufficient health literacy level was determined in both faculties. When the data in Table 5 are examined, it is seen that the health literacy levels of the students of the FAD and FHS are limited and insufficient in the items related to the process of evaluating and using information.

The comparison of the health literacy levels of the participants with the European and the THL-32 studies is shown in Table 6. 44.1 % of the students of the FAD and 51.5 % of the students in the FHS have enough and excellent health literacy level. This rate is 52.5 % in European studies and 30.6 % in THL-32 study. When the average of excellent health literacy levels is examined, the students of the FHS have a rate above the European and THL-32 studies.

The sub-dimensions and information processing processes of the responses given by the participants to the THL-32 scale are shown in Table 7. When a comparison is made according to the sub-dimensions and information processing processes of the FHS and FAD; It was observed that there was a statistically significant difference in health literacy levels in the process of accessing information in treatment and service sub-dimension (p<0.05). In the disease prevention / health promotion sub-dimension, it was observed that there was a statistically significant difference in the processes of accessing, understanding, and evaluating information (p<0.05).

The sub-dimensions and information processing processes of the responses of the FHS students are shown in Table 8 according to their departments. In the FHS, it was observed that there was a statistically significant difference between all departments in the process of accessing information about treatment and service sub-dimension (p<0.05). In the disease prevention / health

Tab. 4: Comparison of Students' "Difficult" and "Very Difficult" Answers with THL-32 Study Data

Nu.	Items	FAD	FHS	THL-32 Study
1	To investigate whether it is a sign of illness or not when you have a complaint about your health.	14.7	4.3	29.0
2	To read and understand any article on this subject (such as brochure, booklet, poster) when you have a complaint about your health.	12.7	5.1	32.5
3	When you have a health complaint, assess whether the advice of your family or friends is reliable.	23.5	23.9	40.0
4	To find out which doctor you should consult when you want to go to a health facility.	21.6	11.6	24.5
5	To make research and find out how to make application (like making an appointment) when you want to go to a health facility.	9.8	5.8	28.0
6	To make an appointment via telephone or internet when you want to go to a health institution.	13.7	8.0	31.7
7	To search and find information about the treatments of the diseases that concern you.	14.7	9.4	37.2
8	To understand your doctor's explanations about your illness.	12.7	9.4	35.0
9	To evaluate the advantages and disadvantages of the different treatment options suggested by your doctor.	27.5	19.6	36.7
10	To use your medicines as recommended by healthcare professionals (such as doctor, pharmacist)	7.8	4.3	18.5
11	To understand the instructions for using the medicine in the medicine box.	7.8	3.6	36.5
12	To decide if you need a second opinion from a different doctor.	30.4	24.6	42.5
13	To understand information about pre-medical test preparations (such as dieting).	5.9	5.1	26.2
14	To search and find the location of the unit (laboratory, polyclinic) where you want to reach in the hospital.	21.6	26.1	29.7
15	To decide what to do in an emergency (such as accident, sudden health problem).	40.2	31.9	47.4
16	To call an ambulance when necessary.	15.7	8.7	17.5
17	To have health follow-ups and check-ups at regular intervals as your doctor recommended.	24.5	24.6	35.5
18	To research and find information about conditions that can be harmful to your health, such as being overweight and having high blood pressure.	4.9	2.2	31.9

Tab. 4: Continued

Nu.	Items	FAD	FHS	THL-32 Study
19	To understand health warnings about conditions (such as being overweight and high blood pressure) that can be harmful to your health.	2	4.3	24.7
20	To research and find information on how to deal with unhealthy behaviors such as smoking and insufficient physical activity.	2.9	3.6	28.2
21	To understand health warnings about how to deal with unhealthy behaviors such as smoking and insufficient physical activity.	5.9	6.5	20.0
22	To research and find information about the health screenings you should have relation according to your age, gender, and health condition (such as breast screening for women and prostate-related diseases for men)	8.8	11.6	36.2
23	To understand the recommendations from resources such as the internet, newspapers, television, and radio for being healthier.	9.8	3.6	25.0
24	To decide whether the information suggested to be made for being healthier in resources such as internet, newspapers, television, and radio is reliable or not.	53.9	37.0	56.2
25	To understand information on food packaging that you think could affect your health.	39.2	33.3	40.7
26	To evaluate the positive and negative characteristics of the environment you live in (such as house, street, neighborhood) that affect health.	14.7	15.9	24.0
27	To find information about what can be done to make the environment you live in (house, street, neighborhood) healthier.	23.5	25.4	30.5
28	To evaluate which of your daily behaviors (such as exercising, eating healthy, not smoking) affects your health.	4.9	3.6	18.8
29	To change your lifestyle (such as exercising, eating healthy, not smoking) for your health.	50.0	49.3	57.5
30	To be able to apply the written diet list given by the dietician.	39.2	39.1	51.8
31	To make suggestions to your family or friends about their health.	14.7	17.4	21.7
32	To interpret health-related policy changes.	36.3	29.7	43.3

Tab. 5: THL-32 Items Index Scores of Students According to Their Faculties

Nu.	Items	FAD (Index)	FHS (Index)
1	To investigate whether it is a sign of illness or not when you have a complaint about your health.	31.21	35.63
2	To read and understand any article on this subject (such as brochure, booklet, poster) when you have a complaint about your health.	31.21	34.18
3	When you have a health complaint, assess whether the advice of your family or friends is reliable.	31.86	28.99
4	To find out which doctor you should consult when you want to go to a health facility.	33.82	39.25
5	To make research and find out how to make application (like making an appointment) when you want to go to a health facility.	40.36	42.39
6	To make an appointment via telephone or internet when you want to go to a health institution.	40.52	41.91
7	To search and find information about the treatments of the diseases that concern you.	31.21	36.23
8	To understand your doctor's explanations about your illness.	36.27	34.3
9	To evaluate the advantages and disadvantages of the different treatment options suggested by your doctor.	27.29	31.04
10	To use your medicines as recommended by healthcare professionals (such as doctor, pharmacist)	40.2	40.2
11	To understand the instructions for using the medicine in the medicine box.	39.22	38.77
12	To decide if you need a second opinion from a different doctor.	26.31	29.35
13	To understand information about pre-medical test preparations (such as dieting).	35.29	37.8
14	To search and find the location of the unit (laboratory, polyclinic) where you want to reach in the hospital.	31.37	33.33
15	To decide what to do in an emergency (such as accident, sudden health problem).	23.69	28.02
16	To call an ambulance when necessary.	28.43	33.82
17	To have health follow-ups and check-ups at regular intervals as your doctor recommended.	29.74	31.28
18	To research and find information about conditions that can be harmful to your health, such as being overweight and having high blood pressure.	27.45	38.89
19	To understand health warnings about conditions (such as being overweight and high blood pressure) that can be harmful to your health.	32.03	38.04

Tab. 5: Continued

Nu.	Items	FAD (Index)	FHS (Index)
20	To research and find information on how to deal with unhealthy behaviors such as smoking and insufficient physical activity.	36.44	39.61
21	To understand health warnings about how to deal with unhealthy behaviors such as smoking and insufficient physical activity.	36.27	39.13
22	To research and find information about the health screenings you should have relation according to your age, gender, and health condition (such as breast screening for women and prostate-related diseases for men)	29.9	35.63
23	To understand the recommendations from resources such as the internet, newspapers, television, and radio for being healthier.	36.93	39.86
24	To decide whether the information suggested to be made for being healthier in resources such as internet, newspapers, television, and radio is reliable or not.	21.73	28.62
25	To understand information on food packaging that you think could affect your health.	25.82	29.35
26	To evaluate the positive and negative characteristics of the environment you live in (such as house, street, neighborhood) that affect health.	30.39	34.3
27	To find information about what can be done to make the environment you live in (house, street, neighborhood) healthier.	25.00	29.83
28	To evaluate which of your daily behaviors (such as exercising, eating healthy, not smoking) affects your health.	40.69	40.34
29	To change your lifestyle (such as exercising, eating healthy, not smoking) for your health.	24.67	26.45
30	To be able to apply the written diet list given by the dietician.	20.75	23.79
31	To make suggestions to your family or friends about their health.	30.72	33.7
32	To interpret health-related policy changes.	14.05	23.79

0-25: unsatisfactory, 25-33: limited, 33-42: adequate, 42-50: excellent

promotion sub-dimension, it was observed that there was a statistically significant difference in the processes of accessing, understanding, and using information ($p<0.05$).

Table 9 shows the sub-dimensions and information processing processes of the answers given by the students of the FAD to the THL-32 scale. In FAD, it was observed that there was a statistically significant difference between all departments in the process of accessing information about the treatment and service sub-dimension ($p<0.05$). In the disease prevention / health promotion

Tab. 6: Comparison of Mean Health Literacy Levels (%)

	European Study	THL-32 Study	FAD	FHS
Insufficient	12.4	27.2	21.6	12.3
Limited	35.2	42.2	34.3	36.2
Enough	36.0	24.8	31.4	31.9
Excellent	16.5	5.8	12.7	19.6

Tab. 7: Health Literacy Index Scores of Students in Sub-dimension and Information Processing Processes According to Their Faculties

Sub-dimension	Information Processing Processes	FAD		FHS		
		n	Index	n	Index	p
Treatment and Service	Accessing Information	102	34.15	138	38.38	*0.00*
	Understanding Information	102	35.50	138	36.26	0.56
	Evaluating Information	102	27.29	138	29.35	0.16
	Using Knowledge	102	35.13	138	36.93	0.22
Prevention from Diseases/ Improving Health	Accessing Information	102	29.70	138	35.99	*0.00*
	Understanding Information	102	32.76	138	36.60	*0.01*
	Evaluating Information	102	26.72	138	31.76	*0.00*
	Using Knowledge	102	26.47	138	28.81	0.15

sub-dimension, it was observed that there was a statistically significant difference in the processes of accessing, evaluating, and using information ($p < 0.05$).

Discussion

Studies have shown that people with enough health literacy can acquire the right information about their health themselves, can solve problems on their own in case of illness, and can make behavioral changes in health promotion (19). In 2016, the Ministry of Health conducted a study on subjects 15 years and older by using THL-32 scale, the general level of health literacy was identified as 29.5 (15). When other studies were examined, it was seen that the average score of general health literacy index in Europe was 33.8. When we examine the health literacy average of some European countries, Bulgaria is 30.5, Austria 32.0, Spain 32.9, Greece 33.6, and Netherlands 37.1 (20). In a study

Tab. 8: Health Literacy Index Scores of Health Sciences Faculty Students in Sub-dimension and Information Processing Processes According to Their Departments

Sub-dimension	Information Processing Processes	ND	PTR	NUR	AUD	HM	p
Treatment and Service	Accessing Information	38.63	38.33	37.5	34.09	39.43	*0.02*
	Understanding Information	38.06	37.92	36.11	31.06	34.45	0.26
	Evaluating Information	30.41	30.42	29.17	21.21	29.67	0.12
	Using Knowledge	37.5	38.23	34.03	31.06	37.4	0.53
Prevention from Diseases/ Improving Health	Accessing Information	38.4	37.08	32.64	25.38	35.87	*0.00*
	Understanding Information	38.85	37.08	34.72	30.68	36.08	0.08
	Evaluating Information	35.25	31.25	24.31	23.86	32.11	*0.00*
	Using Knowledge	33.11	28.54	21.53	19.32	28.66	*0.04*

ND: Nutrition and Dietetics, PTR: Physiotherapy and Rehabilitation, NUR: Nursing,
AUD: Audiology, HM: Health Management

conducted with 300 students at Karabük University, the general health literacy index was found to be 34.53 (21). In our study, the general health literacy level of the FAD and FHS was determined as 32.9. It is 31.0 in FAD and 34.3 in FHS. Although the findings of our study and these studies are close to each other, it is thought that the difference between them may be due to the education levels of the participants in general. Considering the differences between countries it is thought that it may arise from the socio-economic characteristics of each country and its education and health policies.

When a comparison is made according to sub-dimensions and information processing processes of FAD and FHS; It has been concluded that health literacy levels are enough in the process of accessing information in the treatment and service sub-dimension. It is thought that, with the development of technology, students' having easier access to the information they need about health may be the reason for the statistically significant difference.

It has been observed that FAD has a limited level of health literacy and the FHS has enough level of health literacy in the process of accessing and understanding information in the sub-dimension of prevention from diseases/

Tab. 9: Health Literacy Index Scores of FAD Students in Sub-dimension and Information Processing Processes According to Their Departments

Sub-dimension	Information Processing Processes	Industrial Product Design	Interior Architecture and Environmental Design	Architecture	p
Treatment and Service	Accessing Information	31.25	36.46	33.84	*0.02*
	Understanding Information	31.77	37.2	35.7	0.26
	Evaluating Information	23.96	30.51	26.65	0.12
	Using Knowledge	32.55	35.27	35.78	0.53
Prevention from Diseases / Improving Health	Accessing Information	26.82	31.55	29.6	*0.00*
	Understanding Information	30.21	34.97	32.4	0.08
	Evaluating Information	23.7	26.64	27.59	*0.00*
	Using Knowledge	23.44	27.83	26.65	*0.04*

health promotion. This difference can be explained by the fact that health education is predominant in the FHS and that the students of the FHS follow the developments in health and health systems more closely. In the analysis made, it was determined that this difference was statistically significant.

When the health literacy level was examined in terms of departments, statistically significant differences were revealed that the students of Nutrition and Dietetics department had enough health literacy levels. It has been seen that students of the Nutrition and Dietetics department have a higher level of health literacy in the process of accessing information, understanding and using information, especially in the processes of accessing information, understanding and using information, how to deal with unhealthy behaviors, and evaluating health behaviors such as sports and healthy eating.

Physiotherapy and Rehabilitation and Health Management departments in FHS have enough health literacy in the process of accessing information in the sub-dimension of disease prevention / health promotion. In the process of evaluating and using information, it was concluded that health literacy levels are limited in matters such as analyzing health information critically, commenting on these analyzes and making health decisions.

In FAD, limited health literacy was detected in all departments in the process of accessing information, evaluating information, and using information sub-dimension of prevention from diseases / improving health, which was found to have statistically significant differences.

The general index of the health literacy level of the students of the FAD is 30.96, and the general index of the health literacy level of the students of the FHS is 34.25. According to these results, the health literacy level of the students of the FAD is lower than the health literacy level of the students of the FHS.

As a result of the comparison of FAD and FHS according to the sub-dimensions and information processing processes, it was observed that the health literacy levels were limited in the process of accessing, understanding and using information in the treatment and service sub-dimension, and the health literacy level of both faculties was sufficient in the process of information evaluation. It has been concluded that the health literacy level of the FAD is limited and the health literacy level of the FHS is enough in the processes of accessing and understanding information in the prevention of diseases / health promotion sub-dimension. It was found that the health literacy level of both faculties was limited in the process of evaluating and using information.

When we examine the index scores in the sub-dimensions of treatment and service, prevention from diseases / health promotion in the FAD, the department with the highest level of health literacy is the Department of Interior Architecture and Environmental Design. In FHS, the department with the highest level of health literacy is Physiotherapy and Rehabilitation in the treatment and service sub-dimension, and Nutrition and Dietetics in the sub-dimension of prevention / health promotion.

In FHS, the Department of Nutrition and Dietetics has enough health literacy in all processes except for the treatment and service sub-dimension information evaluation process. The level of health literacy in the information evaluation and use processes of the Physiotherapy and Rehabilitation department's disease prevention / health promotion sub-dimension is limited. The health literacy level of the Department of Health Management is limited in the process of evaluating information in both sub-dimensions.

The general health literacy level of FAD and FHS is higher than the THL-32 study. It has been found that the health literacy level of the FHS is higher than the health literacy level of Europe. It was concluded that the proportion of students with inadequate and limited health literacy levels in the FAD and FHS was higher than European studies and lower than THL-32 study. Looking at the average of excellent health literacy levels, students of FHS have a higher rate than European and THL-32 studies.

Conclusion

Studies determining the health literacy levels should be increased. Health literacy scale studies should be conducted for all faculties and the health literacy level of all faculties should be determined.

In-department elective courses for Bahçeşehir University FHS, and non-departmental elective courses for other faculties should be arranged in a way that allows students to understand the concept of health literacy in all aspects and to make positive changes in their own health behaviors.

Seminars on the importance of health literacy, factors affecting health literacy, steps to be taken to increase health literacy and the contribution of adequate health literacy to public health should be organized. The contents of these seminars should be prepared by taking the health literacy levels of students into consideration. Since conducting studies to increase health literacy and developing programs will contribute to the improvement of the life quality of individuals and the society, such studies should be supported.

References

1. Speros, C. (2005). Health literacy: Concept analysis. *Journal of Advanced Nursing, 50*(6), 633-640. doi:10.1111/j.1365-2648.2005.03448.x
2. Yılmaz, M., & Tiraki, Z. (2016). Sağlık okuryazarlığı nedir? Nasıl ölçülür? *Dokuz Eylül Üniversitesi Hemşirelik Fakültesi Elektronik Dergisi, 9*(4), 142-147.
3. World Health Organization (WHO). (1998). *Health promotion glossary.* Geneva.
4. Ertaş, H., Kıraç, R., & Kavuncu, B. (2019). Sağlık bilimleri fakültesi öğrencilerinin sağlık okuryazarlık düzeylerinin belirlenmesi. *Turkish Studies Social Studies, 14*(4), 1459-1469. doi:10.29228/TurkishStudies.24969
5. Kanj, M., & Mitic, W. (2009). *Promoting health and development: Closing the implementation gap.* 7. Global Conference on Health Promotion Nairobi, Kenya: Conference Book; 2009.
6. Kickbusch, I., Wait, S., & Maag, D. (2005). *Navigating health: The role of health literacy.* London: Alliance for Health and the Future, International Longevity Center.
7. Safeer, R., & Keenan, J. (2005). Health literacy: The gap between physicians and patients. *American Family Physician, 72*(3), 463-468.
8. Johnston-Lloyd, L. L., Ammary, N. J., Epstein, L. G., Johnson, R., & Rhee, K. (2006). A transdisciplinary approach to improve health literacy and reduce disparities. *Health Promotion Practice, 7*(3), 331-335. doi:10.1177/1524839906289378

9. Nielsen-Bohlman, l., Panzer, A. M., & Kinding, D. A. (2004). *Health literacy: A prescription to end confusion.* Washington, D.C.: The National Academies Press.

10. World Health Organization (WHO). (2000). *Health promotion report by the secretariat.* A53/16.

11. Yılmazel, G., & Çetinkaya, F. (2016). Sağlık okuryazarlığının toplum sağlığı açısından önemi. *TAF Preventive Medicine Bulletin,* 15(1), 69-74. doi:10.5455/pmb.1-1448870518

12. Okyay, P., Abacigil, F., Harlak, H., Evci-Kiraz, E. D., Karakaya, K., Tuzun H., . . . Beser, E. (2015). A new health literacy scale: Turkish Health Literacy Scale and its psychometric properties. 8th European Public Health Conference: Poster Walks, *European Journal of Public Health,* 25(Supp_3), 357-358.

13. T.C. Kalkınma Bakanlığı. (2014). *Onuncu kalkınma planı 2014/2018. Sağlık hizmetlerinin etkinliğinin artırılması ve mali sürdürülebilirlik: özel ihtisas komisyonu raporu.* Yayın No: KB: 2904-OİK:743.

14. Durusu-Tanrıöver, M., Yıldırım, H. H., Demiray-Ready, F. N., Çakır, B., & Akalın, H. E. (2014). *Türkiye sağlık okuryazarlığı araştırması,* Sağlık-Sen Yayınları, Ankara.

15. T.C. Sağlık Bakanlığı (2016). *Türkiye sağlık okuryazarlığı ölçekleri güvenilirlik ve geçerlilik çalışması.* 1025, Ankara.

16. T.C. Sağlık Bakanlığı Sağlığın Geliştirilmesi Genel Müdürlüğü. (2018). *Türkiye sağlık okuryazarlığı düzeyi ve ilişkili faktörleri araştırması.* 1103, Ankara.

17. T.C. Sağlık Bakanlığı Sağlığın Geliştirilmesi Genel Müdürlüğü. (2018) *Ankara ili Sincan ilçesi birinci basamak sağlık personeli sağlık okuryazarlığı ile ilgili eğitim programı geliştirilmesi.* 1085, Ankara.

18. T.C. Sağlık Bakanlığı. (2019). *2019-2023 stratejik planı,* 1148.

19. Abel, T. (2007). Cultural capital in health promotion. In D. V. McQueen & I. Kickbusch (Eds.), *Health and modernity: The role of theory in health promotion* (pp. 43-73). New York: Springer.

20. HLS-EU Consortium. (2012). *Comparative report of health literacy in eight EU member states.* The European Health Literacy Project 2009-2012, HLS-EU.

21. Yılmaz-Güven, D., Bulut, H., & Öztürk, S. (2018). Sağlık bilimleri fakültesi öğrencilerinin sağlık okuryazarlığı düzeylerinin incelenmesi. *Journal of History Culture and Art Research,* 7(2), 400-409. doi:10.7596/taksad. v7i2.1511

Muzaffer Saraç and Gökay Kurtulan

Difficulties and Challenges in the Field of Nurses Providing Home Care Services

Abstract

Objective: This study was carried out to determine the characteristics of the institution providing home care service, the difficulties that nurses experience in home care service, the difficulties in patient care and their educational needs.

Materials and Methods: The universe of the study consisted of 54 nurses working in the home care unit of İstanbul Metropolitan Municipality as of the study period. Fifty-four home care nurses who worked in the unit between February and March 2018 and agreed to participate in the study were included in the study. Data were collected with a questionnaire form based on literature information and observations. In the first part of the questionnaire form, there are questions about the socio-demographic characteristics of home care nurses and the functioning of their professional and institutional work. In the second part, there are 5-point Likert-type questions under five headings: difficulties related to the institution, difficulties experienced by the nurses, difficulties related to the physical environment at patients' home, difficulties related to patients and their relatives, and difficulties related to the office environment. Percentage distribution, simple and one-way analysis of variance (t-test and One-Way ANOVA) were used to analyze the data.

Results: Most of the nurses are women aged 30 and over, graduated from health-vocational high school and working in the institution for 1-3 years. Eighty-one percent of the nurses have difficulties in providing services. The most difficult patient group is the ones who are angry and refuse treatment/care. The group, which has the most difficulty in communication, is the relatives of the patients. It has been determined that the most difficult problem for nurses is not knowing what they will encounter in the house they go to for the first time. Another difficulty is that patients and their relatives often do not comply with the recommendations.

Conclusion: To strengthen and ensure continuity of services, it is necessary to take precaution to support employees who are effective in-service provision and to eliminate the difficulties they experience.

Keywords: Home Care, Home Care Services, Home Care Nursing

Introduction

Health is one of the basic human rights. Effective health services are an absolute must for the protection of this right. When the history of health care services is examined, in ancient times, health was generally presented at home, in villages or markets, that is, in people's living areas and their proximity. In the current health system, it is seen that hospitalization is preferred primarily compared to home or outpatient treatment. Increasing demand for health-care services and the use of high technology in the diagnosis and treatment of diseases increase health expenditures. In addition to financing problems, the insufficiency of the available number of beds, the inability to provide efficient and quality service, and the increasing trend in costs and expenditures, especially in patients with long-term health needs, direct health policy makers to develop alternative health services to institutional care services. Among these low-cost alternatives, providing health services in the patient's own environment, that is home, is among the priority choices (1,2).

On the other hand, the aging of the population, the increase in disability and chronic diseases have led to an increase in the demand for health services and consequently accumulations in the hospitals. This accumulation in hospitals has revealed the need for home care services and caregivers due to reasons such as expensive services in private hospitals, comfortable home environment for patients and their relatives, and early discharge (1,2).

Home healthcare services are generally providing health and social services at the professional level or by family members in the environment where the patient lives to protect, improve and restore health of the individual (3-5). The cooperation of patients, families and professionals is necessary for home healthcare to be at the desired level (1,2).

Home healthcare can be provided to all patients if necessary medical equipment, materials and personnel are available for the treatment of the disease. Patients with chronic diseases, cancer, physical and mental disabilities, puerperal women who still need care despite being discharged after birth, and the elderly who carry out their daily activities dependent on someone else are suitable patients for home healthcare. To provide home healthcare services, the patient and the patient's family, the conditions of the house where the patient lives and the environment where the house is located must be suitable for providing services (2).

The primary aim of home care nursing is to minimize the effects of disease and disability and to increase the quality of life by achieving maximum treatment efficiency by least affecting the daily living conditions of individuals and families in need of long-term care (6).

Difficulties caused by the patient and family during home care service; the patient and his family changing their treatment in line with their own thoughts, the expectations of the patient and his family from the healthcare personnel do not match the role of the healthcare personnel (such as house-work, the patient's relatives' personal problems, etc.), ethical problems such as misuse of the information provided, the responsibility for the mistakes made by the patient and his family, and the tensions caused by the family members being constantly with the patient. The most important difficulties arising from nurses are the inability to establish an appropriate and effective professional relationship with the patient and the family, and the lack of knowledge and experience about techniques and devices used at home (7-10).

A better-quality service can be provided to patients with solutions such as minimizing the problems experienced by healthcare professionals, planning to eliminate the difficulties in care and training needs, (11,12).

Within the scope of home health services legislation, the "Regulation on the Delivery of Home Care Services", which allows the Ministry of Health to provide home health services by private health institutions at the first stage, and the "Notification on the Presentation of Home Care Services", which was published in the Official Newspaper in 2005 and entered into force. In this way, practices carried out by the private sector are disciplined. In addition, the "Regulation on the Provision of Home Health Care Services by the Ministry of Health and its Affiliates" for the provision of home health services by the health institutions and organizations affiliated to the Ministry of Health was published in the Official Newspaper in 2015 and entered into force. Home care services in Turkey are carried out in accordance with these regulations (3,4,5).

Duties of home care nurse within the scope of the legislation; to receive the written and signed request of the physician for treatment, to record and apply to the nursing forms, to record the results of the application, to support the physician and other team members in the implementation of the special procedures required for the patient, to do the work in the patient care plan, to evaluate and record the vital signs, to report the changes to the physician, to give and record the medicines to be given orally, parenterally and externally to the patient according to the treatment plan, to observe and record the effects and side effects of the medicines applied, to make requests for the equipment and materials that will be required in the services, to provide opinions for their adequate and functional maintenance, cleaning after use, disinfecting and preparing for sterilization when necessary, informing the patient and family about the disease, treatment and care, with pre-determined limits with the physician, patient and family, disease-specific, self-care or assisted care techniques according to their needs matters like and to provide training on general health issues, to apply all practices and procedures in accordance with the ethical rules and in line with patient rights (3,4,5).

Home healthcare services provided by the İstanbul Metropolitan Municipality Health and Social Services Department started with a project established in 2001 with the aim of providing health services to poor and needy patients in their homes in the World Health Organization's "Healthy Cities Project". This service continues to provide health and social services to individuals since 2001 (13).

Materials and Methods

The study was conducted in the İstanbul Metropolitan Municipality Home Care Unit in February and March 2018. The universe of the study was composed of 54 nurses working in the Home Care Unit of the İstanbul Metropolitan Municipality as of the period of study. Fifty-four home care nurses who worked in the unit in question and agreed to participate in the study were included in the study. The data of the study were collected with a questionnaire form prepared based on literature information and observations. The questionnaire form consists of two parts. In the first part, there are 23 multiple-choice questions related to the socio-demographic, vocational and functioning of the home care nurses. In the second part, there are 5-point Likert-type questions under 5 headings such as difficulties related to the institution (18 questions), difficulties experienced by nurses (16 questions), difficulties related to the physical environment at home (7 questions), difficulties related to patients and their relatives (9 questions), and difficulties related to the office environment (6 questions). The initials of the headings (i, n, p, rp and o) related to the difficulties encountered in data entry were coded and made using the SPSS (Version: 20) package program. 95 % confidence interval and one-sided t-test statistics were calculated for each finding. Percentage distribution, simple and one-way analysis of variance (t test and One-Way ANOVA) test were used to analyze the data. Test results showing the homogeneity of variances are shown in Table 1 and Figures 1, 2, 3, 4, and 5, and confidence interval results for variables are shown in Table 2. The mean differences between and within groups were found to be significant with a confidence of 0.95 (Table 3).

Results

When the distribution of the nurses' socio-demographic characteristics is examined; the majority are women (77.8 %), aged 30 and over (70.4 %),

Tab. 1: Homogeneity Test Results of Variances

	Levene's Statistic	df1	df2	Sig.
i_mean	7.395	4	49	.000
n_mean	5.930	4	49	.001
p_mean	7.286	4	49	.000
rp_mean	5.638	4	49	.001
o_mean	12.713	4	49	.000

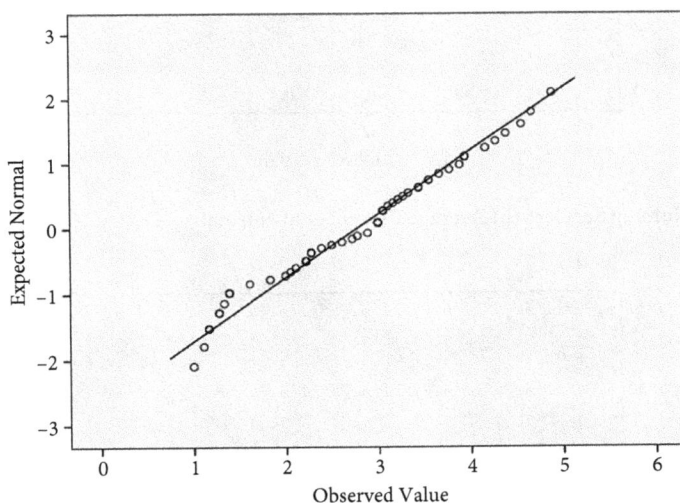

Fig. 1: Institution (i) Average Closeness to Normal

health-vocational high school graduates (50 %) and working in the institution for 1-3 years (44.4 %) (Table 4).

The rate of nurses who need training for home care services is 77.2 %. It was determined that the majority (45.5 %) received in-service training. Considering the content of the training provided, it was seen that the training was received mostly for wound/stoma care (Table 5).

Eighty-one percent of the nurses stated that they had difficulties in providing service. It was stated that the most difficult patient group was the one

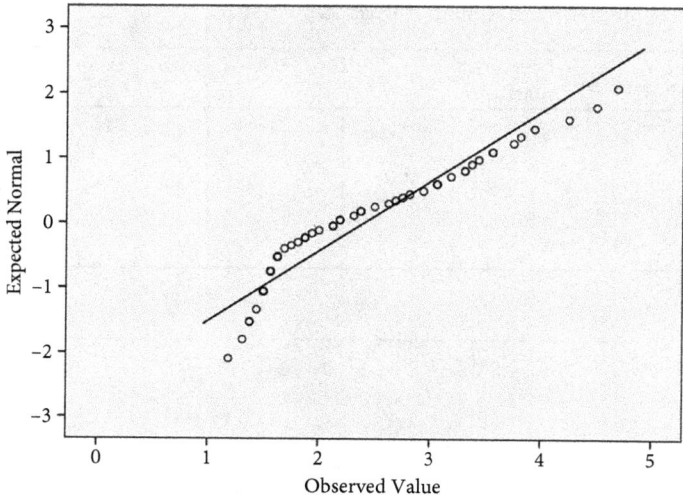

Fig. 2: Nursing Services (n) Average Closeness to Normal

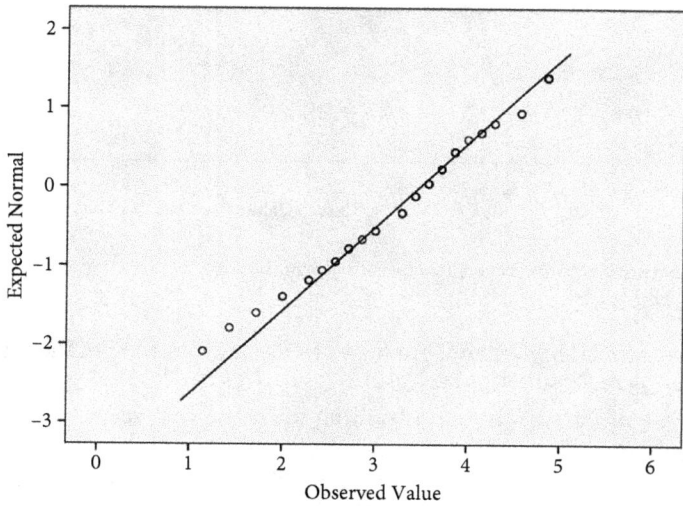

Fig. 3: Physical Environment (p) Average Closeness to Normal

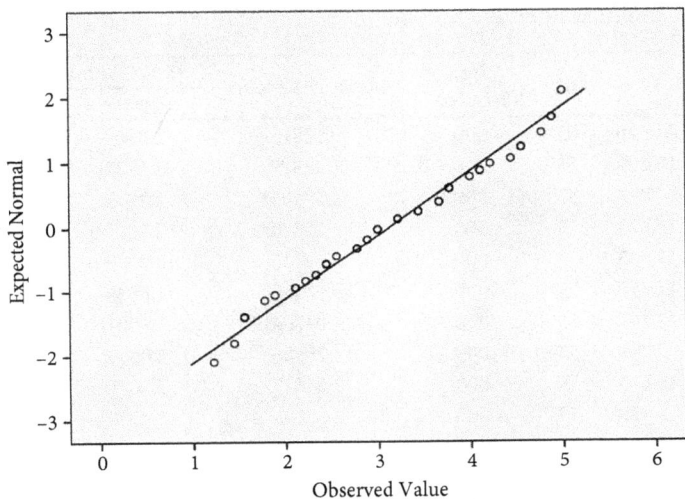

Fig. 4: Relatives of Patients (rp) Average Closeness to Normal

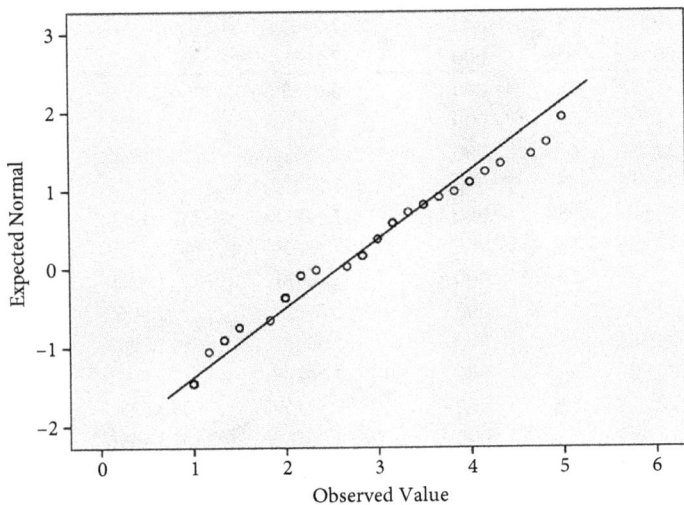

Fig. 5: Office (o) Average Closeness to Normal

Tab. 2: Confidence Interval Results for Variables

	t	df	Sig. (2-tailed)	Mean Difference	95 % Confidence Interval	
					Lower	Upper
i1	23.626	53	.000	3.14815	2.8809	3.4154
i2	18.299	53	.000	2.88889	2.5722	3.2055
i3	17.897	53	.000	2.57407	2.2856	2.8626
i4	16.673	53	.000	2.70370	2.3785	3.0290
i5	17.665	53	.000	2.64815	2.3475	2.9488
i6	13.357	53	.000	1.98148	1.6839	2.2790
i7	17.247	53	.000	2.03704	1.8001	2.2739
i8	17.749	53	.000	2.25926	2.0040	2.5146
i9	15.615	53	.000	2.64815	2.3080	2.9883
i10	15.195	53	.000	2.85185	2.4754	3.2283
i11	14.435	53	.000	2.64815	2.2802	3.0161
i12	24.884	53	.000	3.46296	3.1838	3.7421
i13	33.553	53	.000	3.96296	3.7261	4.1999
i14	24.674	53	.000	2.79630	2.5690	3.0236
i15	18.118	53	.000	2.66667	2.3715	2.9619
i16	17.140	53	.000	2.64815	2.3383	2.9580
i17	19.647	53	.000	3.24074	2.9099	3.5716
i18	20.203	53	.000	2.70370	2.4353	2.9721
n1	17.748	53	.000	3.05556	2.7102	3.4009
n2	14.078	53	.000	1.90741	1.6357	2.1792
n3	14.374	53	.000	2.18519	1.8803	2.4901
n4	14.418	53	.000	1.72222	1.4826	1.9618
n5	16.661	53	.000	1.27778	1.1240	1.4316
n6	17.538	53	.000	2.79630	2.4765	3.1161
n7	12.732	53	.000	1.81481	1.5289	2.1007
n8	15.831	53	.000	2.87037	2.5067	3.2340
n9	12.365	53	.000	1.66667	1.3963	1.9370
n10	20.921	53	.000	3.09259	2.7961	3.3891
n11	20.714	53	.000	3.57407	3.2280	3.9201
n12	12.593	53	.000	4.05556	3.4096	4.7015
n13	15.073	53	.000	2.18519	1.8944	2.4760
n14	13.787	53	.000	2.37037	2.0255	2.7152
n15	12.308	53	.000	1.87037	1.5656	2.1752
n16	12.788	53	.000	2.00000	1.6863	2.3137

Tab. 2:   Continued

	t	df	Sig. (2-tailed)	Mean Difference	95 % Confidence Interval	
					Lower	Upper
p1	33.962	53	.000	3.85185	3.6244	4.0793
p2	24.143	53	.000	3.53704	3.2432	3.8309
p3	26.613	53	.000	3.50000	3.2362	3.7638
p4	32.243	53	.000	3.94444	3.6991	4.1898
p5	27.734	53	.000	3.81481	3.5389	4.0907
p6	24.267	53	.000	3.33333	3.0578	3.6088
p7	15.004	53	.000	2.35185	2.0375	2.6662
rp1	18.975	53	.000	2.77778	2.4842	3.0714
rp2	26.189	53	.000	3.27778	3.0267	3.5288
rp3	26.549	53	.000	3.55556	3.2869	3.8242
rp4	23.224	53	.000	3.25926	2.9778	3.5408
rp5	25.417	53	.000	3.53704	3.2579	3.8162
rp6	25.005	53	.000	3.48148	3.2022	3.7607
rp7	20.196	53	.000	2.94444	2.6520	3.2369
rp8	17.727	53	.000	3.01852	2.6770	3.3601
rp9	14.836	53	.000	2.25926	1.9538	2.5647
o1	19.504	53	.000	3.27778	2.9407	3.6149
o2	16.187	53	.000	2.55556	2.2389	2.8722
o3	14.867	53	.000	2.59259	2.2428	2.9424
o4	12.675	53	.000	2.03704	1.7147	2.3594
o5	16.986	53	.000	2.62963	2.3191	2.9401
o6	15.689	53	.000	2.35185	2.0512	2.6525

One-Sample Test, Test Value=0

who are always angry and refuse treatment/care, and the patients whose daily treatment plan required hospitalization. It was stated that the group with the most difficulties in communication during home care services was patient relatives (Table 6).

Difficulties due to the institution; mostly stated as "high number of daily visits", "late procurement of materials by the institution" and "long and tiring business hours". With 95 % confidence of the general scale mean of the group, the confidence interval was between 3.7261 and 4.1999, and it was observed that it gathers between "mostly" and "always" (Tables 2 and 7).

Tab. 3: One Way ANOVA Test Statistics Results

		Sum Of Squares	df	Mean Square	F	Sig.
	Intergroup	51.196	4	12.799	122.957	.000
i_mean	Intragroup	5.101	49	.104		
	Total	56.297	53			
	Intergroup	40.015	4	10.004	86.337	.000
n_mean	Intragroup	5.678	49	.116		
	Total	45.693	53			
	Intergroup	42.908	4	10.727	134.499	.000
p_mean	Intragroup	3.908	49	.080		
	Total	46.816	53			
	Intergroup	48.794	4	12.198	110.277	.000
rp_mean	Intragroup	5.420	49	.111		
	Total	54.214	53			
	Intergroup	60.417	4	15.104	86.416	.000
o_mean	Intragroup	8.564	49	.175		
	Total	68.981	53			

One Way ANOVA

Tab. 4: Home Care Nurses' Socio-demographic Characteristics

Features		n	%
Age	18-21	1	1.9
	22-25	8	14.8
	26-29	7	13.0
	30 and over	38	70.4
Education Status	Health-Vocational High School	27	50.0
	Undergraduate	12	22.2
	License	14	25.9
	Postgraduate	1	1.9
Work experience	1-3 years	24	44.4
	4-6 years	6	11.1
	6-10 years	12	22.2
	6 years and over	12	22.2
Gender	Female	42	77.8
	Male	12	22.2

Tab. 5: Distribution of Home Care Nurses' Responses Regarding Home Care Nursing Education

Question	Answer	n	%
Do you need training for home care services?	Yes	39	72.2
	No	15	27.8
Have you been trained as home care nursing?	Yes	54	100.0
	No	0	0
When did you receive training? *	Before graduation	9	13.6 %
	Before home care service	11	16.7 %
	Continuously while services continue	16	24.2 %
	In-service training	30	45.5 %
What is the content of the training you received? *	General information about home care	31	13.1
	Medical devices and materials	18	7.6
	Home care nursing and initiatives	26	11.0
	Emergency response	23	9.7
	Patient care (Terminal period-elderly-newborn etc.)	22	9.3
	Interpersonal communication	28	11.9
	Job descriptions	12	5.1
	Institution functioning	16	6.8
	Wound and stoma care	42	17.8
	Registration forms	17	7.2
	Other	1	0.4

* More than one option has been answered.

When the difficulties arising from nursing and nursing services are examined, it was determined that the most difficult problem faced by nurses is not knowing what they will encounter in the houses they go to for the first time. Excessive work responsibility and monitoring of vital signs are among the difficulties experienced in the second and third place. The nurses stated that there was no difficulty in applying oxygen and steam. It was observed that the confidence interval of the group was between 3.2280 and 3.9201 with 95 % confidence regarding the general scale average, and it was observed to be gathered between "occasionally" and "always" (Tables 2 and 8).

When the distribution of difficulties regarding the physical environment is examined, it was found that difficulties were "mostly" experienced. It was determined that the most common difficulties were "not having a suitable environment to give care in the patient's home" and "not ventilating the

Tab. 6: Distribution of Responses Regarding Difficulties Encountered by Home Care Nurses

Question	Answer	n	%
Do you encounter any difficulties in home care nursing service delivery?	Yes	44	81.5
	No	10	18.5
Which patient groups do you experience the most difficulties in home care service? *	Unconscious patients	22	7.8
	Individuals who depend on life support devices and continue their lives with a special care	22	7.8
	Confused / delirium patients	26	9.2
	Terminal individuals	29	10.3
	Patients with sensory loss	17	6.0
	Individuals with a defined level of disability (according to the Disability and Health Classification criteria)	19	6.7
	Seniors (over 65)	18	6.4
	Chronic illnesses	25	8.9
	Patients whose daily treatment plan requires hospitalization	**31**	**11.0**
	Patients with language differences in speaking	24	8.5
	Angry and refusing treatment / care patients	**44**	**15.6**
	Other	5	1.8
Which groups do you have difficulty communicating with in home care services? *	Patient	29	29.0
	Patients' relatives	49	49.0
	Colleagues	2	2.0
	Assistant Staff	7	7.0
	Managers	11	11.0
	Other	2	2.0

* More than one option has been answered.

houses". The least encountered difficulty has been identified as "control of medical waste". With 95 % confidence of the general scale mean of the group, the confidence interval was between 3.2579 and 3.8162, and it was observed that it clustered between "occasionally" and "mostly" (Tables 2 and 9).

Considering the difficulties experienced in patients and their relatives; it has been stated that there is often difficulty in the patients and their relatives not complying with the recommendations. With 95 % confidence of the

Tab. 7: Distribution of Institutional Difficulties

Institutional Difficulties	Never	Very rare	Occasionally	Mostly	Always
	n	n	n	n	n
I am having difficulty due to lack of caring protocols.	4	6	26	14	4
I am having difficulty due to the lack of job descriptions.	10	5	24	11	4
I am having difficulty due to the registration forms not being available for service.	12	9	24	8	1
I am having difficulty due to the large number of registration forms.	11	12	16	12	3
I am having difficulty with the communication with the team during services.	11	9	25	6	3
I am having difficulty due to not knowing who / where to call in an emergency.	24	14	10	5	1
I am having difficulty due to verbal treatment orders.	18	17	18	1	0
I am having difficulty due to feedback to the institution regarding patient care.	12	22	14	6	0
I am having difficulty with the home care institution's surveillance system.	12	13	16	8	5
I am having difficulty due to not getting the wages I deserve for service.	13	10	9	16	6
I am having difficulty in providing personnel for support from the institution when I need it.	15	11	11	12	5
I am having difficulty in procuring materials by the institution.	1	10	14	21	8
I am having difficulty due to the high number of daily visits.	1	3	6	31	13
I am having difficulty reaching the houses.	2	18	24	9	1
I am having difficulty due to management problems.	10	11	22	9	2
I am having difficulties due to insufficient in-service training.	11	11	21	8	3
I am having difficulties due to long and tiring work hours.	7	7	12	22	6
I am having trouble due to inter-team communication and team conflict.	6	16	22	8	2

Tab. 8: Distribution of Difficulties Due to Nursing and Nursing Services

Distribution of Difficulties due to Nursing and Nursing Services	Frequency of Occurrence				
	Never	Very rare	Occasionally	Mostly	Always
	n	n	n	n	n
Vital signs follow-up	10	6	14	19	5
Oral / Parenteral treatment preparation and application	25	13	12	4	-
Catheter application and care	19	15	12	7	1
Feed	27	18	6	3	-
Oxygen and steam application	42	9	3	-	-
Patient positioning	11	9	15	18	1
Wound care	29	12	7	6	-
Meeting the hygienic requirements	10	13	13	10	8
Excretion	32	12	8	-	2
Excessive work responsibilities	6	8	17	20	3
Not knowing what will be encountered at home where the nurses visit for the first time	3	10	11	13	17
Time planning	9	12	21	9	3
Lack of information on prescribed drug side effects, interactions, usage patterns	18	15	15	5	1
Determining the education and consultancy needs of the individual and family	17	16	8	10	3
Registration and evaluation	29	9	12	2	2
Proper planning of care	25	12	11	4	2

general scale mean of the group, the confidence interval was between 3.2579 and 3.8162, and it was observed that it clustered between "occasionally" and "mostly" (Tables 2 and 10).

Considering the difficulties experienced in the office, half of the participants stated that they had difficulties in "noisy office" (Table 11). With 95 % confidence of the general scale mean of the group, the confidence interval was between 2.9407 and 3.6149, and it was observed that it clustered between "occasionally" and "mostly" (Tables 2 and 11).

Discussion

The answers given to the questions about the difficulties experienced by the nurses were evaluated as 1-Never 5-Always. The average value was calculated for each group questions and the analyzes were continued on the means. Significant differences were found between group scale averages and between group averages. Answers given according to education level; It has been concluded that the frequency of difficulties experienced for Health Vocational School graduates is higher than for those who have postgraduate education. Answers given according to education level; it has been concluded that the frequency of difficulties experienced for Health Vocational High School graduates is higher than for those who have postgraduate education.

The data obtained in the study match with some similar studies (1,12,14). It has been determined that the difficulties encountered are focused on the physical environment of the places visited to provide service and the relatives of the patients. Patients who receive home care services and their families often experience many physical, emotional and social problems. This negatively affects the patient's compliance with the treatment and reducing patients' concerns. In addition, patients cannot receive adequate care support from their relatives in diseases such as disc herniation, hypertension, ulcer, migraine, anxiety and especially depression. Increasing psychological support services to patients and their relatives with the support of a psychologist plays an important role in this service, which is a teamwork in order to make the patient feel safe and comfortable and to minimize the problems that may arise in care. In addition, nurses should establish a positive communication with their relatives (15). As there is a study with findings equivalent to our study (16), there is also a study emphasizing that most nurses never had difficulty in communicating with their patients and their relatives (17).

In the evaluation made regarding the difficulties experienced by the nurses related to the institution; It was observed that the high number of daily visits

Tab. 9: Distribution of Physical Environment-Related Difficulties

Physical Environment-Related Difficulties	Frequency of Occurrence				
	Never	Very rare	Occasionally	Mostly	Always
	n	n	n	n	n
Lack of suitable environment for care in patients' home	1	2	11	30	10
In controlling environmental stimuli such as noise, light, ventilation	2	8	13	21	10
Adjusting the heat of the houses	1	7	18	20	8
For ventilation of homes	-	5	8	26	15
In the arrangement of patient rooms	2	3	12	23	14
In safety from being in the house of people she does not know	3	4	27	12	8
In the control of medical waste	17	13	12	12	-

Tab. 10: Distribution of Difficulties Originating from Patients and Their Relatives

Difficulties Originating from Patients and Their Relatives	Frequency of Occurrence				
	Never	Very rare	Occasionally	Mostly	Always
	n	n	n	n	n
Informing patient/relatives about the patient's condition	6	16	20	8	4
In the education of patients / relatives	1	10	20	19	4
Due to the patient and their relatives being intervene in the care	-	7	22	13	12
Patients and their relatives are not satisfied with care	1	12	21	12	8
Patients and their relatives not following the recommendations.	2	6	16	21	9
Increasing expectations of patients / relatives with each visit	-	10	19	14	11
Caring for fully dependent patients	6	11	20	14	3
When requesting service other than job description (housework, etc.)	8	10	16	13	7
Domestic violence, harassment, etc. in encountering situations	18	13	15	7	1

Tab. 11: Distribution of Difficulties Arising from the Office Environment

Difficulties Arising from the Office Environment	Frequency of Occurrence				
	Never	Very rare	Occasionally	Mostly	Always
	n	n	n	n	n
I am having difficulty due to the noise in the center.	7	6	14	19	8
I am having difficulty adjusting the temperature.	11	16	17	6	4
I am having difficulty with ventilation.	14	12	15	8	5
I am having difficulty with lighting.	24	13	11	3	3
I am having difficulties due to insufficient and healthy cleaning and care.	8	20	14	8	4
I am having difficulties due to not placing materials and tools in the proper order of the workflow.	13	20	12	7	2

and vital sign follow-up were positively correlated (sig.=0.00 <0.05). Similarly, in the literature, it has been stated that there are difficulties in home care services due to the lack of nurses (16,17). For an effective study, the number of daily visits should be kept in optimum number by reviewing the data from the regions.

In the evaluation made regarding the difficulties experienced by nurses due to the office environment; It was observed that the noisy office and the excessive work responsibilities were positively related (sig.=0.00 <0.05). Other studies support the same result. It should be kept in mind that the noise of the office may cause nurses to experience difficulties during data collection and data recording.

In the evaluation made regarding the difficulties that nurses experience in terms of nursing services; It was observed that scheduling, intervention of patients and their relatives, and difficulties in reaching homes were positively correlated (sig.=0.00 <0.05). Despite paying attention to the proximity of the residences of the patients to be served and the use of navigation, it has been determined that nurses experience difficulties in reaching their homes due to the traffic jam (16,17).

In the evaluation made regarding the difficulties experienced by the nurses due to the physical environment; It has been observed that ventilation of the houses and insecurity due to being in the houses of unknown people are positively related (sig.=0.00 <0.05). The necessity of controlling environmental stimuli such as noise, light, ventilation, and heating to the patients and their relatives and the importance of ensuring that the patient sleeps and rest should be expressed at each visit with training.

In the evaluation made regarding the difficulties caused by the patients and their relatives, it was observed that the intervention of the patient and their relatives in the care and not knowing what to encounter in the home for the first time were positively related (sig.=0.00 <0.05). Other studies also support this result (16,17).

Conclusion

To strengthen and ensure continuity of services, it is necessary to support employees who are effective in-service delivery and consider the following suggestions.

- While nurses are employed in home care units, nurses with home care nursing certificates should be preferred first.

- Nurses who work as home care nurses but do not have a home care nursing certificate should be directed to certification programs as soon as possible.
- Training of nurses on care for patients who are angry and refuse treatment / care should be improved.
- Hand brochures should be prepared for pre-interview with the patients and their relatives, to get to know the characteristics of the patient and family, and to organize the information activity.
- In-service training should be organized for nurses to fulfill their role as educators and consultants.
- Institution managers should take measures for the difficulties faced by the institution and the difficulties experienced in the office.
- The service control and supervision system should be implemented more actively.
- Home healthcare services should be accepted as a health right. Health and social services should be carried out in coordination with each other.

References

1. Taşdelen, P., & Ateş M. (2012). Evde bakım gerektiren hastaların bakım gereksinimleri ile bakım verenlerin yükünün değerlendirilmesi. *Hemşirelikte Eğitim ve Araştırma Dergisi, 9*(3), 22-29.

2. Coşkun, N. (2014). Evde sağlık hizmeti alan kişilerde yaşam kalitesi ve hasta memnuniyeti. *Hacettepe Sağlık İdaresi Dergisi, 17*(1), 59-75.

3. T.C. Sağlık Bakanlığı. (2005). Evde bakım hizmetleri sunumu hakkında yönetmelik. *Official Newspaper, 25751.*

4. T.C. Sağlık Bakanlığı. (2005). Evde bakım hizmetleri sunumu hakkında tebliğ. *Official Newspaper, 25935.*

5. T.C. Sağlık Bakanlığı. (2015). Sağlık bakanlığı ve bağlı kuruluşları tarafından evde sağlık hizmetlerinin sunulmasına dair yönetmelik. *Official Newspaper, 29280.*

6. İşbaşı, S., & Tütüncüoğlu, G. (1998). Evde bakım sürecine genel bakış. In G. Cimete (Ed.), *I. ulusal evde bakım kongresi kitabı* (pp. 111-113). İstanbul: Marmara University.

7. Arras, J. D. (1995). *Bringing the hospital home: Ethical and social implications of high-tech home care.* Baltimore: The Johns Hopkins University Press.

8. Jaffe, K. B. (1989), Home health care and rehabilitation nursing. *The Nursing Clinics of North America, 24*(1), 171-178.

9. Karamercan, E. (2001). Evde bakım: sağlık hizmetlerinde yeni bir olgu. *Yeni Türkiye Sağlık Özel Sayısı, 39*, 935- 944.

10. Anuk, D. (1998). Tedavi ekibinde stres ve tükenmişlik. In S. Özkan (Ed.). *V. ulusal konsültasyon-liyezon psikiyatri kongresi, kongre kitabı* (pp. 182-187). İstanbul: Novartis İlaçları A.Ş.

11. Luquette, J. (2007). Stress, compassion fatigue, and burnout: Effective self-care techniques for oncology nurses. *Oncology Nursing Forum, 34*(2), 490.

12. Yurtsever, N., & Yılmaz, M. (2016). Evde bakım alanında çalışan hemşirelerin çalışma koşulları, yaşadıkları güçlükler ve eğitim gereksinimlerinin belirlenmesi, *İzmir Kâtip Çelebi Üniversitesi Sağlık Bilimleri Fakültesi Dergisi, 1*(1), 19-25.

13. İstanbul Büyükşehir Belediyesi Başkanlığı. (2019). Evde sağlık hizmeti. Retrieved from https://saglik.ibb.istanbul/saglik-ve-hifzissihha-mudurlugu/evde-saglik-hizmeti/

14. Fesci, H., Doğan, N., & Pınar, G. (2008). İç hastalıkları kliniklerinde çalışan hemşirelerin hasta bakımında karşılaştıkları güçlükler ve çözüm önerilerinin belirlenmesi. *Atatürk Üniversitesi Hemşirelik Yüksekokulu Dergisi, 11*(3), 40-50.

15. Cimete, G. (2008). Evde bakım hemşireliği. *Türk Yoğun Bakım Derneği Dergisi, 6*(4), 47-53.

16. Çoban, S. (2014). *Evde bakım hemşirelerin çalışma alanında karşılaştıkları güçlükler ve bakım vermede duyulan gereksinim alanları.* (Unpublished master's thesis). Dokuz Eylül University, İzmir, Turkey.

17. Kar, G. (2003). *Evde bakım hizmeti veren hemşirelerin hizmetlerde yaşadıkları güçlükler ve iş doyumu düzeyleri.* (Unpublished master's thesis). Marmara University, İstanbul, Turkey.

List of Figures

List of Tables

About the Editors

Prof. Dr. Fatma Eti Aslan

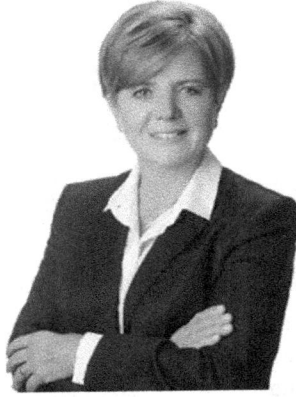

Dean of Faculty of Health Sciences at Bahçeşehir University, İstanbul, Turkey. Professor Dr. Fatma Eti Aslan obtained her nursing license from the İstanbul University Florence Nightingale Nursing School in 1986, her master degree from İstanbul University Institute of Health Sciences Department of Nursing in 1988, her doctoral degree from İstanbul University Institute of Health Sciences Department of Medical Surgical Nursing in 1992. She worked at Cerrahpaşa Hospital as a nurse for three years and then at Marmara University as an assistant professor between 1993 and 1999, as an associate professor between 1999 and 2006 and as a professor between 2006 and 2009. She is still working at Bahçeşehir University Faculty of Health Sciences as a head of Nursing program and as a dean of faculty. Professor Dr. Fatma Eti Aslan managed 49 master's thesis and 7 doctorate theses until now. She is an author of 4 nursing books, editor of 15 books, author of lots of chapters and she also have 40 international SCI, SSCI scientific papers, 98 national papers and 53 international congress participation. She continues to teach continuously.

Assist. Prof. Dr. Gökay Kurtulan

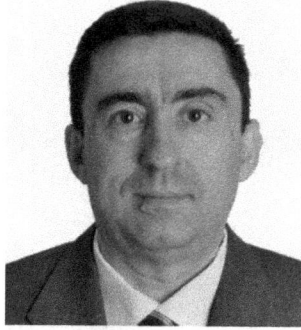

Medical Doctor, Gökay Kurtulan graduated from Gülhane Military Medical Academy, Military Medical Faculty in 1992. He completed his first master's degree in 2005 at Marmara University Institute of Health Sciences, Department of Health Institutions Management. He completed his second master's degree in 2006 at Yeditepe University Department of Atatürk's Principles and Revolution History. He completed his doctorate in 2010 at Marmara University Institute of Health Sciences, Department of Health Institutions Management. Between 1992 and 2016, he served as a military doctor, medical advisor, and senior manager in various positions of the Turkish Armed Forces for 24 years. During the last four years in the Turkish Armed Forces, he served as CEO of military hospital. He participated in NATO missions and World Health Organization activities in Bosnia and Herzegovina in 2003 and Afghanistan in 2005. In 2016, he retired from the Turkish Armed Forces with the rank of "senior colonel" and started to work as an assistant professor at Bahçeşehir University Faculty of Health Sciences. He is currently working as the Head of Health Management Department and Vice Dean of the Faculty of Health Sciences at Bahçeşehir University. He is also a senator of the university senate.

Assist. Prof. Dr. Hayat Yalın

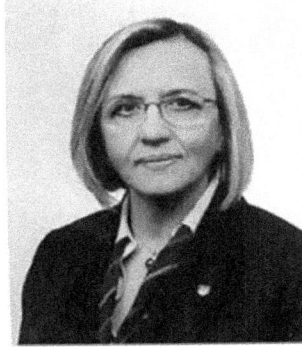

Vice Dean of Faculty of Health Sciences at Bahçeşehir University, İstanbul, Turkey. Asistant Professor Hayat Yalın obtained her nursing license from the İstanbul University Florence Nightingale Nursing School in 1985, her master degree for Internal Diseases Nursing from İstanbul University Institute of Health Sciences in 1995, her master degree for Social Environmental Sciences from Boğaziçi University Institute of Environmental Sciences in 1999, her doctoral degree from Marmara University Institute of Health Sciences Department of Fundamentals of Nursing in 2010. She worked as a nurse at Marmara University Hospital for 25 years and then as an assistant professor at Acıbadem University Faculty of Health Sciences between 2011 and 2015. She is still working at Bahçeşehir University Faculty of Health Sciences as an assistant professor in Nursing program and as a vice dean of faculty. Assistant Professor Hayat Yalın managed 7 master's theses. She is author of chapters in 4 books. She has many scientific papers and congress participations both national and international.

www.ingramcontent.com/pod-product-compliance
Lightning Source LLC
Chambersburg PA
CBHW070745220326
41598CB00026B/3742